CURRENT REVIEW OF

ALLERGIC
diseases

CURRENT REVIEW OF
ALLERGIC
diseases

Edited by

MICHAEL A. KALINER, MD

Professor
Department of Medicine
George Washington University School of Medicine
Institute for Asthma and Allergy
Washington, DC, USA

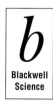

Blackwell Science

Developed by Current Medicine, Inc., Philadelphia

Current Medicine, Inc.

 400 Market Street
Suite 700
Philadelphia, PA 19106

Director of Product Development .... *Lori J. Bainbridge*
Developmental Editor .... *Jennifer Wood*
Cover Design and Layout .... *Jerilyn Bockorick*
Illustrator .... *Lisa Weischedel*
Art Director .... *Paul Fennessy*
Illustration Director .... *Ann Saydlowski*
Production Manager .... *Lori Holland*
Production Assistant .... *Amy Watts*
Indexing .... *Holly Lukens*

ISBN 0-632-04383-0
ISSN 1099-6435

Although every effort has been made to ensure that drug doses and other information are presented accurately in this publication, the ultimate responsibility rests with the prescribing physician. Neither the publishers nor the author can be held responsible for errors or for any consequences arising from the use of the information contained therein. Any product mentioned in this publication should be used in accordance with the prescribing information prepared by the manufacturers. No claims or endorsements are made for any drug or compound at present under clinical investigation.

Printed in the United States by Edwards Brothers
5 4 3 2 1

DISTRIBUTED WORLDWIDE BY BLACKWELL SCIENCE, INC.

Preface

The clinical and basic science of allergic disease is moving and evolving so rapidly that it is nearly impossible to keep up unless you are a bench scientist who spends full time examining T helper 1 and 2 (T_H1 and T_H2) lymphocytes. In order to try to keep abreast of the changes in concept and application of allergic diseases, one can read books and journals and attend lectures and meetings. In the end, the field keeps moving forward and it is a never-ending challenge. It is much better to have a continually updated review of allergic diseases, written over a very limited time period by acknowledged leaders, in order to stay at the edge of knowledge. Such is the concept behind *Current Review of Allergic Diseases*.

The basic science described in this text is stunning in its presentation of the current understanding of allergic mechanisms. The chapters on IgE, mast cells, and lymphocytes are beautifully written and contain well-described sections on how they contribute to the allergic process. If one lost track of this field for only a very brief time, the concepts of cytokines and chemokines, T lymphocytes supporting allergic or delayed hypersensitivity in a nearly opposing manner, the ability to begin to attack IgE on the mast cell as a mechanism of reducing allergic disease, the concept of epitope treatment, and many other exciting advances in the field could be overwhelming. And yet, these concepts will be tomorrow's treatments and the contemporary allergist will be applying them. The only solution is constant upgrading of knowledge, and this book is an excellent means to do so.

The clinical sections take these concepts and apply them to patients' and their diseases. Thus, anaphylaxis, asthma, food allergy, sinusitis, drug allergies, conjunctivitis, allergic dermatosis, urticaria, rhinitis, and others are approached both mechanistically and clinically. The reader will be able to synthesize the advances in basic science into the clinical diseases that are the manifestations of allergy. Our understanding of the inflammatory process in allergic disease is clearly defined in many of these chapters, as is the application of science to clinical treatment. Important topics, such as allergens and immunotherapy, are approached as scientific issues with important clinical applications.

The chapters on treatment modalities bring the latest concepts in the use of leukotriene modifiers, antihistamines, bronchodilators, and immunotherapy to the reader interested in allergic diseases. Each of these chapters is as current as possible and written by a leader in the field. Clinicians will all benefit from these reviews. The chapter on the costs of allergic disease should be required reading for anyone managing the health care system. These diseases are not only very common but also very expensive.

Overall, I am very pleased with this book. We accomplished the creation of a contemporary review written over a 4-month period by experts so that the reader can access the latest concepts and clinical applications. The book is up-to-date, concise, and accurate, and should earn a place in the reading list of all clinicians interested in keeping up with the field.

It is the intention of the editor to publish this book every few years in order to continually update the field. It is certain that there will be new and exciting changes worth documenting, both on the basic science and on the clinical side.

Michael A. Kaliner, MD

Contributors

John A. Anderson, MD

Professor
Department of Pediatrics
Case Western Reserve University
Cleveland, Ohio, USA;
Henry Ford Health System
Detroit, Michigan, USA

Vincent S. Beltrani, MD

Associate Clinical Professor
Department of Dermatology
College of Physicians and Surgeons
Columbia University
New York, New York, USA

Leonard Bielory, MD

Associate Professor
Departments of Medicine, Pediatrics, and Ophthalmology
University of Medicine and Dentistry-New Jersey School of
    Medicine
University of Medicine and Dentistry-New Jersey University
    Hospital
Newark, New Jersey, USA

Michael S. Blaiss, MD

Associate Professor
Department of Pediatrics and Medicine
Division of Clinical Immunology
University of Tennessee
Memphis, Tennessee, USA

Daniel H. Conrad, PhD

Professor
Department of Microbiology and Immunology
Virginia Commonwealth University
Richmond, Virginia, USA

Albert F. Finn, Jr., MD

Clinical Assistant Professor
Department of Medicine, Microbiology, and Immunology
Medical University of South Carolina
Attending Physician
National Urticaria Research and Treatment Center
Charleston, South Carolina, USA

Marianne Frieri, MD, PhD

Associate Professor of Medicine and Pathology
State University of New York at Stony Brook
Stony Brook, New York, USA;
Director of Allergy Immunology Training Program
Nassau County Medical Center
East Meadow, New York, USA

J. Andrew Grant, MD

Professor
Department of Medicine, Microbiology, and Immunology
University of Texas Medical Branch
Galveston, Texas, USA

William R. Henderson, Jr., MD

Professor
Department of Medicine
University of Washington
Seattle, Washington, USA

Noreen R. Henig, MD

Fellow
Department of Medicine
University of Washington
Seattle, Washington, USA

A.B. Kay, MD, PhD

Professor and Head
Department of Allergy and Clinical Immunology, NHLI
Imperial College School of Medicine
Royal Brompton Hospital
London, England

Ann E. Kelly, PhD

Department of Immunology
Jerome Holland Laboratory
American Red Cross
Rockville, Maryland, USA

M. Larché, PhD

Lecturer
Department of Allergy and Immunology, NHLI
Imperial College School of Medicine
London, England

Phillip L. Lieberman, MD

Clinical Professor
Division of Allergy and Immunology
Department of Medicine and Pediatrics
University of Tennessee College of Medicine
Memphis, Tennessee, USA

Richard F. Lockey

Professor of Medicine
Department of Pediatrics and Public Health
Joy McCann Culverhouse Professor in Allergy and Immunology
Department of Allergy and Immunology
University of South Florida College of Medicine
James A. Haley Veterans' Hospital
Tampa, Florida, USA

Shyam S. Mohapatra

Associate Professor of Medicine and Medical Microbiology and
   Immunology
University of South Florida College of Medicine
James A. Haley Veterans' Hospital
Tampa, Florida, USA

Robert A. Nathan, MD

Clinical Professor of Medicine
Department of Asthma and Immunology
University of Colorado Health Sciences Center
Denver, Colorado, USA;
Asthma and Allergy Associates, PC
Colorado Springs, Colorado, USA

Muhammad Rais, MD

Fellow-in-Training
Department of Medicine, Microbiology, and Immunology
University of Texas Medical Branch
Galveston, Texas, USA

William F. Schoenwetter, MD

Clinical Professor
Department of Medicine
University of Minnesota
Park Nicollet Clinic Health System
Minneapolis, Minnesota, USA

Guy A. Settipane, MD

Clinical Professor of Medicine
Department of Medicine
Brown University School of Medicine
Rhode Island Hospital
Division of Allergy and Immunology
Providence, Rhode Island, USA

Russell A. Settipane, MD

Assistant Clinical Professor of Medicine
Department of Medicine
Brown University School of Medicine
Rhode Island Hospital
Division of Allergy and Immunology
Providence, Rhode Island, USA

Reuben P. Siraganian, MD, PhD

National Institutes of Health
Bethesda, Maryland, USA

Richard J. Sveum, MD

Clinical Professor
Department of Medicine
University of Minnesota
Park Nicollet Clinic Health System
Minneapolis, Minnesota, USA

Sheri B. Tinnell, PhD

Department of Microbiology and Immunology
Virginia Commonwealth University
Richmond, Virginia, USA

Martha V. White, MD

Research Director
Institute of Asthma and Allergy
Washington, DC, USA

Tina C. Zecca, DO

Assistant Professor
Department of Pediatric Allergy, Immunology
University of Medicine and Dentistry-New Jersey Medical
   School
University of Medicine and Dentistry-New Jersey University
   Hospital
Newark, New Jersey, USA

Contents

CHAPTER 1

Costs and Trends in the Management of Allergic Diseases

Michael S. Blaiss

Allergic disorders affect a large percentage of the population, and allergic rhinitis and asthma are two of the most common chronic medical conditions. Not only do these diseases lead to high expenditures for medical care; they also generate high indirect costs from work and school absences and decreases in productivity. With the changes occurring in the health care arena and continued decreases in resources, cost considerations must be assessed in addition to clinical efficacy and safety in management of allergic diseases.

This chapter reviews the cost aspects of the two major allergic disorders, allergic rhinitis and asthma, and discusses cost-effective approaches in their treatment.

ALLERGIC RHINITIS

About 20% of the population suffers from allergic rhinitis [1,2]. A majority of allergic rhinitis patients are children and young adults; the prevalence rate in this group is estimated to be as much as 30% [3]. Allergic rhinitis sufferers are rarely, if ever, hospitalized and rarely require surgery or other sophisticated interventions. Because allergic rhinitis does not threaten the patients' day-to-day survival, it may be seen only as a minor nuisance. This is, however, not true. Of allergic rhinitis patients, 50% experience symptoms more than 4 months out of very year and 20% are symptomatic at least 9 months out of the year. This disease accounts for over 10 million office visits to physicians yearly in the United States. It has a major impact on the productivity of the population, leading to an estimated 28 million days of restricted activity yearly in the United States. Allergic rhinitis accounts for over 2 million days of school missed yearly in the United States. This means that on a typical school day, 10,000 children are absent because of allergic rhinitis.

Economic impact

Allergic rhinitis is now recognized as a costly condition in the managed-care setting. Costs of allergic rhinitis can be divided into two major categories: direct and indirect. Direct costs are due to monies consumed in the care of the patient, whereas indirect costs are monies lost due to the disease. An important aspect of allergic rhinitis costs is that this condition can lead to or complicate other high-cost disorders, such as asthma, sinusitis, otitis media with effusion, and nasal polyposis. These conditions can be classified as "hidden" direct costs associated with allergic rhinitis (Table 1-1) [4].

Table 1-1. DIRECT AND INDIRECT COSTS OF ALLERGIC RHINITIS

Direct costs
  Physician/provider consultation
  Laboratory testing: allergy skin tests, RAST
  Costs of specific allergy therapy: environmental control,
    prescription and OTC medications, immunotherapy

"Hidden" direct costs
  Costs for antibiotics, radiographs for treatment, and
    emergency department visits for complicating sinusitis
  Surgical costs for nasal polyposis and sinusitis
  Antibiotic costs for treatment of sinusitis
  Medical and surgical costs for otitis media with effusion
  Costs of worsening asthma and frequent URIs
  Orthodontics costs
  Evaluation and treatment of ocular symptoms

Indirect costs
  Sleep disorders and neuropsychiatric abnormalities
  Activity limitation due to symptoms and effects of first-
    generation antihistamines
  Decreased decision-making capacity
  Impaired psychomotor function
  Poor concentration
  Irritability
  Fatigue
  Decreased functioning at work and school
  Increased motor vehicle accidents and school and
    workplace injuries

OTC—over the counter; RAST—radioallergosorbent test;
URI—upper respiratory infection.
Adapted from *Blaiss* et al. *[4]; with permission.*

Recently, several studies evaluated the cost of allergic rhinitis in the United States. Each of these studies assessed cost in different ways, leading to different cost estimates. McMenamin [5] assessed the costs and prevalence of this condition in 1990 using the National Health Interview Survey to estimate the number of patients with allergic rhinitis and the National Ambulatory Medical Care Survey to estimate the type of physician treatments provided. His results suggested that the prevalence rate of allergic rhinitis was 9.3%, with total costs in 1990 to be $1.8 billion. Direct costs totaled $1.16 billion–$881 million from physician costs and $276 million from medication costs. Indirect costs from allergic rhinitis came to $639 million, estimated from a loss of 3.4 million work days.

Ross [6] assessed the indirect cost of allergic rhinitis in the workplace. Using the data from the United States Public Health Survey, he calculated that allergic rhinitis affected 12.6 million people in the American workforce in 1989. Next, he extrapolated the increase in the work-

force through 1993 and figured the loss of productivity due to allergic rhinitis. For 1993, the loss of productivity in the American labor force due to allergic rhinitis was $2.39 billion in men and $1.4 billion in women. Because such a high percent of the workforce has allergic rhinitis, it is estimated from his data that lost productivity due to hayfever may cost $1000 for each worker in the United States per year.

Malone *et al.* [7] produced another study addressing the burden of allergic rhinitis on the national economy. Using the data from the 1987 National Medical Expenditure Survey, they calculated estimates of resource use, medical expenditures, and lost productivity from allergic rhinitis and extrapolated the data in 1994 dollars. They estimated that 39 million Americans had allergic rhinitis in 1987, but only 12.3% obtained medical care from physicians. Allergic rhinitis accounted for 811,000 missed work days, 824,000 missed school days, and 4,230,000 reduced-activity days in 1987. The total cost of allergic rhinitis in 1994 dollars was $1.23 billion.

Storms *et al.* [8•] conducted a nationwide survey in 1993 to evaluate the costs related to the management of allergic rhinitis in the United States. Patients with ocular or nasal symptoms for 7 days or longer during the previous 12 months were assessed for the amount of medical-care services, including spending on medication, over that 12-month period. Of the respondents, 63% had consulted a physician in the past 12 months with an estimated cost of $1.1 billion dollars. The average per-person expenditure for prescription medications was $56 per year. The same amount was spent on nonprescription medications yearly, giving an estimated total cost in medications for allergic rhinitis to be in the range of $2.4 billion.

Mackowiak [9] developed an employer cost/benefit economic model for allergic rhinitis. Looking at pharmaceutical costs, he obtained data on drug sales from various pharmaceutical companies for his model. The preliminary data shows direct costs of allergic rhinitis at $4.48 billion and indirect costs at $3.37 billion.

These economic studies do not take into consideration complications and secondary costs of rhinitis, such as asthma, sinusitis, otitis media with effusion, and nasal polyposis. Although all of these studies took distinct approaches and used different methodologies to determine costs related to allergic rhinitis, it is clear that this disease has a significant economic impact on the healthcare system.

Cost-effective management

In allergic rhinitis, treatment consists of a threefold approach. First, avoidance procedures are instituted to decrease exposure to harmful allergens. Next, appropriate pharmaceutical agents are prescribed to help alleviate and prevent chronic symptoms. Last, allergen immunotherapy

Table 1-2. ECONOMIC EVALUATIONS IN HEALTHCARE
Cost-effectiveness
Costs are compared to clinical effects produced between different programs or treatments
Cost benefit
Costs are compared with benefits from a program or treatment as defined by society
Cost identification
Costs are compared between different programs or treatments
Cost utility
Costs are compared to quality-adjusted life years attained between different programs or treatment

Animal allergy can be significantly improved by removing the pet from the house. Measures shown to decrease animal dander in homes where pets cannot be removed include use of a filtering device, keeping the pet out of the patient's bedroom, and removing carpet from that room. A major cause of perennial allergic rhinitis is house dust mites [10]. Dust mites grow in hot, humid environments, with the highest concentrations found in carpeting and bedding. Avoidance procedures that have been demonstrated to decrease house dust mite levels include removing all feather objects and wall-to-wall carpeting from the patient's bedroom; encasing the pillow, mattress, and box springs with zipped, impermeable covers; and washing all bedding regularly with hot water.

Medical management

The mainstays of pharmacologic therapy for allergic rhinitis are oral antihistamines and intranasal corticosteroids. Table 1-3 lists some first- and second-generation antihistamines and their daily cost, calculated from their average wholesale cost and recommended daily usage [11]. First-generation antihistamines have been in use for many years. These drugs are all very effective in decreasing the symptoms of allergic rhinitis, such as rhinorrhea, sneezing, nasal itching, and ocular symptoms, and are the least-expensive daily pharmacologic therapy in the management of allergic rhinitis. These agents may not be the most cost effective, however, because many patients

may be necessary to desensitize or possibly eliminate symptoms due to specific allergens. There are many different economic methods used to assess costs between different treatments or programs in the healthcare field (Table 1-2). With the large population of allergic rhinitis sufferers and its high total cost, it is important to be able to determine what treatment measures are truly cost effective in the management of this disease.

Avoidance procedures are probably the most cost-effective means in treating many patients with allergic rhinitis. If one can avoid the allergens that are triggering symptoms, then no other treatments are warranted.

Table 1-3. COST PER DAY FOR ANTIHISTAMINES AT RECOMMENDED DOSAGES*	
Second generation	
Drug	Cost, $
Fexofenadine (Allegra, Hoescht Marion Roussel)	1.77
Loratadine (Claritin, Schering)	2.15
Cetirizine (Zyrtec, Pfizer)	1.81
Astemizole (Hismanal, Janssen)	2.18
First generation	
Drug	Cost, $
Diphenhydramine 25 mg (Benadryl, Wallace)	0.58
Clemastine 1.34 mg (Tavist, Warner Lambert)	0.75
First-generation nasal spray	
Drug	Cost, $
Azelastine (Astelin, Wallace)	1.79

*Based on average wholesale price.
Data from *Amerisource* [11].

experience significant side effects that may impair productivity. These antihistamines cross the blood–brain barrier and may cause significant central nervous system sedation, including depression [12,13]. This sedation may be so pronounced that, in many states, it is illegal to operate heavy machinery or a motor vehicle while using these medications. The first-generation sedating antihistamines have been shown to have a detrimental effect on learning in children [14–16]. Fireman [17], using pharmacy data from a health management organization (HMO), determined that first-generation antihistamine use was associated with statistically significantly elevated work-related injuries compared to control groups. The author estimated the annual cost of lost productivity to employers and society due to allergic rhinitis and use of over-the-counter sedating antihistamines to be greater than $4 billion.

The second-generation antihistamines, which are also shown in Table 1-3, are often thought of as the nonsedating antihistamines. These agents are as effective in relief of symptoms as the first-generation antihistamines [18,19]. The advantages these antihistamines have over the first-generation agents include rare sedation (no higher than placebo at the indicated dosage except cetirizine), no anticholinergic effects, lack of tolerance with prolonged use, and decreased dosing frequency [20,21].

A first-generation antihistamine nasal spray (Table 1-3) is available for treatment of allergic rhinitis. The cost is equivalent to the cost of second-generation antihistamines and has been shown to be equal in efficacy [22,23]. The major side effects observed with this agent are somnolence and bitter taste.

Intranasal corticosteroids

Another important modality in the treatment of allergic rhinitis has been the intranasal corticosteroids. Table 1-4 summarizes the preparations available, along with their daily cost based on the average wholesale price. These drugs have been shown to be extremely effective in patients with moderate to severe allergic rhinitis because of the direct delivery of corticosteroid to the nasal mucosa. Intranasal corticosteroids have been shown to reduce sneezing, nasal itching, nasal congestion, and rhinorrhea. With chronic use at the recommended dose, there is no evidence of systemic corticosteroid side effects, such as adrenal suppression, weight gain, or cataracts. Disadvantages of these medications include local irritation and epistaxis in selected patients; rare complications, such as nasal septal perforation; and patient dislike for corticosteroids in any form.

Comparative studies in pharmacologic management

In general, the daily cost of intranasal corticosteroids is less than that of second-generation antihistamines (Tables

1-2 and 1-3). Several studies have evaluated the cost effectiveness and quality of life of these two major treatments for allergic rhinitis. Bronsky et al. [24] compared an intranasal corticosteroid (fluticasone), a second-generation antihistamine (terfenadine), and placebo for treatment of seasonal allergic rhinitis in 348 patients. Patient-rated total nasal symptom scores throughout treatment and total nasal airflow measured by rhinomanometry were significantly improved ($P < 0.05$) in the fluticasone group compared with the terfenadine group. Other clinical studies have shown that adults and adolescents with seasonal allergic rhinitis had significantly better improvement with fluticasone nasal spray than loratadine tablets [25•,26]. Kozma et al. [27] compared cost-efficacy ratios for intranasal fluticasone propionate and terfenadine tablets within a sample of patients with seasonal allergic rhinitis symptoms due to mountain cedar allergy. Costs measured were the direct costs of the drugs used for therapy; efficacy was assessed using patient ratings of symptoms and their overall assessment of response to treatment. The cost-efficacy ratios for intranasal fluticasone once daily were more favorable than the ratios for terfenadine 60 mg twice daily.

Other intranasal corticosteroids and second-generation antihistamines have been compared in assessing clinical efficacy. Bernstein et al. [28] conducted a multicenter, double-blind, parallel-group study in 239 patients who were randomized to receive either triamcinolone acetonide nasal spray or astemizole tablets. Overall, triamcinolone acetonide spray was more effective than astemizole in reducing total nasal symptoms, nasal stuffiness, nasal itching, and sneezing. Schulz et al. [29] compared the safety and efficacy of intranasal triamcinolone acetonide with oral loratadine in relieving symptoms of ragweed-induced seasonal allergic rhinitis. Improvement in all rhinitis symptoms was significantly

Table 1-4. COST PER DAY FOR INTRANASAL CORTICOSTEROIDS AT RECOMMENDED DOSAGE*

Drug	Cost, $
Beclomethasone (Beconase AQ, Glaxo Wellcome)	1.68
Fluticasone (Flonase, Glaxo Wellcome)	1.54
Triamcinolone acetonide (Nasacort AQ, Rhone-Poulenc Rorer)	1.15
Flunisolide (Nasarel, Dura)	1.46
Budesonide (Rhinocort, Astra)	1.38
Beclomethasone (Vancenase DS, Schering)	1.63
Momentasone (Nasonex, Schering)	1.61

*Based on average wholesale price.
Data from Amerisource [11].

greater with triamcinolone acetonide than with loratadine. Physicians' global evaluations indicated that triamcinolone acetonide provided moderate-to-complete relief in 78% of patients, compared with 58% of loratadine-treated patients ($P < 0.0001$). Schulz et al. [29] also assessed quality of life in patients with allergic rhinitis using triamcinolone nasal spray versus loratadine; at day 14, the patients using triamcinolone spray were significantly better ($P < 0.05$) in several different components and overall quality of life.

In general, these studies tend to indicate that the intranasal corticosteroids are more cost effective than the second-generation antihistamines. It is important to remember that convenience and compliance are factors in chronic use of medication. Oral medications have a higher compliance rate than inhaler agents [30]. Also, these studies evaluated chronic use of these different medications, and many patients only use these agents on an as-needed basis. Informing patients on the pros and cons of each type of medication and allowing them to participate in deciding pharmacologic management may be the best approach for highest compliance.

Role of allergen immunotherapy

Allergen immunotherapy is the administration of low, then sequentially increasing, doses of allergens by subcutaneous injection in patients with IgE-mediated diseases, such as allergic rhinitis, allergic asthma, and insect-sting anaphylaxis [31]. It has been shown to be efficacious in treatment of patients with allergic rhinitis by decreasing or eliminating the condition [32,33•]. Sullivan [34] reported that the average direct cost for immunotherapy at Emory University was $800 for the first year and $170 for the next 2 to 4 years. The estimated costs for immunotherapy based on the Medicare Payment Schedule is $1,640, which includes 24 injections to maintenance dose followed by monthly injections for 3 to 5 years and allergen extract preparation for 10 allergens [35].

In determining the cost effectiveness of allergen immunotherapy, Kumar et al. [36] looked at costs of treatment and quality of life in allergic rhinitis prior to allergen immunotherapy and then assessed these variables yearly over 3 years of immunotherapy. The cost of care in the year prior to immunotherapy was $1129±321 and for the third year of allergen immunotherapy it was $950±352. This study suggests that allergen immunotherapy by the third year is no more costly than allergy treatment without immunotherapy, with significant improvement in quality of life.

ASTHMA

Over 14 million Americans are afflicted with asthma, with an incidence of 4% to 5% of adults and 7% of children [37,38]. Weiss et al. [37] estimated the total cost for asthma care in the United States to be $6.21 billion in 1990. They estimated $3.64 billion for direct costs of asthma care. These include physician costs, medication costs, laboratory procedures, imaging studies, hospitalizations, and emergency-department care. In 1994 dollars, Smith et al. [39] found the total cost of asthma to be $5.8 billion with over one half of the direct costs of asthma due to hospitalizations. A comparison of costs supplied by these studies is shown in Table 1-5. Although hospital charges can vary greatly, a recent study estimated a 3-day stay for status asthmaticus at $3000 [40], whereas another report showed a 4-day charge at $6546 [41]. Yearly costs for each asthmatic child in an HMO in 1992 was $1060.32 compared with $563.81 in the nonasthmatic child [42]. In looking at costs for asthma, more than 70% of the total costs of asthma are generated by about 5% of patients [43].

Weiss et al. [37] computed indirect costs for asthma care at $2.57 billion. This figure represents loss of productivity due to absence from school and work and premature death from asthma. Barnes et al. [44••] reviewed cost studies of asthma from throughout the world. Indirect costs of asthma ranged from 90% of total costs in a study from the United Kingdom to 30% in an Australian report.

Asthma costs are a worldwide burden [44••]. In 1990 US dollars, the cost per year for each asthmatic in Sweden was $1315; in United Kingdom, $1043; and in

Table 1-5. COMPARISON OF ASTHMA CARE COSTS IN 1994 DOLLARS*

	Study	
	Weiss	Smith
Direct costs		
Ambulatory visits	1100	1530
Hospitalizations	2327	2800
Prescribed medicines	1397	817
Total direct costs	4824	5147
Indirect costs		
Housekeeping loss	579	21
Work loss	398	222
School loss	1036	195
Bed days (age, 0–4 y)	N/A	19
Restricted activity loss	N/A	218
Mortality	943	N/A
Total indirect costs	2956	675
Total costs	7780	5822

*in millions
Adapted from Smith et al. [39]; with permission.

Australia, $76 [45]. A recent study estimated the total cost for asthma in Canada during 1990 to be between US $378 and $486 million (US dollars) [46]. Toelle *et al.* [47] evaluated the cost of asthma in children in Australia: the mean annual cost of asthma to the family, in Australian dollars, was $212.48, and 13.4 hours were spent per asthmatic child to obtain treatment.

Environmental control

The components of asthma management include environmental control, objective monitoring, patient education, pharmacologic therapy, and allergen immunotherapy. Environmental allergen-avoidance procedures have been documented to play a role in cost-effective therapy in the allergic asthmatic patient. Studies have shown that early exposure to possible allergens may increase the risk of development of allergic disorders [48]. Initiation of avoidance measures early in life may prevent or delay the development of allergic disorders [49]. Dust-mite avoidance measures, such as removal of carpeting and encasing mattress covers, have been shown to improve pulmonary function and clinical symptomatology in asthmatics sensitive to mites [50,51•,52].

Medication costs

A mainstay of asthma management is appropriate pharmacologic management. With the publication of the National Heart, Lung, and Blood Institute (NHLBI) guidelines for long-term management of asthma, clinicians have a stepwise approach to the use of medication that depends on the severity of the patient's asthma [53]. Short-acting β-agonists, such as albuterol, are the most commonly prescribed medications for the treatment of asthma. They are recommended for acute exacerbations and in the prevention of exercise-induced asthma. According to the NHLBI guidelines, patients requiring the use of short-acting β-agonists more than twice a week are mild-persistent asthmatics and should be placed on a long-term controller anti-inflammatory agent. Anti-inflammatory medications include cromolyn, nedocromil, inhaled corticosteroids, and possibly leukotriene receptor antagonists and leukotriene synthesis inhibitors. Tables 1-6 and 1-7 show cost comparisons of these agents in the management of the mild-persistent asthmatic patient.

In assessing whether a pharmacologic agent is cost effective in asthma therapy, it is important to assess its costs compared with costs for emergency-department visits and hospitalizations. Studies have shown that placing patients on anti-inflammatory agents is an important cost-effective step in overall asthma management. Stempel *et al.* [54] analyzed drug use during 1993 in four HMOs with approximately 673,000 members. Health care costs were identified in asthmatic patients aged 7 years and over who used high doses of inhaled β-adrenergic agonists, defined as more than eight puffs a day. There were a total

of 20,512 asthmatic patients, with 5.3% receiving high doses of an inhaled bronchodilator. This group was then stratified by concurrent use of inhaled anti-inflammatory therapy. Members using high doses of inhaled bronchodilators had annual charges for treatment related to their asthma that were three times higher than the average asthmatic patient ($1346.52 versus $447.42). The high β-agonist users had in-patient hospital and emergency department charges that grew proportionally as a percentage of total annual expenses. Konig and Shaffer [55•] showed that early treatment with anti-inflammatory medication in asthmatic children, using either cromolyn or inhaled corticosteroids rather than as-needed bron-

Table 1-6. COSTS PER DAY OF INHALED CORTICOSTEROIDS FOR TREATMENT OF MILD-PERSISTENT ASTHMA IN ADULTS (MAXIMUM DOSE)*

Drug	Cost, $
Beclomethasone (Beclovent, Glaxo Wellcome)	1.62
Beclomethasone (Vanceril DS, Schering)	2.44
Triamcinolone acetonide (Azmacort, Rhone-Poulenc Rorer)	2.05
Flunisolide (Aerobid, Forest)	2.39
Fluticasone (Flovent, Glaxo Wellcome)	1.33
Budesonide (Pulmicort, Astra)	1.07

*According to National Heart, Lung, and Blood Institute guidelines; based on average wholesale price.
Data from *Amerisource* [11].

Table 1-7. COST PER DAY FOR OTHER CONTROLLER AGENTS FOR TREATMENT OF MILD-PERSISTENT ASTHMA IN ADULTS (MAXIMUM DOSE)*

Drug	Cost, $
Zafirlukast (Accolate, Zeneca)	1.85
Zileuton (Zyflo, Abbott)	2.75
Montelukast (Singulair, Merck & Co.)	2.33
Nedocromil (Tilade, Rhone-Poulenc Rorer)	2.45
Cromolyn (Intal, Rhone-Poulenc Rorer)	2.88
Salmeterol (Serevent, Glaxo Wellcome)	1.94
Theophylline 600 mg (Uni-Dur, Key)	1.17
Generic theophylline	0.43

*According to National Heart, Lung, and Blood Institute guidelines; based on average wholesale price.
Data from *Amerisource* [11].

chodilators alone, improved the long-term prognosis of asthma and may decrease overall total costs. Another study placed 310 adult patients with mild, moderate, or severe asthma on nedocromil sodium for at least 1 year. After initiation of nedocromil sodium therapy, patients showed better asthma control as measured by improvements in pulmonary function scores and by reduced emergency-department visits and hospital admissions [56].

Further data demonstrate that use of inhaled corticosteroid has been shown to reduce hospitalizations in asthmatics, making them a cost-effective method of treatment. A Swedish study documented inhaled corticosteroid use from 1978 to 1991 and showed that increased sales of inhaled corticosteroids significantly correlated ($P < 0.01$) with a reduction in bed-days due to asthma [57]. Rutten-van Molken et al. [58] determined the costs and effects of inhaled terbutaline plus placebo, inhaled terbutaline plus inhaled ipratropium, and inhaled terbutaline plus inhaled beclomethasone. The inhaled terbutaline plus inhaled beclomethasone therapy was more costly, but it was almost matched by the decrease in other costs and the improvement in clinical outcomes compared with bronchodilators only (Fig. 1-1) [58]. This study showed a $201 cost for each 10% improvement in forced expiratory volume and $5 per symptom-free day with inhaled corticosteroid use.

It is important when new agents are approved for treatment of asthma that that they be documented for cost-effectiveness. Suissa et al. [59] evaluated the clinical and economic effectiveness of the leukotriene receptor antagonist zafirlukast compared to placebo for mild-to-moderate asthma in 146 patients. The economic effectiveness outcomes were frequency and type of unscheduled healthcare contacts, use of β-agonist inhalers, consumption of

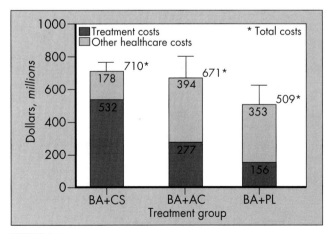

FIGURE 1-1.
Estimated adjusted-mean health care costs for asthma per patient year by treatment group. Error bars indicate upper limit of the 95% confidence interval. AC—anticholinergic; BA—beta agonist; CS—inhaled corticosteroid; PL—placebo. *Adapted from* Rutten-van Molken *et al.* [58]; with permission.)

nonasthma medications, and days of absence from work or school. The subjects in the zafirlukast group had 55% fewer health-care contacts and 55% fewer days of absence from work or school. They used 17% fewer canisters of inhaled β-agonists and 19% fewer nonasthma medications. These data suggest that this medication may have cost-effective benefits in the treatment of asthma, but further data are needed, especially in comparison with other anti-inflammatory agents.

Immunotherapy

Specific allergen immunotherapy as a cost-effective treatment for bronchial asthma has been controversial. Calvo et al. [60] performed a study to attempt to define further the possible contribution of specific immunotherapy in a pediatric asthmatic population. In the study, 166 patients were treated with immunotherapy and 248 received no immunotherapy. The results were compared during 10 years of follow-up in both groups. There was a significant decrease in the number of acute crises in the treated group ($P < 0.05$). However, no differences were seen in the number of hospital admissions or in the quality of life between the treated and untreated groups. The treated group required significantly fewer drugs ($P < 0.05$). Thus, this study illustrates that immunotherapy may be cost-effective by decreasing medication costs over time. Immunotherapy may also represent an effective treatment that changes the natural course of allergic asthma in pediatric patients. Cantani et al. [61] performed a randomized, placebo-controlled trial with dust-mite or pollen immunotherapy in 300 asthmatic children over 3 years. Children who received immunotherapy had significantly decreased drug use, decreased asthma attacks, and improved quality of life.

Abramson et al. [62] performed a meta-analysis of clinical trials of allergen immunotherapy to evaluate the effectiveness of this therapy in asthma. The results extracted included asthmatic symptoms, medication requirements, lung function, and bronchial hyperreactivity. Categorical outcomes were expressed as odds ratios and continuous outcomes as effect sizes. The combined odds of symptomatic improvement from immunotherapy with any allergen were 3.2 (95% confidence interval [CI], 2.2 to 4.9). The odds for reduction in medication after mite immunotherapy were 4.2 (95% CI, 2.2 to 7.9). The authors concluded that allergen immunotherapy is a treatment option for highly selected patients with allergic asthma. Creticos et al. [63] looked at 2-year use of ragweed immunotherapy for adult asthmatics. There were reduced medication costs for asthma with immunotherapy, but these were counterbalanced by the costs of immunotherapy.

Intervention programs in cost-effective management

Many studies have documented the role of asthma intervention programs in producing cost-effective management for children and adults. There have been many different types of programs that show at least short-term efficacy in controlling asthma costs. Bolton *et al.* [64] analyzed the cost effectiveness of a self-management training program in adult asthmatics. The educational sessions cost $85 per person, which was offset by the $628 per person reduction in emergency room charges. A protocol to assess therapeutic benefit and cost saving in the treatment of acute asthma in the emergency department over 1 year was compared with costs prior to implementation of the protocol [65]. Following the protocol decreased the length of stay in the emergency department, the rate of hospitalization, and the frequency of return visits to the emergency department in 24 hours. Charges to patients and third-party payers were consequently reduced by $395,000.

A major emphasis has been the development of intervention programs for the indigent population who primarily use the emergency department for asthma care. An outreach program was developed for an inner-city pediatric asthma population [66]. Patients were scheduled for one-on-one orientation visits with the asthma outreach nurse and an individualized step-care treatment program was outlined for each patient. The outreach nurse maintained personal or telephone contact with the families on a regular basis to ensure compliance. This program resulted in the reduction of emergency department admissions by 79% and hospital admissions by 86%, with estimated savings of approximately $87,000. Kelso *et al.* [67] conceived a major long-term therapeutic and educational intervention program in the emergency department for indigent adult black asthmatics. Outcome measures assessed were emergency department visits and hospitalizations for 1 year after emergency department intervention. These outcomes were compared with a retrospective control group of 22 patients. There was a significant decrease in both emergency department visits and hospitalizations in the intervention group, whereas there was no significant change in either in the control group.

REFERENCES AND RECOMMENDED READING

Recently published papers of particular interest have been highlighted as:
- •   Of interest
- ••   Of outstanding interest

1. Sibbald B, Rink E: Epidemiology of seasonal and perennial rhinitis: clinical presentation and medical history. *Thorax* 1991, 46:895–901.

2. Naclerio R: Allergic rhinitis. *N Engl J Med* 1991, 325:860–869.

3. Arrighi HM, Maler WC, Redding GJ: The impact of allergic rhinitis in Seattle school children [abstract]. *J Allergy Clin Immunol* 1995, 95:192.

4. Blaiss M, Bukstein D, Davis M, Luskin A: Improving allergy and asthma care through outcomes management. *Managed Care Fourth Series*. Edited by Davis M. Milwaukee: American Academy of Allergy, Asthma, and Immunology; 1997: 11.

5. McMenamin P: Costs of hay fever in the United States in 1990. *Ann Allergy* 1994, 73:35–39.

6. Ross RN: Allergic rhinitis: an expensive disease for American business. *Am J Managed Care* 1996, 2:285–290.

7. Malone DC, Lawson KA, Smith DH, *et al.*: A cost of illness study of allergic rhinitis in the United States. *J Allergy Clin Immunol* 1997, 99:22–27.

8•. Storms W, Meltzer EO, Nathan RA, Selner JC: The economic impact of allergic rhinitis. *J Allergy Clin Immunol* 1997, 97:S820–S824.
This article is from a supplement on the prevalence and medical and economic impact of allergic rhinitis. A nationwide survey of 15,000 households was used to assess prescription and over-the-counter medication costs for allergic rhinitis.

9. Mackowiak J: The health and economic impact of rhinitis: a roundtable discussion. *Am J Managed Care* 1997, 3:S8–S18.

10. Platts-Mills TA: How environment affects patients with allergic disease: indoor allergens and asthma. *Ann Allergy* 1994, 72:381–384.

11 *Amerisource*. Paducah, KY: Amerisource; July 3, 1998

12. Nolen TM: Sedative effects of antihistamines: safety, performance, learning, and quality of life. *Clin Ther* 1997, 19:39–55.

13. Storms WW: Treatment of allergic rhinitis: effects of allergic rhinitis and antihistamines on performance. *Allergy Asthma Proc* 1997, 18:59–61.

14. Kemp JP: Special considerations in the treatment of seasonal allergic rhinitis in adolescents: the role of antihistamine therapy. *Clin Pediatr* 1996, 35:383–389.

15. Simons FE: Learning impairment and allergic rhinitis. *Allergy Asthma Proc* 1996, 17:185–189.

16. Vuurman EF, van Veggel LM, Uiterwijk MM, *et al.*: Seasonal allergic rhinitis and antihistamine effects on children's learning. *Ann Allergy* 1993, 71:121–126.

17. Fireman P: Treatment of allergic rhinitis: effect on occupation productivity and work force costs. *Allergy Asthma Proc* 1997, 18:63–67.

18. Busse WW: Role of antihistamines in allergic disease. *Ann Allergy* 1994, 72:371–375.

19. Du Buske LM: Clinical comparison of histamine H_1-receptor antagonist drugs. *J Allergy Clin Immunol* 1996, 98:S307–S318.

20. Adelsberg BR: Sedation and performance issues in the treatment of allergic conditions. *Arch Intern Med* 1997, 157:494–500.

21. Pedinoff AJ: Approaches to the treatment of seasonal allergic rhinitis. *South Med J* 1996, 89:1130–1139.

22. Conde Hernandez DJ, Palma Aqilar JL, Delgado Romero J: Comparison of azelastine nasal spray and oral ebastine in treating seasonal allergic rhinitis. *Curr Med Res Opin* 1995, 13:299–304.

23. Gastpar H, Nolte D, Aurich R, *et al.*: Comparative efficacy of azelastine nasal spray and terfenadine in seasonal and perennial rhinitis. *Allergy* 1994, 49:152–158.

24. Bronsky EA, Dockhorn RJ, Meltzer EO, *et al.*: Fluticasone propionate aqueous nasal spray compared with terfenadine tablets in the treatment of seasonal allergic rhinitis. *J Allergy Clin Immunol* 1996, 97:915–921.

25.• Gehanno P, Desfougeres JL: Fluticasone propionate aqueous nasal spray compared with oral loratadine in patients with seasonal allergic rhinitis. *Allergy* 1997, 52:445–450.
The effectiveness and safety of fluticasone propionate aqueous nasal spray (200 μg once daily for 4 weeks) were compared with those of loratadine (10 mg once daily for 4 weeks) in 114 adults and adolescents with seasonal allergic rhinitis in this multicenter, double-blind, double-dummy, randomized, parallel-group study. In both physician-based and patient-based scoring of clinical symptoms, fluticasone was significantly better than loratadine.

26. Jordana G, Dolovich J, Briscoe MP, et al.: Intranasal fluticasone propionate versus loratadine in the treatment of adolescent patients with seasonal allergic rhinitis. *J Allergy Clin Immunol* 1996, 97:588–595.

27. Kozma CM, Schulz RM, Sclar DA, et al.: A comparison of costs and efficacy of intranasal fluticasone propionate and terfenadine tablets for seasonal allergic rhinitis. *Clin Ther* 1996, 18:334–346.

28. Bernstein DI, Creticos PS, Busse WW, et al.: Comparison of triamcinolone acetonide nasal inhaler with astemizole in the treatment of ragweed-induced allergic rhinitis. *J Allergy Clin Immunol* 1996, 97:749–755.

29. Schulz RM, Smith DH, Lim J: Quality of life in patients with seasonal allergic rhinitis (SAR): triamcinolone acetonide aqueous nasal spray versus loratadine [abstract]. *Ann Allergy Asthma Immunol* 1997, 78:155.

30. Kelloway JS, Wyatt RA, Adlis SA: Comparison of patients' compliance with prescribed oral and inhaled asthma medications. *Arch Intern Med* 1994, 154:1349–1352.

31. Hedlin G: The role of immunotherapy in pediatric allergic disease. *Curr Opin Pediatr* 1995, 7:676–682.

32. Creticos PS: The role of immunotherapy in allergic rhinitis/allergic asthma. *Allergy Proc* 1995, 16:297–302.

33.• Donovan JP, Buckeridge DL, Briscoe MP, et al.: Efficacy of immunotherapy to ragweed antigen tested by controlled antigen exposure. *Ann Allergy Asthma Immunol* 1996, 77:74–80.
This study was designed to evaluate the efficacy of immunotherapy in ragweed-induced rhinoconjunctivitis using an environmental exposure unit. The immunotherapy group, which had been on maintenance injections for 2 years, had combined nasal and ocular scores that were 50% less than in the positive control group after 75 minutes of ragweed pollen exposure (P = 0.039).

34. Sullivan TJ: *Expert Care and Immunotherapy for Asthma.* Chicago: American College of Allergy, Asthma, and Immunology; 1996.

35. American Medical Association: *Medicare RBRVS: The Physician' Guide.* Chicago: American Medical Association; 1995.

36. Kumar P, Kamboj S, Rao P: The cost of care and quality of life in patients with allergic rhinitis on allergen immunotherapy. *Allergy Clin Immunol Int* 1997, 9:133–135.

37. Weiss KB, Gergen PJ, Hodgson TA: An economic evaluation of asthma in the United States. *N Engl J Med* 1992, 326:862–866.

38. Centers for Disease Control: Asthma mortality and hospitalization among children and young adults: United States, 1980–1993. *MMWR* 1996, 45:350–353.

39. Smith D, Malone D, Lawson K: A national estimate of the economic costs of asthma. *Am J Respir Crit Care Med* 1997, 156:787–793.

40. Brillman J, Tandberg D: Observation unit impact on ED admission for asthma. *Am J Emerg Med* 1994, 12:11–14.

41. DeSilva R: A disease management case study on asthma. *Clin Ther* 1996, 18:1374–1382.

42. Lozano P, Fishman P, VonKorff M, Hecht J: Healthcare utilization and cost among children with asthma who were enrolled in a health maintenance organization. *Pediatrics* 1997, 99:757–764.

43. Todd W: New mindsets in asthma: interventions and disease management. *J Care Manage* 1995, 1:2–8.

44.•• Barnes PJ, Jonsson B, Klim JB: the costs of asthma. *Eur Respir J* 1996, 9:636–642.
This excellent paper reviews the current literature on the costs of asthma. The authors assess how effectively money is spent in asthma care. They estimate the proportion of the cost attributable to uncontrolled disease and identify where financial savings might be made in asthma care.

45. The Global Initiative for Asthma: *Global Strategy for Asthma Management and Prevention: NHLBI/WHO Workshop Report.* Bethesda, MD: National Institutes of Health publication 95–3659, 1995.

46. Krahn MD, Berka C, Langlois P, et al.: Direct and indirect costs of asthma in Canada. *Can Med Assoc J* 1996, 154:821–831.

47. Toelle BG, Peat JK, Mellis CM, Woolcock AJ: The cost of childhood asthma to Australian families. *Pediatr Pulmonol* 1995, 19:330–335.

48. Kuehr J, Frischer T, Meinert R, et al.: Sensitization to mite allergens is a risk factor for early and late onset of asthma and for persistence of asthmatic signs in children. *J Allergy Clin Immunol* 1995, 95:655–662.

49. Hide DW, Matthews S, Matthews L, et al.: Effect of allergen avoidance in infancy on allergic manifestations at age two years. *J Allergy Clin Immunol* 1994, 93:842–846.

50. van der Heide S, Kauffman HF, Dubois AE, de Monchy JG: Allergen reduction measures in houses of allergic asthmatic patients: effects of air-cleaners and allergen-impermeable mattress covers. *Eur Respir J* 1997, 10:1217–1223.

51.• Piacentini GL, Martinati L, Mingoni S, Boner AL: Influence of allergen avoidance on the eosinophil phase of airway inflammation in children with allergic asthma. *J Allergy Clin Immunol* 1996, 97:1079–1084.
This study shows that after a 3-month period of antigen avoidance, mite avoidance can significantly reduce the eosinophil phase of airway inflammation, along with bronchial hyperresponsiveness, in patients with asthma.

52. Peroni DG, Boner AL, Vallone G, et al.: Effective allergen avoidance at high altitude reduces allergen-induced bronchial hyperresponsiveness. *Am J Respir Crit Care Med* 1994, 149:1442–1446.

53. Program NAEaP: *Expert Panel Report II: Guidelines for the Diagnosis and Management of Asthma.* Bethesda, MD: National Institutes of Health, 1997.

54. Stempel DA, Durcannin Robbins JF, Hedblom EC, et al.: Drug utilization evaluation identifies costs associated with high use of β-adrenergic agonists. *Ann Allergy Asthma Immunol* 1996, 6:153–158.

55.• Konig P, Shaffer J: The effect of drug therapy on long-term outcome of childhood asthma: a possible preview of the international guidelines. *J Allergy Clin Immunol* 1996, 98:1103–1111.
This retrospective analysis of 75 children followed for a mean of 8.4 years showed that treatment with anti-inflammatory drugs (cromolyn sodium or inhaled corticosteroids) rather than as-needed bronchodilators alone improves the long-term prognosis of asthma.

56. Thomas P, Ross RN, Farrar JR: A retrospective assessment of cost avoidance associated with the use of nedocromil sodium metered-dose inhaler in the treatment of patients with asthma. *Clin Ther* 1996, 18:939–952.

57. Gerdtham UG, Hertzman P, Jonsson B, Boman G: Impact of inhaled corticosteroids on acute asthma hospitalization in Sweden 1978 to 1991. *Med Care* 1996, 34:1188–1198.

58. Rutten-van Molken MP, Van Doorslaer EK, Jansen MC, *et al.*: Costs and effects of inhaled corticosteroids and bronchodilators in asthma and chronic obstructive pulmonary disease. *Am J Respir Crit Care Med* 1995, 151:975–982.

59. Suissa S, Dennis R, Ernst P, *et al.*: Effectiveness of the leukotriene receptor antagonist zafirlukast for mild-to-moderate asthma: a randomized, double-blind, placebo-controlled trial. *Ann Intern Med* 1997, 126:177–183.

60. Calvo M, Marin F, Grob K, *et al.*: Ten-year follow-up in pediatric patients with allergic bronchial asthma: evaluation of specific immunotherapy. *J Invest Allerg Clin Immunol* 1994, 4:126–131.

61. Cantani A, Arcese G, Lucenti P, *et al.*: A three-year prospective study of specific immunotherapy to inhalant allergens: evidence of safety and efficacy in 300 children with allergic asthma. *J Invest Allerg Clin Immunol* 1997, 7:90–97.

62. Abramson MJ, Puy RM, Weiner JM: Is allergen immunotherapy effective in asthma? A meta-analysis of randomized controlled trials. *Am J Respir Crit Care Med* 1995, 151:969–974.

63. Creticos PS, Reed CE, Norman PS, *et al.*: Ragweed immunotherapy in adult asthma. *N Engl J Med* 1996, 334:501–506.

64. Bolton MB, Tilley BC, Kuder J, *et al.*: The cost and effectiveness of an education program for adults who have asthma. *J Gen Intern Med* 1991, 6:401–407.

65. McFadden ER Jr, Elsanadi N, Dixon L, *et al.*: Protocol therapy for acute asthma: therapeutic benefits and cost savings. *Am J Med* 1995, 99:651–661.

66. Greineder DK, Loane KC, Parks P: Reduction in resource utilization by an asthma outreach program. *Arch Pediatr Adolesc Med* 1995, 149:415–420.

67. Kelso TM, Self TH, Rumbak MJ, *et al.*: Educational and long-term therapeutic intervention in the ED: effect on outcomes in adult indigent minority asthmatics. *Am J Emerg Med* 1995, 13:632–637.

CHAPTER 2

Mast Cells and Basophils

Reuben P. Siraganian

Mast cells and basophils were first recognized more than 100 years ago because they stained metachromatically with certain basic dyes. Although mast cells and basophils have many similarities, they are distinct cell types (Table 2-1). Mast cells are found in connective tissues, whereas basophils are present in the circulation. Both mast cells and basophils synthesize and store histamine, proteoglycans, and proteases within their granules and have surface receptors (FcεRI) that bind IgE with high affinity. The binding of multivalent antigen to this cell-bound IgE results in degranulation and the release of mediators. The physiological effects of immediate hypersensitivity and inflammation are due to the response of other cells to the mediators released from the basophils and mast cells. IgE-mediated reactions, besides resulting in immediate wheal and erythema reactions, also induce a late-phase response, which occurs within 4 to 8 hours after challenge. Such reactions are clearly mediated by IgE-antigen interactions and require the presence of mast cells in the tissues. The release of cytokines from mast cells recruits basophils, neutrophils, eosinophils, and macrophages to these sites where mast cells are degranulating. The cytokines released from the mast cells also activate the resident and recruited cells to release other cytokines and inflammatory mediators. Recent data have implicated these late responses for the inflammation that is prominent in asthma and other allergic diseases.

Mast cells, by controlling neutrophil influx, play an important role in host defense against bacterial infection. In this pathway, mast cells are activated independently of IgE to release tumor necrosis factor (TNF)-α, which is chemotactic for neutrophils [1,2•]. Experiments also suggest that IgE and non-IgE–mediated pathways involving basophils and mast cells may play a role in eliminating parasitic infestations.

CHARACTERISTICS OF BASOPHILS AND MAST CELLS
Development

Mast cells are derived from pluripotential stem cells in the bone marrow. The precursors enter the circulation and appear as nongranulated lymphoid cells that are CD34+, c-Kit+, Ly 1+, CD14- and CD17-. These precursors undergo differentiation after entering a particular tissue and their phenotypic characteristics depend on the local microenvironment. The interaction between the receptor tyrosine kinase, c-Kit, and its ligand stem cell factor (SCF, also called c-Kit ligand) is essential for mast cell development [3]. SCF is produced by fibroblasts, bone marrow stromal cells, and endothelial cells, whereas c-Kit is present on mast cells and mast cell precursors. SCF occurs both as a membrane-associated form and as a soluble secreted product. Both forms are biologically active and the local level of this factor regulates the number of mast cells at sites of inflammation. Mast cells are distributed in connective tissues, often adjacent to blood vessels and beneath epithelial surfaces (*eg*, gastrointestinal and respiratory tracts, skin). Mature mast cells normally do not circulate, are long-lived, and appear to retain the capacity to proliferate.

Basophils, like the other members of the granulocytes, differentiate and mature in the bone marrow before entering into the circulation, where they constitute less than 0.5% of the total leukocytes. Like mast cells, they develop from a common bone-marrow–derived hematopoietic CD34+ precursor cell. Interleukin (IL)-3 appears to be important for the development of basophils. In contrast to mast cells that mature in the tissues where they finally reside, basophils differentiate in the bone marrow and enter the circulation as mature,

functionally active cells. Basophils have the capacity for chemotaxis and are recruited into tissues during inflammatory reactions. However, even in tissues they can be identified as basophils; they do not transform into mast cells. Basophils are smaller than mast cells, are short-lived (< 2 weeks), and are probably end-cells. Basophils contain less histamine than most mast cells. There are several other differences between basophils and mast cells, as shown in Table 2-1. Unlike mast cells, chondroitin monosulfates are the major proteoglycan of basophils. There are also differences in the surface proteins found on basophils compared to those on mast cells.

Ultrastructural studies

Ultrastructurally, mast cells have many long, thin projections that appear as villi by scanning electron microscopy. The nucleus is round and not segmented; there are some mitochondria, but the endoplasmic reticulum and the Golgi apparatus are not prominent. Mast cells also contain intermediate filaments and lipid bod-

Table 2-1. COMPARISON OF BASOPHILS AND MAST CELLS

Characteristics	Basophil	Mast cells
General		
Origin	Bone marrow	Bone marrow
Progenitor cell	CD34+	CD34+
Site of maturation	Bone marrow	Peripheral tissue
Location	Circulation	Peripheral tissue
Life span	Short (days)	Long (weeks to months)
Growth factor	IL-3	SCF
Surface adhesion molecules		
PECAM-1 (CD31)	Positive	Negative
β_1 integrins (VLA/CD29/49)	Positive	Positive
β_2 integrins (CD11/CD18)	Positive	Probably negative or low
Receptors		
FcεRI	Yes	Yes
FcεR	Yes	Yes
Activating stimuli		
IgE antigen	Yes	Yes
C5a	Yes	Yes
Formal peptides	Yes	No
Basic molecules (*eg*, morphine)	No	Some types
Mediators		
Histamine	<1 pg/cell	2 to 3 pg/cell
Proteoglycan	Chondroitin sulfate A	Heparin, chondroitin sulfate E
Neutral proteases		Tryptase
Lipid mediators	LTC_4	$PGD_2 > LTC_4$
Cytokines	TNF-α, IL-4	TNF-α

IL—interleukin; LTC$_4$—leukotriene C$_4$; PECAM—platelet/endothelial cell adhesion molecule; PGD$_2$—prostaglandin D$_2$; SCF—stem cell factor; TNF—tumor necrosis factor.

ies. The granules are heterogeneous in substructural pattern; some have a scroll-like appearance, whereas others have an amorphous electron-dense matrix.

Human basophils have a segmented nucleus with condensed nuclear chromatin and absent nucleoli. They have little endoplasmic reticulum and free ribosomes. The cytoplasm contains a large number of granules that are heterogeneous in size but are less numerous than in mast cells. By electron microscopy some granules are filled uniformly with electron-dense material, whereas others lack this dense material. When antigen is added in vitro, the basophils lose their oriented motility and extend pseudopodia. The degranulating basophils develop small cytoplasmic "vesicles," which rapidly increase in size and coalesce. The granular membranes fuse with the plasma membrane, resulting in the development of narrow openings between the outside of the cell and individual granules. This results in the extrusion of membrane-free granular material through multiple openings in the circumference of the cell. However, some rare, interconnected chains of granules open to the exterior at a single point on the cell surface. The granule matrix is released as a whole to the outside, but the granule membrane is left behind. Frequently, membrane-free granular contents are seen attached to the cell exterior. In contrast to basophils, where most of the granules fuse directly with the plasma membrane, the degranulation of mast cells is of the compound type, with granules fusing with each other and then opening to the outside.

Basophils infiltrate and occasionally constitute a significant proportion of the total cells at reactions of the delayed hypersensitivity type. These reactions have been termed *cutaneous basophil hypersensitivity*. At these sites, mononuclear cells probably release chemokines that are chemotactic for basophils and might also induce the basophils to degranulate slowly; the granules never fuse with the cell membrane and they lose their matrix in "piecemeal" manner over a period of days. Small packages of granular content appear to bud from granule membranes, traverse the cytoplasm, and fuse with the plasma membrane, leaving completely degranulated cells.

Heterogeneity of mast cells

The concept of heterogeneity of mast cells developed from studies in rodents. Two populations of mast cells have been described: the mucosal type, which is considered immature, and the connective tissue type, which is considered more mature [4–6]. The two types vary in many characteristics, such as tissue distribution, morphology, histamine content, staining, and growth factor requirements. Although both cell types respond to IgE-receptor–mediated activation, they respond differently to other secretagogues and release different arachidonic acid metabolites.

Although not as clearly defined, two types of mast cells have been identified in human tissues. The majority of the mast cells on mucosal surfaces, such as the intestinal mucosa and lung alveolar wall, contain tryptase (MC_T). In contrast, the majority of mast cells in the connective tissue and in the dermis contain tryptase, chymase, and carboxypeptidase (MC_{TC}). There are also some differences in the response of mast cells from different sites to different stimuli, although these have not been as clearly defined as with rodent tissues. The heterogeneity of human mast cell populations is shown in Table 2-2.

MEDIATORS FROM MAST CELLS AND BASOPHILS

The secretory granules of these cells contain pre-formed mediators that are released when the cells are stimulated. Histamine is the major biogenic amine present in the secretory granules of human basophils and mast cells. Histamine is produced from the amino acid L-histidine by the cytoplasmic enzyme histidine decarboxylase. Histamine is then stored in the granules complexed to proteoglycans. Human mast cells contain 2 to 3 pg of histamine per cell. Histamine released from cells dissociates from the proteins it is complexed with and has local effects. The effects of histamine are due to its binding to specific histamine receptors (H_1, H_2, or H_3) on cells. H_1 receptors mediate immediate allergic reactions and inflammation. These receptors are present on smooth muscle cells in the venules and bronchi and stimulation results in vasodilation, enhanced permeability of postcapillary venules, contraction of bronchial and gastrointestinal smooth muscles, and mucous secretion. Classical antihistamines, such as chlorpheniramine, block these

Table 2-2. HETEROGENEITY OF HUMAN MAST CELL POPULATIONS

Characteristics	MC_{TC}	MC_T
Unique sites of distribution	Skin	Alvelolar wall; intestinal mucosa
Granule morphology	Grating/lattice, scroll poor	Scroll rich
Granule content		
Tryptase	Yes	Yes
Chymase	Yes	No
Carboxypeptidase	Yes	No
Cathepsin G	Yes	No
Heparin	Yes	Yes
Chondroitin sulfate E	Yes	Yes

MC_T—mast cell containing tryptase; MC_{TC}—mast cell containing tryptase, chymase, and carboxypeptidase.

receptors. H_2 receptors are prominent on parietal gastric cells, where stimulation results in increased gastric acid production. However, H_2 receptors may regulate the function of other cells, such as lymphocytes and eosinophils, and may play a role in allergic inflammation. H_3 receptors are thought to be important for control of neuroreceptors. The histamine that is released by cells has a short half life because it is rapidly degraded by either diamine oxidase or methyl transferase, which first results in the formation of methyl histamine that is then deaminated by monoamine oxidase.

Neutral proteases are also a major component of the secretory granules of mast cells. They cleave peptide bonds, a process resulting in the degradation of proteins. Several different proteases have been found in mast cells including tryptase, chymase, and carboxypeptidase. The presence or absence of these enzymes has been used as markers to distinguish different populations of mast cells. *Tryptase* is a trypsin-like serine-class protease present in mast cells but essentially absent in basophils. It is stored as an active molecule in the secretory granule, although the acidic pH of granules suppresses its enzymatic activity. It is released parallel to histamine from mast cells. Tryptase results in inflammation by acting on smooth muscles and fibroblasts, thereby inducing an increase in airway hyperresponsiveness [7–9]. Because tryptase is uniquely present in mast cells, measurement of its level in serum or other fluids can be used as a marker for mast cell activation and degranulation. *Chymase, cathepsin G,* and *carboxypeptidase* are present in mast cells but not in basophils. When released, they may also play a role in causing inflammation.

The characteristic metachromatic staining of mast cells or basophils with basic dyes is due to the presence of sulfated *proteoglycans* in their granules. Proteoglycans are composed of a protein core covalently linked with a glycosaminoglycan side chain. Human mast cells contain heparin and chondroitin sulfate E, whereas basophils have chondroitin sulfate A. Proteoglycans are involved in packaging pre-formed mediators, such as histamine, and neutral proteases in granules. Heparin is an anticoagulant and has several other biological effects, including effects on cell adhesion and proliferation. A number of other enzymes, including β-hexosaminidase, β-glucuronidase, β-D-galactosidase, arylsulfatase, superoxide dismutase, and peroxidase, are present and released from the secretory granules. Chemotactic factors for eosinophils, neutrophils, and monocytes are also released from mast cells or basophils.

A number of *lipid mediators* are generated when mast cells or basophils are stimulated. During secretion, arachidonic acid is released from phospholipids due to the activation of phospholipase enzymes. The arachidonic acid is then metabolized, either along the cyclooxygenase pathway with the formation of prostaglandins (predominantly prostaglandin D_2 [PGD_2], but also thromboxanes) or by the lipoxygenase pathway, with the formation of monhydroxyl fatty acids and leukotrienes (LT) (predominantly the cysteinyl leukotriene C_4, and the two peptidolytic products LTD_4 and LTE_4). These lipid mediators have potent inflammatory activities. Mast cells make more PGD_2 than LTC_4, whereas basophils produce LTC_4 but not PGD_2. Platelet activating factor is a low–molecular-weight phospholipid generated from alkyl phospholipids in these cells.

Mast cells and basophils synthesize and release *cytokines* when stimulated. Cytokines are a group of proteins synthesized and released by activated cells that then have effects on other cells. Cytokines induce or enhance the inflammatory reaction, are chemotactic for other cells, and can modulate the function of cells. These effects of cytokines on cells are due to their binding to specific cell surface receptors that induce intracellular signals, which results in changes in adherence of the cells, secretory events, and the induction of new gene expression. Unlike the rapid release (within minutes) of pre-formed mediators, release of most cytokines from mast cells or basophils is a slow process that usually requires several hours. This slow synthesis and release of cytokines is probably the mechanism that underlies the late-phase responses that are characteristic of IgE-mediated allergic reactions.

TNF-α is present as a pre-formed molecule in mast cells. Antibodies to TNF-α inhibit the mast cell or IgE-mediated infiltration of leukocytes at sites of inflammation [10]. Other cytokines that are either released or the synthesis of whose mRNA is increased after stimulation are the following: IL-1, IL-3, IL-4, IL-5, IL-6, IL-8, IL-9, IL-13, IL-16, granulocyte-macrophage colony-stimulating factor (GM-CSF), interferon (IFN)-γ, macrophage inflammatory protein (MIP)-1a, MIP-1b, basic fibroblast growth factor, and other chemokines. Some of these conclusions are based on studies with human or rodent cell lines or purified cells. Most of these studies have been with mast cells; however, at least IL-4 and IL-13 are produced by human basophils.

The cytokines released from basophils or mast cells are biologically important. By acting on the local endothelial cells, cytokines induce changes in the expression or activity of cell surface adhesion molecules, such as P-selectin, E-selectin, or CD31, that allow cells in capillaries to be trapped and to migrate into tissues. Several of the cytokines, such as TNF-α, IL-16, and lympotaxin, are potent chemotactic factors and therefore contribute to the recruitment of cells. Some cytokines (*eg*, chemokines) can directly induce other cells to release inflammatory mediators. Cytokines also promote the maturation and development of cells, such as eosinophils (*eg*, IL-5). IL-4 and IL-13 may also promote the class switching that is required for the production of IgE. Basophils and mast cells have the CD40 ligand and therefore can functionally present antigen to B cells for the production of IgE [11].

HIGH-AFFINITY RECEPTOR FOR IMMUNOGLOBULIN E

There are two types of receptors for IgE on cells: mast cells and basophils, which have a high-affinity receptor for monomeric IgE (FcɛRI); and other cells (*eg*, lymphocytes, eosinophils, macrophages), which have receptors that bind IgE with much lower affinity (FcɛRII) (Table 2-3). Structurally, the two receptors are different. Recent studies have shown that FcɛRI is present at low levels on monocytes, platelets, skin Langerhan's cells and dendritic cells.

The FcɛRI receptor consists of four polypeptide chains: an IgE-binding α chain of 45 to 60 kD, a 33 kD β subunit and a homodimer formed of disulfide-linked γ chains [12]. The different receptor subunits are not covalently linked, but associate closely in the membrane. The binding of IgE to FcɛRI is a simple, reversible reaction with a high affinity and is not inhibited by immunoglobulins of other classes. FcɛRIs are distributed diffusely over the surface of the cell, and monomeric IgE-receptor complexes are freely mobile in the membrane. There are a large number of receptors on basophils and mast cells (best estimates are over 10^5 per cell).

The FcɛRI subunits lack any known enzymatic activity; thus, this receptor depends on associated molecules for transducing intracellular signals. The extracellular domain of the α chain of FcɛRI binds IgE, whereas its relatively short cytoplasmic domain probably does not play a role in cell signaling. This interaction is with the third constant domain of the FcɛRI portion of IgE (Cɛ3) [13•]. The carboxy-terminal cytoplasmic domains of both the β and the γ subunits are important in FcɛRI-mediated signal transduction. The cytoplasmic domains of the β and the γ subunits of FcɛRI contain a sequence of amino acids called the immunoreceptor tyrosine-based activation motif (ITAM) that is critical for signal transduction (Fig. 2-1). This motif is also present in subunits of the T-cell and B-cell antigen receptor complexes. The γ component of FcɛRI appears to be the essential receptor subunit for signaling cells for secretion, whereas the β subunit functions as an amplifier [14•].

It was reported some time ago that the number of FcɛRI on basophils correlates directly with the serum concentration of IgE. Recent studies have found that IgE appears to regulate the expression level of FcɛRI on basophils and mast cells both in vitro and in vivo [15•–17•]. For example, the baseline expression of FcɛRI on basophils and mast cells is dramatically reduced in genetically IgE-deficient mice, and this can be up-regulated by the in vitro culture of the cells with IgE. In allergic patients treated with monoclonal anti-IgE, there is a dramatic decrease in the total serum IgE

level and a greater than 90% decrease in FcɛRI number on basophils, although anti-IgE–induced histamine release is not dramatically decreased. This regulation of the FcɛRI expression level could be an important mechanism for regulating the release of mediators from basophils or mast cells and therefore the extent of immediate hypersensitivity or inflammatory responses.

STIMULI FOR MAST CELLS OR BASOPHIL SECRETION

The physiologically important stimulation of basophils and mast cells is through FcɛRI (Table 2-4). The IgE binds through Fc portion of the molecule, whereas the two Fab domains are available for interacting with anti-

Table 2-3. HIGH-AFFINITY IMMUNOGLOBULIN E RECEPTOR (FcɛRI)	
Subunit	**Characteristics**
α	IgE binding component
	One transmembrane domain and short cytoplasmic tail
β	Signal transducer or signal amplification component for the receptor
	Four transmembrane domains; both ends in the cytoplasm
	Has an ITAM sequence, is tyrosine phosphorylated after FcɛRI aggregation
	Binds signaling molecules:
	Quiescent cells: Lyn, protein kinase C$_\gamma$
	Activated cells: Syk, phospholipase Cγ, Shc, SHIP and SHP-2
γ	Signaling component
	Covalently linked homodimer each with short extracellular domain, one transmembrane domain
	Has an ITAM sequence, is tyrosine-phosphorylated after FcɛRI aggregation
	Binds Syk after tyrosine phosphorylation

ITAM—immunoreceptor tyrosine-based activation motif; SHIP—Src homology 2 (SH2) domain containing inositol-polyphosphate 5-phosphatase; SHP-2—SH2 domain containing protein tyrosine phosphatase 2.

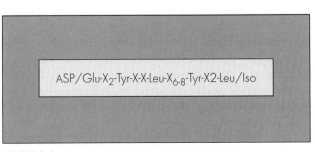

ASP/Glu-X$_2$-Tyr-X-X-Leu-X$_{6-8}$-Tyr-X2-Leu/Iso

FIGURE 2-1.

The immunoreceptor tyrosine activation motif (ITAM).

Table 2-4. STIMULATION OF MAST CELL/BASOPHIL FOR SECRETION

FcεRI-mediated
   Cell-bound IgE
     Antigen
     Anti-IgE
     Lectins (eg, concanavalin A)
   Anti-FcεRI
IgG receptor
C5a receptor
Lymphokines/cytokines/chemokines
Formyl methionine peptides
Eosinophil granule major basic protein
Other compounds: polymyxin, morphine, substance P

gen. Activation of the cell is due to aggregation of the IgE molecules by antigen. Receptor-bound IgE can also be cross-linked with anti-IgE antibodies or mitogens. A large percentage of patients with chronic urticaria or autoimmune diseases have antibodies that react with the α subunit of FcεRI and induce degranulation [18•,19•]. Besides FcεRI, mast cells have FcγRII and FcγRIII that bind IgG with much lower affinity than the binding of IgE to the FcεRI. These receptors for IgG may activate or regulate mast cell secretion [20•,21,22•]. Mast cells and basophils can also be activated to release by other secretagogues, some of which act by binding to surface receptors. These secretagogues include the complement component C5a (anaphylatoxin), formyl methionine–containing small peptides that are related to bacterial chemotactic factors, members of the IL-8 family of chemokines, the eosinophilic granule major basic protein, the ionophores, phorbol myristate acetate, polycationic compounds (eg, polymyxin B or compound 48/80), neuropeptides (eg, substance P), basic peptides, and some drugs (eg, contrast media or morphine). Several lymphokines (eg, SCF or IL-3) modulate IgE-mediated histamine release at low concentrations and induce degranulation at high concentrations [23]. Histamine-releasing factors are released from many different cells, such as monocytes, B cells, and platelets [24•]. Some of these are chemokines that bind to specific receptors [25]. However, one of the factors is an IgE-dependent histamine releasing factor [26•]. This protein, p23, induces histamine release from human basophils that express a particular type of human IgE (called IgE+). The nature of this difference in the IgE has not been determined.

There are differences in the response of basophils to different stimuli compared with mast cells. For example, the rate of histamine release with human mast cells is faster than with human basophils, and mast cells require higher concentrations of anti-IgE for activation than basophils. When tested with various stimuli, differences have been observed between mast cells and basophils. Basophils and skin mast cells respond to C5a and f-met peptides, whereas lung mast cells do not release with these stimuli. Basophils also release when activated with the phorbol esters, whereas this has no effect on lung mast cells. Similarly, the lipoxygenase product hydroperoxyeicosatetraenoic acid (5HPETE) releases histamine from basophils but not from lung mast cells. There are also differences in mast cells isolated from different tissues; skin mast cells respond to compound 48/80, bradykinin, substance P, and morphine. However, lung, intestinal, and synovial mast cells do not respond to these compounds. Even in cells from one tissue there is some heterogeneity; human basophils separated by density show functional differences in response to FcεRI and non–receptor-mediated activation. There is also density heterogeneity of human lung mast cells, with some differences in the quantitative but not the qualitative response to secretagogues. These variations could be due to differences in the stage of maturation of the cells.

There are also differences in the capacity of pharmacologic agents to inhibit FcεRI-mediated secretion from basophils compared to mast cells. Inhibitors of the cyclooxygenase pathway enhance release from basophils but not from mast cells. The H_2 agonists inhibit release from basophils but have no effect on mast cells, whereas PGD_2 enhances the release from human basophils but is without effect on mast cells. Other differences include the effect of dexamethasone that inhibits mediator release from human basophils but not from human mast cells. Adenosine inhibits the basophil release but slightly enhances the release from mast cells. Some of these differences in the effects of pharmacologic agents could be due to the presence or absence of agonist-specific receptors on these cells.

BIOCHEMICAL MECHANISMS FOR THE RELEASE OF MEDIATORS BY MAST CELLS OR BASOPHILS

Mast cells are stimulated to secrete mediators by antigen reacting with IgE molecules bound to receptors on the cell surface (Fig. 2-2). The release is a rapid, noncytotoxic secretory process. Optimal conditions for the reaction depend on the concentration of IgE on the basophil/mast cell surface, the concentration of the antigen, and the affinity of the IgE for the antigen. The bridging of two IgE molecules on the cell surface initiates the cell-triggering signal. The cross-linking of a very small proportion of the total surface IgE is necessary for cell activation (probably bridging less than 100 IgE molecules, representing 1% of the total receptors on the cell surface).

A number of morphologic changes occur during basophil or mast cell secretion [27]. The bridging of receptors transforms the microvillous surface of basophils to a plicated appearance; the cells spread and become more adherent. The degranulation of human mast cells results in the swelling of individual granules, a change in the electron-dense granular contents, and the formation of interconnected granules with the granule closest to the cell surface fusing with the plasma membrane and thus open to the extracellular medium. An ion exchange mechanism then results in the release of the biogenic amines [28]. The biochemical events unfolding during IgE-mediated basophil/mast cell secretion are listed in Table 2-5.

Many intracellular processes are regulated by the phosphorylation-dephosphorylation of proteins, and molecules involved on FcɛRI signaling are described in Table 2-6. Protein tyrosine phosphorylation is an early and critical signal for FcɛRI-induced degranulation [29,30•]. FcɛRI associates and activates several nonreceptor protein tyrosine kinases. Lyn, a member of the Src family of kinases, is associated with the inner surface of

the plasma membrane and with the β subunit of FcɛRI in nonstimulated cells, where its function is regulated by Csk [31]. Aggregation of the receptor results in activation of Lyn. This activation may be due to the dephosphorylation of Lyn at its regulatory site by a protein tyrosine phosphatase, possibly CD45. The activation of Lyn results in autophosphorylation of Lyn and in the phosphorylation of the tyrosine residues in the ITAMs of both the β and γ subunits of the FcɛRI. This is due to a transphosphorylation reaction where Lyn, associated with one FcɛRI, phosphorylates the ITAM of another FcɛRI, both of which have been brought together by aggregation [32]. Other members of the Src family of tyrosine kinases can replace Lyn function [33•]. Phosphorylation of the two tyrosines in the ITAM causes more Lyn binding to FcɛRI and also renders both the β and γ subunits accessible for interacting with Src homology 2 domain (SH2)-containing molecules. Tyrosine phosphorylation of the γ subunit appears to be essential for propagating the signal for degranulation. The phosphorylated ITAMs recruit the cytoplasmic tyrosine kinase Syk that binds by its two SH2 domains pre-

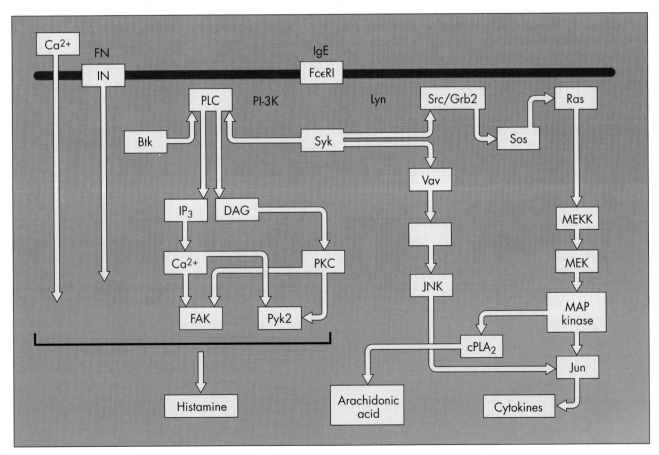

FIGURE 2-2.

Signaling pathways and molecules in basophils and mast cells. BtK—Bruton's tyrosine kinase; cPLA$_2$—cytoplasmatic phospholipase A$_2$; DAG—diacylglycerol; FAK—focal adhesion kinase;

FN—fibronectin; IN—integrins; JNK—c-Jun NH$_2$-terminal kinase; MAP—mitogen-activated protein; MEK—MAP kinase; MEKK—MEK kinase; PKC—protein kinase C; PLC—phospholipase C.

Table 2-5. BIOCHEMICAL EVENTS DURING IMMUNOGLOBULIN E-MEDIATED BASOPHIL/MAST-CELL SECRETION

Binding of IgE to receptors on cell surface

Interaction of multivalent antigen with cell-bound IgE

Aggregation of the IgE-receptor complex

Activation of Lyn protein tyrosine kinase

Phosphorylations of FcεRI subunits on Tyr residues in the ITAM

Recruitment and activation of protein tyrosine kinase Syk

Tyrosine phosphorylation of substrates (eg, phospholipase Cγ)

Hydrolysis of phosphatidyl inositides, with the generation of

   $InsP_3$: releases Ca^{2+} from intracellular sources

   2,4 DAG: activates PKC

Influx of extracellular Ca^{2+}

Phosphorylation of proteins on Ser and Thr residues

Activation of Ras pathway to MAP kinase

Activation of phospholipase A_2 and D

   Release of arachidonic acid

Activation of other enzymes

   FAK and Bruton's tyrosine kinase

Changes in the cytoskeleton

   Morphological changes

   Fusion of the granular membrane to the plasma membrane

Opening of the granule to the extracellular space

   Release of granular contents

DAG—diacylglycerol; FAK—focal adhesion kinase; $InsP_3$—inositol 1,4,5-trisphosphate; ITAM—immunoreceptor tyrosine-based activation motif; MAP—mitogen-activated protein; PKC—protein kinase C.

dominantly to the γ subunit of the receptor. This results in conformational changes in Syk, in its autophosphorylation and activation [34].

The Syk protein tyrosine kinase is essential for inducing degranulation in mast cells [35•]. Downstream of Syk is the tyrosine phosphorylation of phospholipase C-γ1 and phospholipase C-γ2 that results in increased catalytic activity of these two phospholipases. These phospholipases catalyze the hydrolysis of phosphatidylinositol 4,5-bisphosphate resulting in the generation of inositol 1,4,5-trisphosphate and 1,2-diacylglycerol. These second messengers release Ca^{2+} from internal stores and activate protein kinase C (PKC), respectively. Both events are essential for FcεRI-mediated secretion.

Following FcεRI aggregation, there is an increase in the cytoplasmic calcium concentration due to the mobilization of Ca^{2+} as a result of the binding of inositol 1,4,5-trisphosphate to specific intracellular receptors [36]. This initial rise in intracellular calcium is followed by the sustained influx of Ca^{2+} from extracellular medium [37•,38]. The increase in intracellular calcium regulates Ca^{2+}/calmodulin-dependent events. One of these downstream enzymes is calcineurin, a calcium/calmod-

ulin-dependent serine phosphatase that is sensitive to the immunosuppressive drug cyclosporin.

Aggregation of FcεRI also activates other cytoplasmic protein tyrosine kinases. One of these is Bruton's tyrosine kinase, which associates with and is phosphorylated by PKC. Others include focal adhesion kinase (FAK) and Pyk2, members of the FAK family [39,40], kinases that are present in many cells and are activated by adhesion. FAK is tyrosine phosphorylated after cell adherence and by FcεRI aggregation, and may play an essential role in the late steps of degranulation [41•]. The aggregation of FcεRI also induces the tyrosine phosphorylation of many other proteins, some of which may function as regulators or adaptors [42,43]. Among these are the SH2 domain containing inositol-polyphosphate 5-phosphatase (also called SHIP), the SH2 domain containing protein tyrosine phosphatases (SHP-1 and SHP-2) and Cbl [44•,45]. These molecules may regulate the extent of signaling initiated by FcεRI [46,47•]

The early tyrosine phosphorylation events activate the Ras protein kinase cascade. In this pathway, the adaptor protein Shc binds to the tyrosine phosphorylated FcεRI components and recruits Grb2, which in turn recruits Sos (the mammalian homologue of the Drosophila son of sevenless) [48,49]. Sos is constitutively associated with Grb2 in a complex that is cytosolic but becomes membrane-associated after cell activation. Sos is a guanine nucleotide exchange factor that activates Ras to the guanosine triphosphate (GTP) form by the promotion of guanine nucleotide exchange. Vav also may have similar guanine nucleotide exchange factor activity and links FcεRI through Rac1 to the c-Jun NH_2-terminal kinase (JNK) pathway [50•,51,52]. Activation of Ras by the dissociation of guanosine diphosphate and the binding of GTP results in stimulation of downstream kinases. Ras is deactivated by GPTase-activating proteins, which results in the hydrolysis of GTP. In mast cells, Ras activates the Raf pathway. Activated Ras binds Raf, a cytosolic serine/threonine kinase, and recruits it to the plasma membrane. This results in Raf activation. Raf then activates mitogen-activated protein (MAP)-kinase kinases by phosphorylating them on Ser residues. The MAP-kinase kinases then activate MAP kinase by phosphorylating them on both Tyr and Thr residues. The substrates of the MAP-kinases include transcription factors such as c-Jun, c-Fos and cytoplasmic phospholipase A_2 ($cPLA_2$). Phosphorylation of the transcription factors of the c-Jun and c-Fos families by the MAP-kinase and JNK allows their nuclear migration and the induction of new genes. The Ras pathway thus leads to both the release of arachidonic acid and to nuclear events, such as the induction of cytokine genes [53].

The PKC family of molecules phosphorylates proteins on serine or threonine residues, and some members of this family of molecules are essential transducers of signals for

Table 2-6. MOLECULES INVOLVED IN FCεRI SIGNALING

Molecule	Type of molecule	Characteristics
Lyn	Tyrosine kinase	Member of Src family of protein tyrosine kinases; associated with the plasma membrane and with FcεRI
Syk	Tyrosine kinase	Member of Syk/ZAP70 family of protein tyrosine kinases; cytosolic kinase that binds to and is activated by the tyrosine phosphorylated ITAM of the γ subunit of FcεRI; essential to secretion
Btk and Itk	Tyrosine kinase	Members of Bruton's tyrosine kinase family; cytosolic kinases activated by FcεRI aggregation; translocate to the membrane; interact with PKC
FAK and Pyk2	Tyrosine kinase	Members of focal adhesion kinase family; cytosolic; activated and tyrosine phosphorylated by both integrin and FcεRI aggregation; associated with other signaling molecules
CD45	Tyrosine phosphatase	Has an extracellular domain and two intracellular phosphatase domains; mast cells from KO mice do not release with FcεRI stimulation
Phospholipase C$_\gamma$	Phospholipase	Tyrosine-phosphorylated after cell activation; translocate to the membrane; hydrolyze inositol phospholipids results in formation of InsP$_3$ and DAG; two isoforms, PLCγ1 and PLCγ2 present
InsP$_3$ receptor	Intracellular receptor for InsP$_3$	Ca^{2+} channel protein; binding of InsP$_3$ opens channel and releases Ca^{2+} to the cytosol
PKC	Family of Ser/Thr kinases	PKC β and δ critical for secretion; α and ε inhibit secretion; activated by DAG and calcium
PI-3K	Lipid kinase	Generates phospholipids that recruit other molecules to the membrane
Vav	Adaptor protein, exchange factor for Rac	Binds to activated receptors and is itself tyrosine-phosphorylated after FcεRI aggregation; activates the small G proteins Rac, leading to JNK activation
Shc	Adaptor protein	Associates with β subunit of FcεRI; tyrosine-phosphorylated in nonstimulated RBL-2H3 cells
Ras	Small GTP-binding protein	Activation leads to MAP kinase pathway
MAP kinase	Ser/Thr kinase	Activated by dual phosphorylation on Tyr and Ser by MEK; substrates include cPLA$_2$, transcription factors, RSK kinase
cPLA$_2$	Phospholipase	Phosphorylated by MAP kinase; translocates to the membrane in activated cells; releases arachidonic acid
Rho, Rac	Small GTP-binding protein	Participates in changes in the cytoskeleton; Rho essential for stress fiber formation; Rac essential for membrane ruffles
Cbl	Adaptor protein	Associates with many other proteins; overexpression downregulates secretion
SHP-1, SHP-2	Tyrosine phosphatase	Cytosolic molecules with two SH2 domain associates with FcεRI; may negatively regulate cell signaling
SHIP	Phospholipid phosphatase	Cytosolic phosphatase has SH2 domain associates with FcεRI; may negatively regulate cell signaling
Paxillin	Cytoskeletal protein	Accumulates at focal adhesion sites; associates or interacts with many other proteins
Myosin	Cytoskeletal protein	Light chain and heavy chain of myosin phosphorylated by PKC on Ser by cell activation

cPLA$_2$—cytoplasmic phospholipase A$_2$; DAG—diacylglycerol; FAK—focal adhesion kinase; GTP—guanosine trisphosphate; InsP$_3$—inositol 1,4,5-trisphosphate; ITAM—immunoreceptor tyrosine-based activation motif; JNK—c-Jun NH$_2$-terminal kinase; KO—knockout; MAP—mitogen-activated protein; MEK—MAP kinase kinase; PI-3K—phosphoinositide 3-kinase; PKC—protein kinase C; PLC—phospholipase C; RSK—ribosomal S6 kinase; SH2—Src homology 2 domain; SHIP—SH2 domain containing inositol-polyphosphate 5-phosphatase; SHP—SH2 containing protein tyrosine phosphatase.

secretion. The RBL-2H3 mast cells contain the α, β, δ, ε and ζ isoforms of PKC. After FcεRI aggregation PKC translocates to the membrane fractions. The β or δ isozymes of PKC isozymes are required for optimal FcεRI-mediated secretion, whereas the α and ε isozymes inhibit the receptor-induced hydrolysis of inositol phospholipids. Activated PKC phosphorylates several proteins, including myosin light chain and the γ subunit of FcεRI.

Cytoskeletal reorganization plays a role in the movement of granules and in the degranulation process. These changes are secondary to the rise in intracellular calcium, phosphorylation of cellular proteins, and activation of GTP-binding proteins. Ras-related small GTPases, such as Rho, Rac and Rab3, appear to play a role in secretion [54•,55,56]. The cytoskeleton is also involved in the large-scale clustering and capping of aggregated FcεRI.

The activation of phospholipase C (PLC) and phospholipase A$_2$ (PLA$_2$) in stimulated cells results in the release of arachidonic acid from cellular phospholipids. The activity of cPLA$_2$ is regulated by phosphorylation by MAP kinase and PKC. Either the cyclooxygenase or the lipoxygenase pathway metabolizes the arachidonic acid released. The products of the lipoxygenase pathway are the leukotrienes (LTC$_4$, LTD$_4$, LTE$_4$, LTB$_4$), whereas the cyclooxygenase pathway results in the formation of PGD$_2$. There is also the formation of some thromboxane A$_2$ and prostacyclin.

MODULATION OF THE SECRETORY RESPONSE OF BASOPHILS OR MAST CELLS

Releasability

Releasability of basophils is a term that refers to the variation in the extent of in vitro histamine release from the cells of different donors. The extent of this release from the basophils of any one individual can vary from no different than background to values as high as 90% to 100% of the total cellular histamine. The releasability of the same cells can also vary with different secretagogues. There is no correlation between the number of IgE molecules present on the surface of basophils and releasability. Recent evidence suggests that these differences in secretion are regulated by intracellular factors. For example, the cells of donors who are high responders release histamine with chemically cross-linked IgE dimers, whereas the cells of the donors who are low responders release with chemically cross-linked trimers, but very poorly with dimers. The sensitivity of cells to different stimuli can be modified by factors, such as adherence of the cells to other cells or extracellular matrix proteins, by lymphokines, by steroids, or by dietary lipids that are incorporated into the membranes [57•]. Nerve growth factor and several lymphokines, such as IL-3, IL-5, IFN-γ, SCF, G-CSF, or M-CSF, enhance both FcεRI and non–receptor-mediated histamine release from human basophils [58–61]. Some of these cytokines affect the spectrum of mediators that are released from the cells. These effects are due to changes in intracellular signaling pathways [62].

Adhesion receptors

Both basophils and mast cells have surface adherence receptors that can mediate binding to other cells and to the extracellular matrix [63–66]. Adherence not only regulates the migration of cells into sites of inflammation but also results in intracellular signals that modulate developmental, cellular, and immunological processes and the response of cells to other stimuli [67]. Integrins are one class of adhesion molecules present on basophils and mast cells [65]. Growth factors induce changes in the expression of integrins on mast cells, suggesting that these changes occur during differentiation [68]. There is also enhanced adherence of basophils and mast cells after stimulation that may be related to tyrosine phosphorylation of adhesion molecules [69•,70].

Adherence of cells results in the aggregation of adhesion receptors and the transduction of intracellular signals, such as protein tyrosine phosphorylation, phosphatidylinositol hydrolysis, changes in intracellular calcium, and the expression of new genes [67]. These signals result in the reorganization of the cytoskeleton and changes in intracellular signaling and degranulating capacity of the cells. For example, culture of mature human or rat mast cells on fibroblasts maintains or changes their phenotype, viability, and secretory function. Fibroblasts may also influence the phenotype of the mast cells in culture, due to the interaction of the fibroblast product, SCF, with its receptor (c-Kit) on mast cells [6]. The adherence of mast cells results in changes in the cytoskeleton, cell spreading, and the redistribution of secretory granules to the periphery of the cell [71]. These changes may play an important role in intracellular signaling and degranulation. Thus, there is enhanced secretion from cultured mast cells that are adherent to surfaces coated with fibronectin, which may be due to change in the activation or tyrosine phosphorylation of the nonreceptor protein tyrosine kinase pp125^{FAK} [39, 71, 72]. Thus, adherence may regulate the extent of mast cell and basophil degranulation by modulating intracellular protein tyrosine phosphorylations.

Secretory desensitization

As discussed in the previous sections, FcεRI aggregation results in the activation of enzymes that induce secretion of mediators. However, some of these biochemical reactions also regulate the extent of the release reaction by a process called *cell desensitization*. Experimentally, desensitization is initiated by addition of the secretagogue under conditions that do not result in secretion. After a defined incubation period, the permissive conditions are restored [73•]. Desensitization is an active process blocked by some pharmacologic agents and is secretagogue-specific. The IgE-receptor–mediated desensitization requires receptor aggregation and can be specific to either the one antigen or for all IgE-mediated release reactions. At low-cell-surface IgE densities there is antigen-specific desensitization, whereas at high-surface IgE levels there is desensitization for all IgE-mediated reactions. Desensitization is not due to the loss of cell-surface antigen-specific IgE caused by endocytosis or shedding of IgE-antigen complexes. It is probably due to the decay of an unstable intermediate or the activation of negative regulatory molecules during the cascade initiated by receptor aggregation. The degree of desensitization probably regulates the extent of the release process. Recent interest has focused on several molecules present on basophils or mast cells that can inhibit FcεRI-mediated reactions; some of these, such as FcγRIIB or gp49B, have to be cross-linked with the receptor for this inhibition [74•,75].

CONCLUSIONS

Studies during the past 10 years have added tremendously to our knowledge of the biology of basophils and mast cells. This knowledge on the development of these cells and the intracellular pathways may lead to better methods of inhibiting allergic reactions.

REFERENCES AND RECOMMENDED READING

Recently published papers of particular interest have been highlighted as:

- • Of interest
- •• Of outstanding interest

1. Malaviya R, Ikeda T, Ross E, et al.: Mast cell modulation of neutrophil influx and bacterial clearance at sites of infection through TNF-α. *Nature* 1996, 381:77–80.

2.• Galli SJ, Wershil BK: The two faces of the mast cell. *Nature* 1996, 381:21–22.
This short paper reviews recent data that suggest that mast cells may play a role in innate immune protection against bacterial or parasitic diseases.

3. Galli SJ, Zsebo KM, Geissler EN: The kit ligand, stem cell factor. *Adv Immunol* 1994, 55:1–96.

4. Schwartz LB: Basophils and mast cells. In *Allergy*. Edited by Kaplan AP. Philadelphia: WB Saunders; 1997:133–148.

5. Kitamura Y: Heterogeneity of mast cells and phenotypic change between subpopulations. *Annu Rev Immunol* 1989, 7:59–76.

6. Swieter M, Mergenhagen SE, Siraganian RP: Microenvironmental factors that influence mast cell phenotype and function. *Proc Soc Exp Biol Med* 1992, 199:22–33.

7. Blair RJ, Meng H, Marchese MJ, et al.: Human mast cells stimulate vascular tube formation: tryptase is a novel, potent angiogenic factor. *J Clin Invest* 1997, 99:2691–2700.

8. Gruber BL, Kew RR, Jelaska A, et al.: Human mast cells activate fibroblasts: tryptase is a fibrogenic factor stimulating collagen messenger ribonucleic acid synthesis and fibroblast chemotaxis. *J Immunol* 1997, 158:2310–2317.

9. Huang CF, Wong GW, Ghildyal N, et al.: The tryptase, mouse mast cell protease 7, exhibits anticoagulant activity in vivo and in vitro due to its ability to degrade fibrinogen in the presence of the diverse array of protease inhibitors in plasma. *J Biol Chem* 1997, 272:31885–31893.

10. Wershil BK, Wang ZS, Gordon JR, et al.: Recruitment of neutrophils during IgE-dependent cutaneous late phase reactions in the mouse is mast cell–dependent: partial inhibition of the reaction with antiserum against tumor necrosis factor-alpha. *J Clin Invest* 1991, 87:446–453.

11. Gauchat JF, Henchoz S, Mazzei G, et al.: Induction of human IgE synthesis in B cells by mast cells and basophils. *Nature* 1993, 365:340–343.

12. Metzger H: Receptor for IgE and initiation of allergic reactions. In *Allergy*. Edited by Kaplan AP. Philadelphia: WB Saunders; 1997:92–98.

13.• Henry AJ, Cook JD, McDonnell JM, et al.: Participation of the N-terminal region of Cε3 in the binding of human IgE to its high-affinity receptor FcεRI. *Biochemistry* 1997, 36:15568–15578.
This report uses mutagenesis of IgE to define the sites that are important for interaction with FcεRI. The better definition of such sites will only come when the crystal structure of IgE and FcεRI are determined.

14.• Lin SQ, Cicala C, Scharenberg AM, et al.: The FcεRβ subunit functions as an amplifier of FcεRIγ-mediated cell activation signals. *Cell* 1996, 85:985–995.
Using transfection into cell lines, this paper reports that the presence of the β subunit and of the ITAM sequence in FcγRI enhances early signaling events, including tyrosine phosphorylation of the γ subunit and of Syk.

15.• Yamaguchi M, Lantz CS, Oettgen HC, et al.: IgE enhances mouse mast cell FcεRI expression in vitro and in vivo: evidence for a novel amplification mechanism in IgE-dependent reactions. *J Exp Med* 1997, 185:663–672.
This work demonstrates that the increase in the serum level of IgE in mice enhances the expression of FcεRI on basophils and mast cells.

16.• Lantz CS, Yamaguchi M, Oettgen HC, et al.: IgE regulates mouse basophil FcεRI expression in vivo. *J Immunol* 1997, 158:2517–2521.
Another work demonstrating that the increase in the serum level of IgE in mice enhances the expression of FcεRI on basophils and mast cells.

17.• MacGlashan DW Jr, Bochner BS, Adelman DC, et al.: Downregulation of FcεRI expression on human basophils during in vivo treatment of atopic patients with anti-IgE antibody. *J Immunol* 1997, 158:1438–1445.
This article reports that in patients treated with anti-IgE there is a decrease in IgE and in the number of FcεRI on basophils.

18.• Tong LJ, Balakrishnan G, Kochan JP, et al.: Assessment of autoimmunity in patients with chronic urticaria. *J Allergy Clin Immunol* 1997, 99:461–465.
This work extends recent observations that patients with chronic urticaria have IgG antibodies to FcεRI. Such antibodies are also present in the serum of patients with other autoimmune diseases. These antibodies could play a role in these diseases.

19.• Fiebiger E, Hammerschmid F, Stingl G, et al.: Anti-FcεRIα autoantibodies in autoimmune-mediated disorders: identification of a structure-function relationship. *J Clin Invest* 1998, 101:243–251.
Another work on IgE antibodies to FcεRI in patients with chronic urticaria.

20.• Daeron M, Malbec O, Latour S, et al.: Regulation of high-affinity IgE receptor-mediated mast cell activation by murine low-affinity IgG receptors. *J Clin Invest* 1995, 95:577–585.
Data are presented to suggest that cross-linking FcγR to FcεRI on basophils/mast cells results in decreased degranulation. This would suggest that, after immunotherapy, the binding of IgG antibodies to the allergen would form a complex that can bridge the IgE and the FcγR on the cell surface and decrease cell activation.

21. Daeron M: Fc receptor biology. *Annu Rev Immunol* 1997, 15:203–234.

22.• Vivier E, Daeron M: Immunoreceptor tyrosine-based inhibition motifs. *Immunol Today* 1997, 18:286–291.
This work reviews the concept that the immunoreceptor tyrosine-based inhibition motifs (ITIM), a sequence of amino acids, is present on the cytoplasmic domain of many transmembrane proteins, including FcγRIIB, gp49B1, and mast cell function associated antigen on mast cells. ITIMs recruit negative signaling molecules that down-modulate receptor mediated signaling.

23. Lin TJ, Befus AD: Differential regulation of mast cell function by IL-10 and stem cell factor. *J Immunol* 1997, 159:4015–4023.

24.• MacDonald SM: Histamine-releasing factors. *Curr Opin Immunol* 1996, 8:778–783.
Review of information on histamine-releasing factors including chemokines, interleukins, and the IgE-dependent histamine-releasing factor.

25. Uguccioni M, Mackay CR, Ochensberger B, et al.: High expression of the chemokine receptor CCR3 in human blood basophils. Role in activation by eotaxin, MCP-4, and other chemokines. *J Clin Invest* 1997, 100:1137–1143.

CHAPTER 3

T Lymphocytes

M. Larché

A.B. Kay

Allergic diseases, including asthma, are among the most common causes of chronic ill health in developed countries. They are of considerable socioeconomic importance and substantially impair the quality of life. Allergic tissue reactions in both humans and experimental animals consist of an immediate, acute response dependent on IgE and mast cells as well as on a chronic inflammatory component with a prominence of eosinophils and T lymphocytes (Fig. 3-1). It is now established that CD4+ T lymphocytes are critical to the orchestration of eosinophil recruitment and activation and to the triggering of IgE synthesis in B lymphocytes [1–3]. In particular, allergen-specific CD4+ T-helper-2 (T_H2)-type T cells play a pivotal role in baseline asthma [4] and in allergen-induced late asthmatic, skin, and nasal responses [5,6]. Furthermore, corticosteroids, the most effective anti-inflammatory treatment for asthma, inhibit CD4 T-cell activation and production of interleukin (IL)-4 and IL-5 in the airway. Clinical efficacy of the immunosuppressive agent cyclosporin A in severe steroid-dependent asthma [7] has also been demonstrated. Recently, it has been shown that a single infusion of monoclonal antibodies to CD4 produces significant improvement in lung function in chronic corticosteroid-dependent asthmatics [8].

LYMPHOCYTES

Inflammation occurs in vascularized tissue in response to mechanical or biologic insult. Inflammatory lesions are characterized by both cell-mediated and humoral responses, which, in the case of biologic insult, are orchestrated by lymphocytes, the antigen-specific component of the immune system. Lymphocyte antigen receptors are generated in a stochastic fashion via recombination of multiple gene segments. B-cell receptors occur as both membrane-bound and secreted soluble molecules (immunoglobulins [Ig]). Several classes of Ig exist; their individual structural differences are related to effector function. T-cell receptors occur in membrane-bound form and are not secreted. Recognition of antigen by T-cell receptors differs from the process in B-cell receptors because T-cell receptors recognize small fragments of antigen presented by molecules that are encoded by the class I and II regions of the major histocompatibility complex (MHC) and related molecules. In general, T-cell receptors recognize peptide fragments of antigen coupled to MHC, although in some cases, they may be able to interact with glycolipids bound to nonclassic MHC molecules, such as the CD1 family [9]. In addition to MHC-restricted recognition of peptides and

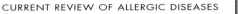

glycolipids, MHC-independent recognition of carbohydrate moieties from pollen allergens has also recently been suggested [10•].

The response of B lymphocytes to the majority of antigens is T-lymphocyte–dependent, requiring interaction between cell surface structures, such as CD40 on the surface of B cells and its ligand found on activated T cells. In addition, soluble factors secreted by T cells act on B cells, directing their choice of Ig heavy-chain gene segments and, thus, the ultimate class of Ig produced. The cytokines produced by T lymphocytes have been used to identify separate populations of cells whose products promote qualitatively different effector responses to antigen encounter. Cell-mediated immunity is generated primarily through cells secreting interferon-γ (IFN-γ), which are known as T_H1 cells. Induction of T_H1 responses has been demonstrated to be dependent on IL-12 produced by monocytic and dendritic antigen-presenting cells. The specificity of IL-12 action on T_H1 cells may be explained by the observation of Rogge *et al.* [11•] that the β-2 subunit of the IL-12 receptor is expressed by T_H1 but not T_H2 cells. In addition, reduced production of IL-12 and IL-12–dependent IFN-γ has recently been demonstrated in patients with allergic asthma [12•]. Humoral immunity has been ascribed to T_H2 cells, which produce cytokines characteristic of those found in allergic inflammation, such as occurs with IL-4 and IL-5. Induction of T_H2 cells has been demonstrated to be dependent on the presence of IL-4 during priming of naive cells. More recently, additional subpopulations of T lymphocytes have been identified, which are described in more detail later in the chapter. Although absolute divisions between T_H1 and T_H2 responses may be more demonstrable in vitro than in vivo, it is clear that, in general terms, allergic inflammation is driven by T_H2-type cytokines, notably by IL-4 and IL-5.

T-HELPER 1 AND T-HELPER 2 RESPONSES
Nature of allergens

The pathogenesis of allergic diseases is multifactorial. Both genetic (*eg*, identification of polymorphisms in the β chain of the FcεRI receptor and the β-adrenoceptor) and environmental (*eg*, increased exposure to allergens and pollutants) influences have been identified as contributing factors in the development of IgE-mediated hypersensitivity. Because production of IgE is dependent on a T_H2-type response to particular antigens, the question arises why, within populations equivalently exposed to allergenic material, such as house dust, animal dander, and pollens, are there individuals who mount a normal (protective) T_H1 response and others who mount a T_H2 response? Attention has been paid to the biochemical nature of molecules that commonly elicit allergic T_H2-type responses. Many allergenic proteins, such as Der p 1 and 2, have enzymatic activity, and it has been suggested that these properties may directly enhance IgE production [13]. For example, Hewitt *et al.* [14] have recently demonstrated the ability of the Der p 1 protein to cleave CD23 from the surface of B cells. Because soluble CD23 can act as an up-regulator of IgE production, such observations have clear and important implications for the development and amplification of allergic disease.

Effects of antigen and allergen dose

Data from a number of animal models have led to the conclusion that almost any protein antigen can be allergenic, but the induction of T_H1 versus T_H2 T-cell respons-

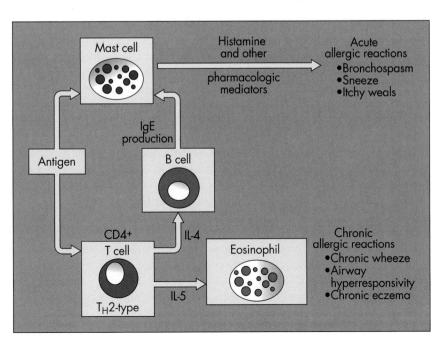

FIGURE 3-1.

A diagrammatic representation of immunologic mechanisms in acute and chronic allergic reactions. Acute allergic reactions involve mast cells, IgE, and pharmacologic mediators, such as histamine. Chronic allergic reactions are dependent on CD4+ T_H2 cells and eosinophils. IL—interleukin; T_H—T-helper cell.

Table 3-1. FACTORS AFFECTING T HELPER CELL DEVELOPMENT*

Factor	Effect	Study
Antigen dose	Low dose induces T_H2 development	Hosken et al. [17••]
	Moderate-to-high dose induces T_H1 development	
	High dose may induce apoptosis in T_H1 cells while allowing outgrowth of T_H2 cells	Constant and Bottomly [19]
Peptide/MHC affinity	Substitutions that increase peptide affinity induce IFN-γ production on a background of IL-4 production	Kumar et al. [21••]
	Strong T-cell receptor–MHC interactions lead to T_H1 responses, weak interactions lead to T_H2 responses	Pfeiffer et al. [16•]
Route/duration of antigen administration	Constant low doses of antigen over prolonged peroids in the absence of adjuvant (via miniosmotic pump) leads to T_H2 responses	Guery et al. [18•]
Genetic susceptibility	Certain strains of mice make T_H2 responses (BALB/c, BALB/b), whereas others mount T_H1 responses (CDA, C57B1/6) when challenged with the same antigen	Pfeiffer et al. [16•] Guery et al. [18•]
Expression of cytokine receptor chains	Lack of expression of the IL-12 receptor $\beta2$ chain on T cells leads to the development of T_H2 responses	Rogge et al. [11•]
Production of IL-12	Reduced levels of IL-12 production in atopic asthmatics	Van der Pauw Kraan et al. [12•]

*Data derived from murine and human systems. IFN-γ—interferon-γ; IL-4—interleukin-4; MHC—major histocompatibility complex; T_H—T helper cell.

es may be more related to the genetic background of the host and to the dose of antigen administered (Table 3-1). Furthermore, dose, as related to affinity of T-cell receptor interaction and numbers of receptors ligated, may be the primary determining factor in the generation of cytokine phenotype. Factors affecting commitment to either T_H1 or T_H2 phenotype include genetic predisposition, antigen dose and route of administration, strength of T-cell receptor interaction with peptide MHCs, and differential expression of cytokines and their receptors. Murray et al. [15] analyzed the response of several inbred strains of mice to immunization with the same peptide. They found that the peptide was capable of inducing T_H1 responses in certain strains (H-2^s) and T_H2 responses in others. These findings emphasize the importance of genetics in allergic diseases in humans in cases in which clear familial associations with atopy have been observed. Several investigators have addressed the issue of dose by immunizing mice with varying amounts of antigen and observing the subsequent effect on T-cell maturation into T_H1 or T_H2 subsets. Pfeiffer et al. [16•] demonstrated that immunization of peptide determinants from human collagen led to T_H1 responses at a high dose (50 µg) and to T_H2 responses at a lower dose (2 µg). Similar studies done by Hosken et al. [17••] used mice carrying a transgenic T-cell receptor specific for an ovalbumin peptide to analyze the effect of antigen dose in T-cell priming for T_H1 and T_H2 responses. At very low (< 0.05 µM) and very high (> 10 µM) doses of peptide, T_H2 responses predominated, whereas midrange concentrations (0.3 to 0.6 µM) led to T_H0/T_H1 responses. In an attempt to mimic natur-

al exposure to low-dose antigens, such as aeroallergens, Guery et al. [18•] administered low doses of soluble antigen continuously, using a miniosmotic pump. Prolonged inhibition of proliferative responses resulted, and this correlated with inhibition of T_H1-type responses in these mice and a strong T_H2 response characterized by high levels of IL-4 and IL-5 production. In this model, the effect of mouse strain was also analyzed, with BALB/c mice demonstrating enhanced T_H2 responses compared with other strains such as DBA/2, C3H, and C57BL/6. In contrast, the inhibition of IFN-γ responses was found to occur equally in all strains analyzed. These data suggest that the ability to inhibit T_H1 responses with soluble antigen is not under the same genetic control as the ability of certain genetic backgrounds to promote T_H2 responses. A consistent finding in murine models of T_H2 induction is that administration of anti–IL-4 antibodies during priming of naive cells completely abrogates the T_H2 response, highlighting the dependence of this maturation pathway on the presence of this cytokine. Why both very low and very high doses of antigen give rise to T_H2-type responses remains unclear. It has been suggested, however, that the relatively higher susceptibility of T_H1 cells to activation-induced apoptosis at high antigen dose may result in lower numbers of T_H1 cells surviving in cultures, thus allowing outgrowth of T_H2 cells in the absence of inhibitory cytokines such as IFN-γ [19].

Altered peptide ligands

Changing the affinity of interaction between antigenic peptide and MHC or T-cell receptor molecules can have dramatic effects both on the proliferative capacity and on the cytokine production profile of T cells. By altering peptide residues, which interact with either the T-cell receptor or the MHC, alterations in proliferative capacity and cytokine production have been observed in several systems. Evavold and Allen [20] provided the initial demonstration that altering peptide antigen can lead to a dissociation between the ability to produce cytokines (IL-4 in this example) and the ability to proliferate, which was lost in their model. More recently, altered peptide ligands have been used to investigate the role of changing affinity on the ability of peptides to induce proliferative responses and T_H1 or T_H2 cytokine production. Kumar et al. [21••] analyzed a series of peptides derived from the myelin basic protein N-terminal peptide (Acl-9). A panel of peptides substituted at position 4 was assessed for affinity for the restricting I-A^u allele and for their ability to induce proliferation and cytokine production. They found a 10,000-fold range in the ability of peptides to bind to I-A^u. In addition, the ability of the analogues to induce proliferative responses correlated with peptide-MHC affinity; the higher-affinity peptides induced the strongest proliferation. Furthermore, cytokine production also correlated with peptide affinity. High-affinity peptides could be shown to induce fivefold more IFN-γ production than low-affinity binders. In contrast, the frequency of cells producing IL-4 and IL-5 was similar between high- and low-affinity peptides. To assess the combined effects of dose and affinity, the authors increased the dose of low-affinity peptide by 50- to 100-fold and found that the frequency of cells producing IL-5 increased by tenfold in the absence of a concomitant increase in IFN-γ–producing cells.

The conclusions to be drawn from these and many other studies of the effects of antigen dose, affinity of T-cell receptor interaction with peptide antigen, and genetic background may be that, in genetically susceptible individuals, low-dose chronic exposure to allergen may lead to T_H2-type responses and thus ultimately to atopy. Encouraging observations, such as the induction of T_H1 responses by increasing the affinity of peptide ligands, may hold promise for future therapy in allergic diseases.

ANIMAL MODELS OF ALLERGIC ASTHMA

A number of murine models of "asthma" have been developed. Protocols vary, but most rely on priming with antigen and adjuvant followed by inhalation challenge, which results in airway hyperresponsiveness, eosinophil infiltration, and antigen-specific IgE synthesis. Results obtained from such models vary considerably and are often contradictory. These discrepancies may be due, at least in part, to the different sensitization protocols adopted. Takeda et al. [22] have shown that

airway hyperresponsiveness and pulmonary eosinophilia can be induced in mast-cell–deficient mice following airway challenge, indicating that mast cell activation is not required for induction of these inflammatory processes. Mehlhop et al. [23] sensitized mice with the naturally occurring aeroallergen Aspergillus fumigatus and demonstrated the persistence of airway hyperresponsiveness and pulmonary eosinophilia. Although this suggests that IgE may be redundant in this model, keep in mind that, in the mouse, IgG is also capable of sensitizing and activating mast cells. The respective roles of IL-4 and allergen-specific Ig in the induction of bronchial hyperresponsiveness and airway eosinophilia following bronchial challenge with ovalbumin have been addressed by Hogan et al. [24•]. In IL-4–deficient mice, no IgE or IgG1 was detectable, although other IgG subclasses were present. Eosinophil accumulation in the airways was diminished but not abolished, although the latter could be effected by the administration of antibodies to IL-5 prior to challenge with aerosolized allergen. In CD40-deficient mice, Ig class switching did not occur, and allergen-specific IgE, IgG, and IgA isotypes were not detected. Bronchial hyperresponsiveness, however, was unaffected. Taken together, these results suggest that airway hyperresponsiveness and eosinophil accumulation are related primarily to the production of T_H2-type cytokines, particularly IL-5 by T cells, which is in agreement with the findings of Foster et al. [25] in IL-5–deficient mice. Contrasting results were obtained by Hamelmann et al. [26] using both wild-type and B-cell–deficient mice; both developed increased production of T_H2 cytokines and airway eosinophilia following airway sensitization. Only wild-type mice or ovalbumin-specific, IgE-reconstituted, B-cell–deficient mice developed airway hyperresponsiveness, however, indicating that, in this model, IgE contributes to its development. This agrees with other data from the same group addressing the role of allergen-specific IgE in the induction of bronchial hyperresponsiveness by passive sensitization [27]. Recently, Kuperman et al. [28•] demonstrated that disruption of signal transducer and activator factor 6 (STAT6) (activated following IL-4 signaling) results in a failure to develop bronchial hyperresponsiveness following allergen challenge, indicating a prominent role for IL-4 in asthma. This agrees with the findings of earlier studies done by Corry et al. [29] and Renz et al. [30]. Furthermore, murine models have shown that depletion of CD4 T cells abolishes antigen-induced airway hyperresponsiveness and that airway hyperresponsiveness to inhaled antigen can be transferred by adoptive transfer of CD4 T cells [31•]. Animal models have also allowed testing of potential therapeutic strategies, such as blocking anti–IL-5 antibodies [32,33,34••], blocking T-cell co-stimulation [35], and T-cell–directed peptide therapy

[36,37]. Although animal models have been useful for establishing the principles of immunologic intervention, T-cell–directed peptide therapy is not ready for clinical testing in humans.

T-HELPER-2-TYPE CYTOKINES IN ASTHMA

Interleukin-4 is a pleiotropic cytokine produced by a variety of cell types, including T cells, mast cells, and bone marrow stromal cells. In the context of allergic responses including asthma, the most prominent role of IL-4 is in the switching of antibody isotype to the IgE subclass. Production of sterile germline transcripts of the epsilon heavy-chain gene segment can be demonstrated in B cells following incubation with IL-4 and also with the related cytokine IL-13. Concomitant signals via the CD40/CD40L pathway and IL-4 (IL-13) are required for IgE production [38]. Studies in atopic individuals have revealed a direct correlation between serum IgE concentrations and the quantity of IL-4 produced by T cells from the peripheral blood. Intriguingly, in the context of allergic disease, it has recently been suggested that mast cells, which synthesize IL-4 and express CD40L, may also have the capacity to effect isotype switching of B cells to the IgE subclass, providing a T-cell–independent mechanism for amplification of the allergic response [39].

Interleukin-5 is less pleiotropic, and its actions are primarily confined to eosinophils and basophils. This cytokine, for which the T cell is an important source, promotes terminal differentiation of the committed eosinophil precursor, releases mature eosinophils from the bone marrow, and enhances the effector capacity of the mature eosinophil [40]. IL-5 also prolongs the survival of eosinophils in vitro, and anti–IL-5 inhibits allergen-induced bronchial hyperresponsiveness and eosinophilia in a primate model of asthma [34••]. More IL-5 mRNA+ cells were found in endobronchial mucosal biopsy specimens from asthmatics than were found in control subjects [41]. In the subjects who demonstrated detectable IL-5 mRNA, there was a correlation between IL-5 mRNA expression and the number of CD25+ and EG2+ cells and total eosinophil counts. This study supported the concept that in the bronchial mucosa of asthmatics, T-cell–derived cytokines regulate eosinophil accumulation and function.

In further studies examining the wider cytokine profile in atopic asthma, Robinson et al. [42] showed that, in patients with asthma, there were increased numbers of bronchoalveolar lavage (BAL) cells encoding mRNA+ for IL-3, IL-4, IL-5, and granulocyte-macrophage colony-stimulating factor (GM-CSF). This pattern is compatible with predominant activation of the T_H2-type T-cell population, compared with cells from nonatopic control subjects. For IL-4 and IL-5, mRNA was localized to T

cells within the BAL-cell population. These findings were confirmed using CD4+- and CD8+-enriched peripheral blood T cells isolated from patients with severe asthma [43]. These individuals showed spontaneous expression of mRNA for T_H2-type cytokines localized to CD4+ cells but not CD8+ cells. This was accompanied by spontaneous elaboration of the eosinophil-active cytokines IL-3, IL-5, and GM-CSF. These results were confirmed in part by Kamei et al. [44], who observed allergen-induced release of IL-5 and GM-CSF protein from blood T cells of asthmatics. Similarly, Del Prete et al. [45] found that T-cell clones raised in vitro from bronchial mucosal biopsy specimens from asthmatics predominantly had the type 2 T_H cytokine profile.

Further studies showed that atopic asthma provoked by allergen inhalation was associated with local increases in activated T cells, eosinophils, and cells expressing mRNA for IL-4, IL-5, and GM-CSF [46,47]. Again, these data supported the hypothesis that allergen-induced late asthmatic responses are accompanied by T-cell activation, increased expression of cytokines, such as IL-5 and GM-CSF, and local recruitment and activation of eosinophils in the bronchial mucosa.

Conversely, prednisolone treatment in asthmatics was associated with reduction in BAL cells expressing mRNA for IL-4 and IL-5 [48,49•]. This was accompanied by decrease in BAL eosinophils and clinical improvement, as shown by an increase in the methacholine PC_{20}. Interestingly, there was an increase in the number of cells expressing mRNA for IFN-γ, indicating that prednisolone treatment favors enhancement of a cytokine that down-regulates IgE production.

Using the technique of in situ hybridization, it was shown that, in a group of atopic asthmatics with a range of disease severity, there were significant associations between the numbers of cells expressing mRNA for IL-4, IL-5, and GM-CSF, and airflow restriction, bronchial hyperresponsiveness, and an asthma symptom score [50]. These results have recently been confirmed (in the case of IL-5) using a more precise semiquantitative reverse transcription polymerase chain reaction (RT-PCR) technique [51••]. Furthermore, Virchow et al. [52], using segmental allergen challenge, found a correlation between IL-5 concentrations, eosinophil numbers, and activated T cells, again supporting the hypothesis that T-cell–derived IL-5 is involved in tissue eosinophilia in allergic asthma.

Although several authors have now confirmed that asthma is characterized by increased expression, at either the mRNA or the protein level, of several cytokines including IL-4 and IL-5, there has been some debate regarding the principal cellular source of these cytokines. Using the technique of double in situ hybridization/immunohistochemistry, researchers showed that T cells were the major source of mRNA encoding IL-4 and IL-5 in bronchial biopsy specimens obtained from asthmatics at baseline [53]. Eosinophils and mast cells also contribute to the overall cytokine profile, although the number of mRNA+ cells was about one fifth of the number of CD3+ T cells. Furthermore, using a combination of semi-quantitative PCR, in situ hybridization, and immunohistochemistry, we have been able to establish that IL-4 and IL-5 expression was similar in bronchial biopsy specimens taken from atopic and nonatopic asthmatics. In general, the expression of IL-5 was significantly higher in asthmatics compared with atopic nonasthmatic normal controls, whereas the expression of IL-4 was increased in asthmatics and atopic nonasthmatics compared with normal nonatopic controls [51••]. The detection of increased expression of IL-4 mRNA-bearing cells in bronchial mucosal biopsy specimens from atopic nonasthmatics obtained by the sensitive technique of RT-PCR raises the possibility that, in general, IL-5 is related more closely to clinical expression of asthma and IL-4 is related to overproduction of IgE. In both atopic and nonatopic asthmatics, mRNA for IL-4 and IL-5 colocalized predominantly to CD4+, but it also localized to CD8+ T cells, major basic protein (MBP)-positive eosinophils, and tryptase-positive mast cells (Fig. 3-2) [54•]. These findings were in agreement with those of Till et al. [55], who found that CD8+ as well as CD4+ T-cell lines from BAL specimens from asthmatics elaborated the IL-5 protein. Thus, T-cytotoxic type-2 lymphocytes (T_C2) may play a role in allergic inflammation at mucosal surfaces.

Our finding of increased IL-4 expression at both mRNA and protein levels in intrinsic asthma was in contrast to the finding of Walker et al. [56], who measured

protein product in concentrated BAL fluid. These authors detected increased concentrations of IL-2 and IL-5 (but not IL-4) in BAL fluid from nonatopic asthmatics compared with control subjects, whereas IL-4 and IL-5 were increased in atopic asthmatics. There is, at present, no satisfactory explanation for these apparent discrepancies. The role of T_H2-type cells in intrinsic asthma, as well as that of local IgE-dependent mechanisms as suggested by Humbert et al. [57], is unlikely to be resolved until the putative antigen(s) has been identified.

Maestrelli et al. [58] cloned T cells using cells isolated from bronchial biopsy fragments from patients with asthma induced by toluene di-isocyanate. They found that the majority of clones were IL-5– and IFN-γ–producing CD8+ cells. Whether these findings are related specifically to this form of occupational asthma or to the method of cloning is unclear. Thus, the relative contributions of CD4 and CD8 T cells and the precise cytokine profile of different forms of asthma have yet to be firmly established.

In contrast to mRNA, the expression of the IL-4 and IL-5 protein product in bronchial biopsy specimens from atopic and nonatopic asthmatics appeared to be associated more with eosinophils and mast cells than with T cells [54•]. It is difficult to demonstrate intracytoplasmic staining of cytokines in nongranular cells, such as T cells, presumably because of the sensitivity limitations of current immunostaining methods. On the other hand, the eosinophil appears to concentrate several cytokines in its cell granule, and granule-associated cytokines are readily detectable by immunocytochemistry [59,60]. Despite the limitations of immunocytochemical detec-

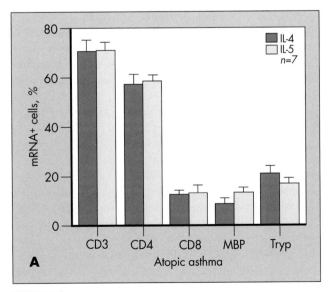
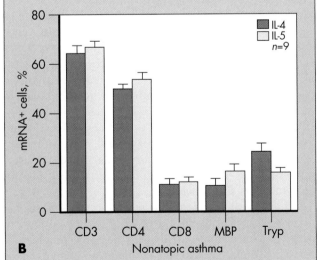

FIGURE 3-2.
The phenotype of cells expressing mRNA for interleukin-4 and interleukin-5 as shown by double immunohistochemistry and in situ hybridization. Bronchial biopsy specimens were obtained from atopic (extrinsic, **A**) and nonatopic (intrinsic, **B**) asthmatics.

IL-4 and IL-5 were colocalized to CD3+, CD4+, and CD8+ lymphocytes, major basic protein (MBP)+ eosinophils, and tryptase+ mast cells. IL—interleukin; Tryp—tryptase. (*Adapted from* Ying et al. [54•]; with permission.)

tion of cytokines, it seems likely that T cells are an important source of IL-4 and IL-5 in asthma, although the relative contribution of the different cell types to the overall cytokine profile remains uncertain.

T CELLS AND LATE-PHASE ALLERGIC REACTIONS

Allergen inhalation challenge of atopic asthmatics in the clinical laboratory results in an early asthmatic reaction (EAR) followed by a delayed late asthmatic reaction (LAR). The airway narrowing of EAR occurs within minutes of exposure to allergen, is maximal 10 to 15 minutes after exposure, and usually returns to near baseline by 1 hour. EAR is dependent on the IgE-mediated release of mast-cell–derived mediators, such as histamine and leukotrienes [61–63]. In contrast, LAR reaches a maximum at 6 to 9 hours after exposure and is believed to represent, at least in part, the cellular inflammatory component of the asthmatic response. In this sense, it has served as a useful model of chronic asthma. LAR is characterized by airway infiltration with activated eosinophils and CD4 T cells, with increased numbers of T cells expressing mRNA for the T_H2-type (IL-4 and IL-5) and eosinophil-active cytokines (IL-3, IL-5, and GM-CSF) [5,54•]. The importance of the T-cell component of LAR was also suggested by our observation that cyclosporin A attenuated LAR but not EAR when provoked by allergen inhalation (Fig. 3-3) [64•].

In an attempt to induce the counterpart of murine experimental T-cell tolerance in individuals allergic to cats, Norman *et al.* [65••] also observed asthma-like symptoms that began several hours after administration of the 27 amino acid peptides IPC1/IPC2 derived from the sequence of the major cat allergen Fel d 1 (although there was no local redness or swelling at the site of injection), which may have been due to T-cell activation causing an isolated late response. To determine whether T-cell peptides, which did not cross-link IgE, could indeed

induce an isolated LAR, we designed Fel d 1 chain-1–derived peptides (FC1P) of 16 or 17 residues. We first established that a mixture of three short overlapping peptides produced statistically significant proliferative responses but did not release histamine from basophil-enriched mononuclear cells. Following intradermal injection of 80 µg of FC1P, 9 of 35 asthmatics allergic to cats experienced a fall in the 1-second forced expiratory volume that started 3 to 4 hours after injection and reached a plateau by 6 hours. In none of the 35 subjects were immediate skin or lung reactions observed. We believe that this provided firm evidence that T-cell activation, as an initiating event, can provoke asthma in susceptible individuals.

T-CELL ACTIVATION AND HYPORESPONSIVENESS

In addition to recognition of peptide antigen presented by MHC molecules, productive T-cell responses resulting in proliferation or cytokine production also require co-stimulation through such pathways as CD28 interacting with CD80 or CD86 [66]. In addition, the presence of an innate immune response may amplify the T-cell response through production of such factors as tumor necrosis factor-α and IL-1α. As previously discussed, cytokines are important determinants of the nature of the T-cell response: IL-4 favors T_H2 T-cell responses, and IL-12 drives a T_H1 phenotype (IFN-γ and IL-2). In recent years, much attention has been focused on the possibility of functional inactivation of such T-cell responses leading to "tolerance." Presentation of antigen to high-affinity T-cell receptors during thymic maturation leads to death of the responding T cells in a process termed thymic deletion or central tolerance. Peripheral T-cell tolerance is also described and may result from a number of mechanisms including deletion, inhibition of migration, and active suppression. Presentation of peptide in the absence of co-stimulation leads to T-cell unre-

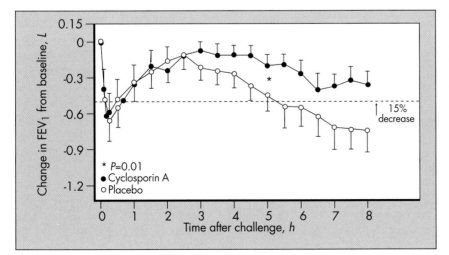

FIGURE 3-3.
Inhibition of the late-phase but not the early-phase asthmatic reaction to inhaled allergen with a single dose of oral cyclosporin A. FEV₁—forced expiratory volume in one second. (*Adapted from Sihra et al.* [64•]; with permission.)

sponsiveness ("anergy") to rechallenge, which may result from failure of certain T-cell signaling pathways [67,68]. It is well established in murine models that injection of peptides produces T-cell anergy or nonresponsiveness through as-yet-unexplained mechanisms [35]. In humans and in experimental animals, in vitro experiments have shown that different concentrations of peptides can be either tolerogenic or stimulatory, depending on dose [68]. There is good evidence of peptide-induced nonresponsiveness of human CD4 cells in vitro. For example, clonal anergy was induced with supraoptimal concentrations of cognate peptide in human CD4+ T-cell clones reactive to house dust mite [69,70]. This resulted in down-regulation of IL-2 and IL-4 and maintenance of IFN-γ secretion. This approach has been used in animal models of allergen challenge to induce tolerance. Briner et al. [36] showed decreased production of IgG and IL-2 by lymphocytes from Fel-d-1–primed mice following multiple injections of a peptide fragment of the priming allergen. Hoyne et al. [37] demonstrated that intranasal administration of peptides from the house dust mite allergen, Der p 1, could not only prevent sensitization but also inhibit lymphocyte responses in previously sensitized mice.

ALLERGEN-SPECIFIC IMMUNOTHERAPY, TOLERANCE, AND ANERGY

Recent data have suggested that conventional allergen immunotherapy for the treatment of human allergic disease, which has been practiced for many years, may also act by modulating T-cell responsiveness. Double-blind studies have shown that conventional immunotherapy with allergen extracts for grass pollen and cat rhinitis or asthma can be highly efficacious [71–73]. Questions continue to be raised about safety, however, particularly in relation to immediate IgE-mediated anaphylactic reactions. We and others have shown that one mechanism of successful immunotherapy may be modulation of the T-cell phenotype with increased numbers of T cells producing IFN-γ and IL-2, increased local production of IL-12, and variable down-regulation of IL-4– and IL-5–positive cells [72,74,75•,76]. More recently, epitope-specific T-cell nonresponsiveness to phospholipase A₂ has been demonstrated after whole-allergen immunotherapy for bee-sting allergy [77•]. Thus, as indicated previously, an attractive modification of allergen immunotherapy might be the use of peptides derived from T-cell epitopes of allergen proteins, which could inactivate T-cell responses in the absence of the IgE-binding epitopes of the whole allergen, avoiding the potential for anaphylaxis.

The studies of Norman et al. [65••] and Simons et al. [78] involved injecting individuals allergic to cats sub-

cutaneously with two T-cell reactive peptides, IPC1 and IPC2. The peptides were originally designed on the basis of patterns of epitope recognition of short overlapping peptides by Fel-d-1–reactive T-cell lines [79–81]. It was found that peptides derived from chain 1 showed greater in vitro proliferative responses than those from chain 2, with the majority of activity associated in the N terminal region of chain 1. IPC1 and IPC2 were considerably longer (27 amino acids each) than most previously defined T-cell epitopes [79–81]. This may have been partly responsible for the immediate-type (presumed IgE-mediated) hypersensitivity reactions observed in some patients following administration [65••]. Although the peptides gave limited protection against natural exposure to cats, large doses (4 × 750 μg) were required to achieve a significant clinical effect [65••]. The choice of peptides for therapy was based on reactivity of secondary T-cell lines derived from a large number of individuals allergic to cats and did not take into account primary T-cell reactivity (ie, ex vivo), which may be more sensitive, or, more important, MHC class-II haplotype.

Recently, much attention has focused on T cells that may regulate the immune response. A number of these regulatory T-cell populations have been described in animal studies. Weiner et al. [82•] have defined a murine "T$_H$3" population of cells producing transforming growth factor-β (TGF-β), IL-4, and IL-10 that may be responsible for oral tolerance, and Powrie et al. [83•] showed that suppression of colitis by CD45RB^{lo} cells could be blocked by anti–TGF-β antibodies. An additional regulatory population of murine and human T-cell clones producing IL-10, termed Tr1, and a T-cell population producing TGF-β, IL-2, and IFN-γ–inhibited T$_H$2-dependent autoimmune disease in rats have been described [84•,85•]. The mechanisms by which these cells modulate T$_H$1 or T$_H$2 responses require further clarification, but TGF-β is likely to be an important factor in this "suppression" (Fig. 3-4). TGF-β inhibited both T$_H$1 and T$_H$2 development from naive CD4+ T cells in vitro [86–90]. Linked suppression is a phenomenon, demonstrated in animal models, in which administration of a single epitope from a protein modifies responses of nontolerant T cells specific for other epitopes within the same protein and, in some models, epitopes derived from other proteins ("bystander suppression") [91]. In transplantation models, CD4+ T cells from animals treated with anti-CD4 at the time of transplantation could transfer allograft tolerance to naive recipient animals, a phenomenon termed infectious tolerance [92]. This may also be mediated by regulatory T cells.

The mechanisms of linked suppression vary from model to model. In a human in-vitro system, Lombardi et al. [93] found that anergic T-cell clones competed for

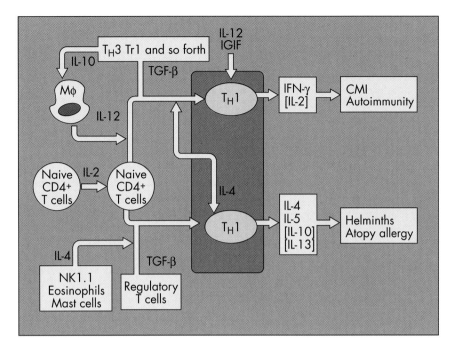

FIGURE 3-4.
The regulation of $T_H 1$ and $T_H 2$ responses. CMI—cell-mediated immunity; IFN—interferon; IGIF—interferon-gamma–inducing factor; IL—interleukin; M—macrophage; NK—natural killer; TGF-β—transforming growth factor-β; T_H—T-helper cell; Tr—regulatory T cell. (*Adapted from* O'Garra [86]; with permission.)

local IL-2 production. In a murine model of experimental allergic encephalomyelitis (EAE), Chen *et al.* [94] demonstrated enhanced production of TGF-β, IL-10, and IL-4 by MBP-specific T-cell clones that could downregulate responses to proteo lipid protein (PLP). Induction of nonresponsiveness to whole proteins following administration of a single peptide epitope has been demonstrated in a number of models [36,95,96,97•,98,99]. Hoyne *et al.* [100••] have demonstrated linked suppression in T-cell responses to epitopes within the same allergen protein after inhalation challenge of a single immunodominant epitope. Although such an approach to the amelioration of allergic diseases holds promise for human therapy, it is likely to be confounded by the outbred nature of the population, making identification of individual "dominant" epitopes more difficult but perhaps not impossible. Following their work in murine EAE, Fukaura *et al.* [101••] have succeeded in inducing increased frequencies of circulating $T_H 3$ cells producing TGF-β1 in human subjects with multiple sclerosis receiving orally administered bovine MBP [101••]. This work has important implications for intervention in human allergic diseases because TGF-β has been shown to inhibit both $T_H 1$ and $T_H 2$ responses [83•,85•,87] and has also been shown to inhibit IgE production [38].

CONCLUSIONS

There is now persuasive evidence to support the hypothesis that activation of $T_H 2$ or $T_C 2$ cells is pivotal in atopic allergic inflammation and the asthma process.

The hypothesis is supported by numerous lines of evidence, particularly studies of bronchial, skin, and nasal biopsy specimens from subjects with allergic diseases; treatment studies; and experimental animal models.

The T-cell hypothesis has led to the possibility of several novel therapeutic approaches, particularly in chronic asthma, for which present treatment is unsatisfactory (Fig. 3-5). Such approaches include strategies to inhibit co-stimulatory pathways (*eg*, cytotoxic T lymphocyte antigen 4 [CTLA4] Ig and anti–B7-2); agents that modulate the $T_H 2$ response (*eg*, IL-12); humanized antibodies against CD4 (shown to have efficacy in rheumatoid arthritis); anticytokine antibodies, particularly against IL-4 and IL-5 and cytokine receptor antagonists (*eg*, IL-1 receptor antagonist, which has been shown to modulate human cutaneous late responses to allergen); and a range of immunosuppressive drugs, including FK506, rapamycin, and mycophenalate mofetil, all of which are active in inhibiting mitogen-driven T cells from corticosteroid-resistant asthmatics in vitro.

A number of important questions still remain unanswered. What initiates the $T_H 2$ response in asthma and other allergic diseases? How does asthma differ from atopy alone at the immunopathologic level? (Not all atopics have asthma.) What proportion of activated T cells in the bronchial mucosa is allergen- (or antigen-) specific? What is the role of CD8 T cells in asthma? How is T-cell response regulated in asthma and allergic diseases? It is anticipated that with advances in molecular pathologic techniques and more precise and selective therapy, many of these questions can be answered.

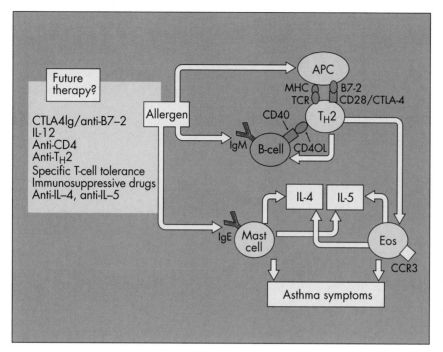

FIGURE 3-5.

Possible therapeutic strategies in asthma based on the T-cell hypothesis. Approaches include blocking of co-stimulation with agents such as CTLA4 Ig, which may inhibit T-cell activation, or coadministration of interleukin-12, possibly together with allergen immunotherapy, which may enhance switching from T_H2 to a T_H1-predominant T-cell response. Direct blocking of IL-4 and IL-5 may also have therapeutic efficacy. Other possible strategies include T-cell–directed antibody therapy with monoclonal antibodies directed against CD4, putative targets on T_H2-type cells, or immunosuppressants such as FK-506, rapamycin, and mycophenolate mofetil. The use of T-cell peptide epitope vaccines to develop specific T-cell tolerance is also under development. APC—antigen-presenting cell; CCR3—CC chemokine receptor 3; CTLA4—cytotoxic T lymphocyte antigen 4; Eos—eosinophil; Ig—immunoglobulin; IL—interleukin; MHC—major histocompatibility complex; TCR—T-cell receptor; T_H—T helper cell.

REFERENCES AND RECOMMENDED READING

Recently published papers of particular interest have been highlighted as:
• Of interest
•• Of outstanding interest

1. Jeffery PK, Wardlaw AJ, Nelson FC, et al: Bronchial biopsies in asthma: an ultrastructural, quantitative study and correlation with hyperreactivity. *Am Rev Respir Dis* 1989, 140:1745–1753.

2. Azzawi M, Bradley B, Jeffery PK, et al.: Identification of activated T lymphocytes and eosinophils in bronchial biopsies in stable atopic asthma. *Am Rev Respir Dis* 1990, 142:1407–1413.

3. O'Hehir RE, Bal V, Quint D, et al.: An in vitro model of allergen-dependent IgE synthesis by human B lymphocytes: comparison of the response of an atopic and a nonatopic individual to *Dermatophagoides* spp. (house dust mite). *Immunology* 1989, 66:499–504.

4. Robinson DS, Hamid Q, Ying S, et al.: Predominant T_H2-like bronchoalveolar T-lymphocyte population in atopic asthma. *N Engl J Med* 1992, 326:298–304.

5. Bentley AM, Meng Q, Robinson DS, et al.: Increases in activated T lymphocytes, eosinophils, and cytokine mRNA expression for interleukin-5 and granulocyte/macrophage colony-stimulating factor in bronchial biopsies after allergen inhalation challenge in atopic asthmatics. *Am J Respir Cell Mol Biol* 1993, 8:35–42.

6. Durham SR, Ying S, Varney VA, et al.: Cytokine messenger RNA expression for IL-3, IL-4, IL-5 and GM-CSF in the nasal mucosa after local allergen provocation: relationship to tissue eosinophilia. *J Immunol* 1992, 148:2390–2394.

7. Alexander AG, Barnes NC, Kay AB: Trial of cyclosporin A in corticosteroid-dependent chronic severe asthma. *Lancet* 1992, 339:324–328.

8. Kon OM, Sihra BS, Compton CH, et al.: A double-blind, placebo-controlled trial of a chimeric anti-CD4 monoclonal antibody, keliximab (IDEC CE9.1), in chronic severe asthma. *Lancet* 1998: in press.

9. Moody DB, Reinhold BB, Guy MR, et al.: Structural requirements for glycolipid antigen recognition by CD1b-restricted T cells. *Science* 1997, 278:283–286.

10.• Corinti S, Palma RD, Fontana A, et al.: Major histocompatibility complex-independent recognition of a distinctive pollen antigen, most likely a carbohydrate, by human CD8+ alpha/beta T cells. *J Exp Med* 1997, 186:899–908.
A description of CD8+ T-cell recognition of a carbohydrate moiety on a pollen allergen that appears to be independent of MHC, indicating a nonclassic lymphocyte response to certain allergens.

11.• Rogge L, Barberis-Maino L, Biffi M, et al.: Selective expression of an interleukin 12 receptor component by human T helper 1 cells. *J Exp Med* 1997, 185:825–831.
Messenger RNA for the β2 chain of the IL-12 receptor was detected in naive cells 24 hours after stimulation with mitogen. Induction of the β2 chain was observed following culture with IL-12 and type I but not type II interferons. No expression was observed in cells cultured with IL-4. Phosphorylation of STAT4 did not occur in T_H2 cells, indicating unresponsiveness to this cytokine.

12.• Van der Pauw Kraan TCTM, Boeije LCM, de Groot ER, et al.: Reduced production of IL-12 and IL-12–dependent IFN-γ release in patients with allergic asthma. *J Immunol* 1997, 158:5560–5565.
Production of IL-12 and IL-12–dependent IFN-γ was examined in 15 allergic asthmatics compared with that in 15 normal controls in cultures of whole blood stimulated with Staphylococcus aureus. Significantly lower levels of IL-12 p70 (P < 0.005) and IL-12–dependent IFN-γ (P < 0.005) were found in the asthmatics, although the ratio of IFN-γ to IL-12 was unaltered. The results could not be explained by increased production of IL-10 in the asthmatic group.

13. Stewart GA, Thompson PJ: The biochemistry of common aeroallergens. *Clin Exp Allergy* 1996, 26:1020–1044.

14. Hewitt CR, Brown AP, Hart BJ, Pritchard DI: A major house dust mite allergen disrupts the immunoglobulin E network by selectively cleaving CD23: innate protection by antiproteases. *J Exp Med* 1995, 182:1537–1544.

15. Murray JS, Pfeiffer C, Madri J, Bottomly K: Major histocompatibility complex (MHC) control of CD4 T cell subset activation, II: a single peptide induces either humoral or cell-mediated responses in mice of distinct MHC genotype. *Eur J Immunol* 1992, 22:559–565.

16.• Pfeiffer C, Stein J, Southwood S, *et al.*: Altered peptide ligands can control CD4 T lymphocyte differentiation in vivo. *J Exp Med* 1995, 181:1569–1574.
This study demonstrates that alterations in epitope sequence can give rise to T_H1 or T_H2 responses. Results indicate that strong interactions between T-cell receptor and MHC or peptide lead to T_H1 responses and that weak interactions favor T_H2.

17.•• Hosken NA, Shibuya K, Heath AW, *et al.*: The effect of antigen dose on CD4+ T helper cell phenotype development in a T cell receptor-alpha beta-transgenic model. *J Exp Med* 1995, 182:1579–1584.
A peptide-specific T-cell receptor transgenic mouse model is used to investigate the effects of challenge with low, intermediate, or high doses of peptide. The results indicate that low and high doses of antigen may preferentially give rise to T_H2-type responses, whereas intermediate doses may favor T_H1 responses.

18.• Guery JC, Galbiati F, Smiroldo S, Adorini L: Selective development of T helper (T_H)2 cells induced by continuous administration of low dose soluble proteins to normal and beta(2)-microglobulin-deficient BALB/c mice. *J Exp Med* 1996, 183:485–497.
Mice were exposed (using miniosmotic pumps) to chronic low-level antigen in the absence of adjuvant to mimic natural exposure to allergen. T_H2-type responses predominated.

19. Constant SL, Bottomly K: Induction of T_H1 and T_H2 CD4+ T cell responses: the alternative approaches. *Annu Rev Immunol* 1997, 15:297–322.

20. Evavold BD, Allen PM: Separation of IL-4 production from T_H cell proliferation by an altered T cell receptor ligand. *Science* 1991, 252:1308–1310.

21.•• Kumar V, Bhardwaj V, Soares L, *et al.*: Major histocompatibility complex binding affinity of an antigenic determinant is crucial for the differential secretion of interleukin 4/5 or interferon gamma by T cells. *Proc Natl Acad Sci USA* 1995, 92:9510–9514.
The ability to induce INF-γ production on a background of T_H2 cytokine production to a single peptide by increasing the affinity of the peptide-MHC interaction is described. The findings of this study may have important implications for the design of peptide-based therapeutics for modulation of T_H2 responses in allergic diseases.

22. Takeda K, Hamelmann E, Joetham A, *et al.*: Development of eosinophilic airway inflammation and airway hyperresponsiveness in mast cell-deficient mice. *J Exp Med* 1997, 186:449–454.

23. Mehlhop PD, van de Rijn M, Goldberg AB, *et al.*: Allergen-induced bronchial hyperreactivity and eosinophilic inflammation occur in the absence of IgE in a mouse model of asthma. *Proc Natl Acad Sci USA* 1997, 94:1344–1349.

24.• Hogan SP, Mould A, Kikutani H, *et al.*: Aeroallergen-induced eosinophilic inflammation, lung damage, and airways hyperreactivity in mice can occur independently of IL-4 and allergen-specific immunoglobulins. *J Clin Invest* 1997, 99:1329–1339.
Airway hyperreactivity and eosinophila were investigated in both IL-4–deficient and CD40-deficient mice. In CD40-deficient mice, no allergen-specific IgE, IgG, or IgA was detected, but airway hyperreactivity remained unaltered following allergen challenge. In IL-4–deficient mice, a partial reduction in the degree of airway eosinophilia was observed, but airway hyperreactivity remained unattenuated.

25. Foster PS, Hogan SP, Ramsay AJ, *et al.*: Interleukin-5 deficiency abolishes eosinophilia, airways hyperreactivity, and lung damage in a mouse asthma model. *J Exp Med* 1996, 183:195–201.

26. Hamelmann E, Vella AT, Oshiba A, *et al.*: Allergic airway sensitization induces T cell activation but not airway hyperresponsiveness in B-cell–deficient mice. *Proc Natl Acad Sci USA* 1997, 94:1350–1355.

27. Hamelmann E, Oshiba A, Schwarze J, *et al.*: Allergen-specific IgE and IL-5 are essential for the development of airway hyperresponsiveness. *Am J Respir Cell Mol Biol* 1997, 16:674–682.

28.• Kuperman D, Schofield B, Wills-Karp M, Grusby MJ: Signal transducer and activator of transcription factor 6 (STAT-6)-deficient mice are protected from antigen-induced airway hyperresponsiveness and mucus production. *J Exp Med* 1998, 187:939–948.
Airway responsiveness was investigated in wild-type or STAT6-deficient mice following challenge with allergen. STAT6-deficient mice failed to develop airway hyperreactivity, in contrast to wild-type mice. No antigen-induced increase in mucus-secreting cells was observed in STAT6-deficient mice. A 50% reduction in airway eosinophila was also observed.

29. Corry DB, Folkesson HG, Warnock ML, *et al.*: Interleukin-4, but not interleukin-5 or eosinophils, is required in a murine model of acute airway hyperreactivity. *J Exp Med* 1996, 183:109–117.

30. Renz H, Bradley K, Enssle K, *et al.*: Prevention of the development of immediate hypersensitivity and airway hyperresponsiveness following in vivo treatment with soluble IL-4 receptor. *Int Arch Allergy Immunol* 1996, 109:167–176.

31.• De Sanctis GT, Itoh A, Green FHY, *et al.*: T-lymphocytes regulate genetically determined airway hyperresponsiveness in mice. *Nature Med* 1997, 3:460–462.
Transfer of bone marrow from a mouse strain genetically susceptible to nonatopic airway hyperreactivity into a nonsusceptible strain results in airway hyperresposiveness, which can be prevented by T-cell depletion of bone marrow prior to transplant or the administration of anti–T-cell monoclonal antibodies. The results indicate that in the model selected, T cells alone can transfer airway hyperreactivity.

32. Hamelmann E, Oshiba A, Loader J, *et al.*: Anti–interleukin-5 antibody prevents airway hyperresponsiveness in a murine model of airway sensitization. *Am J Respir Crit Care Med* 1997, 155:819–825.

33. Mauser PJ, Pitman A, Witt A, *et al.*: Inhibitory effect of the TRFK-5 anti-IL-5 antibody in a guinea pig model of asthma. *Am Rev Respir Dis* 1993, 148:1623–1627.

34.•• Mauser PJ, Pitman AM, Fernandez X, *et al.*: Effects of an antibody to interleukin-5 in a monkey model of asthma. *Am J Respir Crit Care Med* 1995, 152:467–472.
Cynomolgus monkeys were sensitized to Ascaris, and airway reactivity to histamine was measured together with eosinophil and neutrophil influx. Increased airway reactivity was suppressed following treatment with 0.3 mg/kg of a monoclonal antibody to IL-5. Eosinophil and neutrophil influx was reduced but not totally abrogated. Inhibition of bronchial hyperresponsiveness and pulmonary eosinophilia was seen for up to 3 months following treatment.

35. Tsuyuki S, Tsuyuki J, Einsle K, *et al.*: Co-stimulation through B7-2 (CD86) is required for the induction of a lung mucosal T helper cell 2 (T_H2) immune response and altered airway responsiveness. *J Exp Med* 1997, 185:1671–1679.

36. Briner TJ, Kuo MC, Keating KM, *et al.*: Peripheral T-cell tolerance induced in naive and primed mice by subcutaneous injection of peptides from the major cat allergen Fel d I. *Proc Natl Acad Sci USA* 1993, 90:7608–7612.

37. Hoyne GF, O'Hehir RE, Wraith DC, *et al.*: Inhibition of T cell and antibody responses to house dust mite allergen by inhalation of the dominant T cell epitope in naive and sensitized mice. *J Exp Med* 1993, 178:1783–1788.

38. Vercelli D: Molecular regulation of the IgE immune response. *Clin Exp Allergy* 1995, 25(suppl):43–45.

39. Burd PR, Thompson WC, Max EE, Mills FC: Activated mast cells produce interleukin-13. *J Exp Med* 1995, 181:1373–1380.

40. Wardlaw AJ, Moqbel R, Kay AB: Eosinophils: biology and role in disease. *Adv Immunol* 1996, 60:151–266.

41. Hamid Q, Azzawi M, Ying S, *et al.*: Expression of mRNA for interleukin-5 in mucosal bronchial biopsies from asthma. *J Clin Invest* 1991, 87:1541–1546.

42. Robinson DS, Hamid Q, Ying S, *et al.*: Predominant T_H2-type bronchoalveolar lavage T-lymphocyte population in atopic asthma. *N Engl J Med* 1992, 326:298–304.

43. Corrigan CJ, Hamid Q, North J, *et al.*: Peripheral blood CD4, but not CD8 T lymphocytes in patients with exacerbation of asthma transcribe and translate messenger RNA encoding cytokines which prolong eosinophil survival in the context of a T_H2-type pattern: effect of glucocorticoid therapy. *Am J Respir Cell Mol Biol* 1995, 12:567–578.

44. Kamei T, Ozaki T, Kawaji K, *et al.*: Production of interleukin-5 and granulocyte/macrophage colony-stimulating factor by T cells of patients with bronchial asthma in response to *Dermatophagoides farinae* and its relation to eosinophil colony-stimulating factor. *Am J Respir Crit Care Med* 1993, 9:378–385.

45. Del Prete GF, De Carli M, D'Elios MM, *et al.*: Allergen exposure induces the activation of allergen-specific T_H2 cells in the airway mucosa of patients with allergic respiratory disorders. *Eur J Immunol* 1993, 23:1445–1449.

46. Robinson DS, Hamid Q, Bentley A, *et al.*: Activation of CD4+ T cells, increased T_H2-type cytokine mRNA expression, and eosinophil recruitment in bronchoalveolar lavage after allergen inhalation challenge in atopic asthmatics. *J Allergy Clin Immunol* 1993, 92:313–324.

47. Bentley AM, Meng Q, Robinson DS, *et al.*: Increases in activated T lymphocytes, eosinophils and cytokine messenger RNA for IL-5 and GM-CSF in bronchial biopsies after allergen inhalation challenge in atopic asthmatics. *Am J Respir Cell Mol Biol* 1993, 8:35–42.

48. Robinson DS, Hamid Q, Ying S, *et al.*: Prednisolone treatment in asthma is associated with modulation of bronchoalveolar lavage cell interleukin-4, interleukin-5 and interferon-γ cytokine gene expression. *Am Rev Respir Dis* 1993, 148:401–406.

49.• Bentley AM, Hamid Q, Robinson DS, *et al.*: Prednisolone treatment in asthma: reduction in the numbers of eosinophils, T cells, tryptase-only positive mast cells, and modulation of IL-4, IL-5, and interferon-gamma cytokine gene expression within the bronchial mucosa. *Am J Respir Crit Care Med* 1996, 153:551–556.
Confirmation of the use of bronchial biopsy specimens and demonstration of prednisolone-induced down-regulation of tryptase-positive mast cells.

50. Robinson DS, Ying S, Bentley AM, *et al.*: Relationships among numbers of bronchoalveolar lavage cells expressing messenger ribonucleic acid for cytokines, asthma symptoms, and airway methacholine responsiveness in atopic asthma. *J Allergy Clin Immunol* 1993, 92:397–403.

51.•• Humbert M, Durham SR, Ying S, *et al.*: IL-4 and IL-5 mRNA and protein in bronchial biopsies from atopic and non-atopic asthmatics: evidence against "intrinsic" asthma being a distinct immunopathological entity. *Am J Respir Crit Care Med* 1996, 154:1497–1504.
Extrinsic and intrinsic asthma have comparable expression of IL-4 and IL-5 mRNA and protein in bronchial biopsy specimens.

52. Virchow JC Jr, Walker C, Hafner D, *et al.*: Cells and cytokines in bronchoalveolar lavage fluid after segmental allergen provocation in atopic asthma. *Am J Respir Crit Care Med* 1995, 151:960–968.

53. Ying S, Durham SR, Corrigan CJ, *et al.*: Phenotype of cells expressing mRNA for T_H2-type (interleukin-4 and interleukin-5) and T_H1-type (interleukin-2 and interferon-γ) cytokines in bronchoalveolar lavage and bronchial biopsies from atopic asthmatics and normal control subjects. *Am J Respir Cell Mol Biol* 1995, 12:477–487.

54.• Ying S, Humbert M, Barkans J, *et al.*: Expression of IL-4 and IL-5 mRNA and protein product by CD4+ and CD8+ T cells, eosinophils, and mast cells in bronchial biopsies obtained from atopic and non-atopic (intrinsic) asthmatics. *J Immunol* 1997, 158:3539–3544.
IL-4 and IL-5 mRNA colocalizes predominantly to CD4+ T cells in bronchial biopsy specimens obtained from patients with atopic extrinsic or nonatopic intrinsic asthma.

55. Till S, Li B, Durham S, *et al.*: Secretion of the eosinophil-active cytokines interleukin-5, granulocyte/macrophage colony-stimulating factor and interleukin-3 by bronchoalveolar lavage CD4+ and CD8+ T-cell lines in atopic asthmatics, and atopic and nonatopic controls. *Eur J Immunol* 1995, 25:2727–2731.

56. Walker C, Bode E, Boer L, *et al.*: Allergic and nonallergic asthmatics have distinct patterns of cytokine production in peripheral blood and bronchoalveolar lavage. *Am J Respir Dis* 1992, 146:109–115.

57. Humbert M, Grant JA, Taborda-Barata L, *et al.*: High affinity IgE receptor (FcεRI)-bearing cells in bronchial biopsies from atopic and nonatopic asthma. *Am J Respir Crit Care Med* 1996, 153:1931–1937.

58. Maestrelli P, Del Prete GF, De Carli M, *et al.*: CD8 T-cell clones producing interleukin-5 and interferon-gamma in bronchial mucosa of patients with asthma induced by toluene di-isocyanate. *Scand J Work Environ Health* 1994, 20:376–381.

59. Levi-Schaffer F, Lacey P, Severs NJ, *et al.*: Association of granulocyte-macrophage colony-stimulating factor with the crystalloid granules of human eosinophils. *Blood* 1995, 85:2579–2586.

60. Moqbel R, Ying S, Barkans J, *et al.*: Identification of mRNA for interleukin-4 in human eosinophils with granule localization and release of the translated product. *J Immunol* 1995, 155:4939–4947.

61. Metzger WJ, Zavala D, Richerson HB, *et al.*: Local allergen challenge and bronchoalveolar lavage of allergic asthmatic lungs: description of the model and local airway inflammation. *Am Rev Respir Dis* 1987, 135:433–440.

62. Sedgwick JB, Calhoun WJ, Gleich GJ, *et al.*: Immediate and late airway response of allergic rhinitis patients to segmental antigen challenge: characterization of eosinophil and mast cell mediators. *Am Rev Respir Dis* 1991, 144:1274–1281.

63. Liu MC, Hubbard WC, Proud D, *et al.*: Immediate and late inflammatory responses to ragweed antigen challenge of the peripheral airways in allergic asthmatics: cellular, mediator, and permeability changes. *Am Rev Respir Dis* 1991, 144:51–58.

64.• Sihra BS, Durham SR, Walker S, *et al.*: Effect of cyclosporin A on the allergen-induced late asthmatic reaction. *Thorax* 1997, 52:447–452.
Cyclosporin A inhibits the early but not the late-phase allergen-induced asthmatic reaction.

65.•• Norman PS, Ohman JL Jr, Long AA, et al.: Treatment of cat allergy with T-cell reactive peptides. Am J Respir Crit Care Med 1996, 154:1623–1628.
Results are presented from a multicenter study of the effects of subcutaneous administration of two peptides derived from the major cat allergen Fel d 1. Three doses were evaluated in a total of 95 patients (including control group). Patients received weekly injections for 4 weeks, and lung and nasal symptoms were evaluated. Patients were also exposed to allergen in a "cat room" before and after treatment, and symptom scores were evaluated. Six weeks after treatment, symptom scores compared with baseline were significantly reduced at the highest dose of peptides.

66. Schwartz RH: Co-stimulation of T lymphocytes: the role of CD28, CTLA-4, and B7/BB1 in interleukin-2 production and immunotherapy. Cell 1992, 71:1065–1068.

67. Schwartz RH: T cell clonal anergy. Curr Opin Immunol 1997, 9:351–357.

68. Lamb JR, Skidmore BJ, Green N, et al.: Induction of tolerance in influenza virus-immune T lymphocyte clones with synthetic peptides of influenza hemagglutinin. J Exp Med 1983, 157:1434–1447.

69. O'Hehir RE, Garman RD, Greenstein JL, Lamb JR: The specificity and regulation of T-cell responsiveness to allergens. Annu Rev Immunol 1991, 9:67–95.

70. Higgins JA, Lamb JR, Marsh SG, et al.: Peptide-induced non-responsiveness of HLA-DP restricted human T cells reactive with Dermatophagoides spp. (house dust mite). J Allergy Clin Immunol 1992, 90:749–756.

71. Varney VA, Gaga M, Frew AJ, et al.: Usefulness of immunotherapy in patients with severe summer hay fever uncontrolled by antiallergic drugs. BMJ 1991, 302:265–269.

72. Varney VA, Hamid QA, Gaga M, et al.: Influence of grass pollen immunotherapy on cellular infiltration and cytokine mRNA expression during allergen-induced late-phase cutaneous responses. J Clin Invest 1993, 92:644–651.

73. Varney V, Gaga M, Frew AJ, et al.: The effect of a single oral dose of prednisolone or cetirizine on inflammatory cells infiltrating allergen-induced cutaneous late-phase reactions in atopic subjects. Clin Exp Allergy 1992, 22:43–49.

74. Secrist H, Chelen CJ, Wen Y, et al.: Allergen immunotherapy decreases interleukin-4 production in CD4+ T cells from allergic individuals. J Exp Med 1993, 178:2123–2130.

75.• Hamid QA, Schotman E, Jacobson MR, et al.: Increases in IL-12 messenger RNA+ cells accompany inhibition of allergen-induced late skin responses after successful grass pollen immunotherapy. J Allergy Clin Immunol 1997, 99:254–260.
Messenger RNA levels for IL-12 were noted in skin biopsy samples from allergen-induced late-phase reactions from patients who had undergone 4 years of pollen immunotherapy. The samples were compared with findings in untreated controls. Significant increases in IL-12 message were observed in the treated group, which correlated with IFN-γ+ cells. The results suggest that successful immunotherapy may be accompanied by increased IL-12 production from macrophages, which gives rise to a concomitant increase in IFN-γ production.

76. Jutel M, Pichler WJ, Skrbic D, et al.: Bee venom immunotherapy results in decrease of IL-4 and IL-5 and increase of IFN-gamma secretion in specific allergen-stimulated T cell cultures. J Immunol 1995, 154:4187–4194.

77.• Akdis CA, Akdis M, Blesken T, et al.: Epitope-specific T cell tolerance to phospholipase A₂ in bee venom immunotherapy and recovery by IL-2 and IL-15 in vitro. J Clin Invest 1996, 98:1676–1683.
Patients successfully desensitized to bee venom phospholipase A₂ after 2 months of RUSH immunotherapy with whole bee venom were investigated for phospholipase A₂–specific and peptide-epitope–specific peripheral tolerance by culture of peripheral blood mononuclear cells. Following immunotherapy, proliferative and cytokine responses to both phospholipase A₂ and peptide epitopes were abolished. TH2 responses and TH1-type cytokines were inhibited. Proliferative responses and TH1-type cytokines were rescued by addition of IL-2 or IL-15 to cultures. In contrast, TH2-type responses remained suppressed unless cultures were treated with IL-4, which partially reversed suppression.

78. Simons FE, Imada M, Li Y, et al.: Fel d 1 peptides: effect on skin tests and cytokine synthesis in cat-allergic human subjects. Int Immunol 1996, 8:1937–1945.

79. Rogers BL, Bond JF, Craig SJ, et al.: Potential therapeutic recombinant proteins comprised of peptides containing recombined T cell epitopes. Mol Immunol 1994, 31:955–966.

80. Counsell CM, Bond JF, Ohman JL Jr, et al.: Definition of the human T-cell epitopes of Fel d 1, the major allergen of the domestic cat. J Allergy Clin Immunol 1996, 98:884–894.

81. Morgenstern JP, Griffith IJ, Brauer AW, et al.: Amino acid sequence of Fel d 1, the major allergen of the domestic cat: protein sequence analysis and cDNA cloning. Proc Natl Acad Sci USA 1991, 88:9690–9694.

82.• Weiner HL, Inobe J, Kuchroo V, Chen Y: Induction and characterisation of TGF-β secreting TH3 cells. FASEB J 1996, 10:A1444.
The first description of the TH3 cell, a regulatory population of T cells secreting TGF-β.

83.• Powrie F, Carlino J, Leach MW, et al.: A critical role for transforming growth factor-β but not IL 4 in the suppression of T helper type 1-mediated colitis by CD45RB (low) CD4+ T cells. J Exp Med 1996, 183:2669–2674.
Demonstration that memory T cells secreting TGF-β are capable of preventing the induction of colitis by previously naive T cells in a murine model.

84.• Groux H, O'Garra A, Bigler M, et al.: A CD4+ T-cell subset inhibits antigen-specific T-cell responses and prevents colitis. Nature 1997, 389:737–742.
The first description of the Tr1 population of regulatory T cells secreting IL-10 and IL-5 and generated by culture in IL-10.

85.• Bridoux F, Badou A, Saoudi A, et al.: Transforming growth factor beta (TGF-beta)–dependent inhibition of T helper cell 2 (TH2)-induced autoimmunity by self-major histocompatibility complex (MHC) class II-specific, regulatory CD4(+) T cell lines. J Exp Med 1997, 185:1769–1775.
A study suggesting that TH2 as well as TH1 cells can be negatively regulated by populations secreting TGF-β.

86. O'Garra A: Cytokines induce the development of functionally heterogeneous T helper cell subsets. Immunity 1998, 8:275–283.

87. Swain SL, Huston G, Tonkonogy S, Weinberg A: Transforming growth factor-beta and IL-4 cause helper T cell precursors to develop into distinct effector helper cells that differ in lymphokine secretion pattern and cell surface phenotype. J Immunol 1991, 147:2991–3000.

88. Sad S, Mosmann TR: Single IL-2-secreting precursor CD4 T cell can develop into either TH1 or TH2 cytokine secretion phenotype. J Immunol 1994, 153:3514–3522.

89. Wahl SM, Hunt DA, Wong HL, et al.: Transforming growth factor-beta is a potent immunosuppressive agent that inhibits IL-1–dependent lymphocyte proliferation. J Immunol 1988, 140:3026–3032.

90. Holter W, Kalthoff FS, Pickl WF, et al.: Transforming growth factor-beta inhibits IL-4 and IFN-gamma production by stimulated human T cells. Int Immunol 1994, 6:469–475.

91. Davies JD, Leong LYW, Mellor A, et al.: T cell suppression in transplantation tolerance through linked suppression. J Immunol 1996, 156:3602–3607.

92. Qin S, Cobbold SP, Pope H, et al.: "Infectious" transplantation tolerance. Science 1993, 259:974–977.

93. Lombardi G, Sidhu S, Batchelor R, Lechler R: Anergic T cells as suppressor cells in vitro. *Science* 1994, 264:1587–1589.

94. Chen Y, Kuchroo VK, Inobe J, *et al.*: Regulatory T cell clones induced by oral tolerance: suppression of autoimmune encephalomyelitis. *Science* 1994, 265:1237–1240.

95. Gaur A, Wiers B, Liu A, *et al.*: Amelioration of experimental autoimmune encephalomyelitis by myelin basic protein synthetic peptide-induced anergy. *Science* 1992, 258:1491–1494.

96. Ku G, Kronenberg M, Peacock DJ, *et al.*: Prevention of experimental autoimmune arthritis with a peptide fragment of type II collagen. *Eur J Immunol* 1993, 23:591–599.

97.• Vaysburd M, Lock C, McDevitt H: Prevention of insulin-dependent diabetes mellitus in nonobese diabetic mice by immunogenic but not tolerated peptides. *J Exp Med* 1995, 182:897–902.
Development of diabetes in nonobese diabetic mice can be prevented by a peptide that binds to the I-A^g molecule. This article describes a mechanism other than direct major histocompatibility complex competition or blockade for the efficacy of this peptide, which is related to the ability of the peptide to elicit an immune response in the mouse. This may modulate the T_H1 versus T_H2 status of the animal or may generate a population of regulatory cells.

98. Staines NA, Harper N, Ward FJ, *et al.*: Mucosal tolerance and suppression of collagen-induced arthritis (CIA) induced by nasal inhalation of synthetic peptide 184-198 of bovine type II collagen (CII) expressing a dominant T cell epitope. *Clin Exp Immunol* 1996, 103:368–375.

99. Clayton JP, Gammon GM, Ando DG, *et al.*: Peptide-specific prevention of experimental allergic encephalomyelitis. *J Exp Med* 1989, 169:1681–1691.

100.••Hoyne GF, Jarnicki AG, Thomas WR, Lamb JR: Characterisation of the specificity and duration of T cell tolerance to intranasally administered peptides in mice: a role for intramolecular epitope suppression. *Int Immunol* 1997, 9:1165–1173.
Intranasal administration of peptides derived from house dust mite proteins was previously shown to induce tolerance to the whole molecule. In this study, the effect of administration of one peptide epitope on the T-cell response to a distinct epitope within the same protein is investigated.

101.••Fukaura H, Kent SC, Pietrusewicz MJ, *et al.*: Induction of circulating myelin basic protein and proteolipid protein-specific transforming growth factor-β1 secreting T_H3 T cells by oral administration of myelin in multiple sclerosis patients. *J Clin Invest* 1996, 98:70–77.
T-cell lines were investigated from 34 patients with relapsing-remitting multiple sclerosis. Seventeen received oral bovine myelin for at least 2 years, and 17 remained untreated. An increased frequency of TGF-β–producing T-cell lines specific for either myelin basic protein or proteolipid protein was found in the actively treated group, with no change in the frequency of IFN-γ or in the frequency of TGF-β–producing lines specific for the recall antigen tetanus toxoid.

CHAPTER 4

Immunoglobulin E

Daniel H. Conrad
Sheri B. Tinnell
Ann E. Kelly

Immunoglobulin (Ig) E is found only in mammals and is one of the five classes of antibody recognized in humans. It is generally recognized as having a role in parasitic infections common in undeveloped countries; however, in developed countries, where parasitic diseases in humans are more largely controlled, IgE is considered to have little beneficial function. Indeed, the primary activity observed for IgE in developed countries relates to type I allergic disease. Allergic diseases affect more than 20% of the population; their rise in prevalence has led to their designation as the "number-one environmental disease" [1]. IgE constitutes a minuscule fraction of the total antibody titer in human serum (50 to 300 ng/mL compared with mg/mL concentrations of IgG). Their action is mediated by interaction with specific Fc receptors for IgE. Fc receptors are cell-surface glycoproteins that have a significant affinity for the Fc region of Ig molecules. Fc receptors have been implicated in various immune functions, including phagocytosis, antibody-dependent cell-mediated cytotoxicity, and release of inflammatory mediators. The high-affinity receptor for IgE, FcεRI, is classically known for its presence on mast cells and basophils, although more recent studies have found expression of the FcεRI on other cell types as well. Cross-linking of the IgE bound to the FcεRI on mast cells or basophils sets into motion the series of events that ultimately develops into allergic disease. A second receptor for IgE, termed FcεRII or CD23, is found on lymphocytes and other hematopoietic cells and interacts with IgE with an affinity lower than the FcεRI. This chapter is concerned primarily with IgE, including a brief discussion of the two Fc receptors for IgE mentioned above [2–5].

HISTORICAL PERSPECTIVE

The experiments of Prausnitz and Kustner [6] in 1921 demonstrated that the serum of allergic individuals contained a humoral factor that could transfer specific allergen sensitivity to nonallergic individuals. This serum factor, known for decades as *reagin*, was conclusively identified in the late 1960s as a unique class of Ig and was given the name IgE. Shortly after IgE was discovered, it was found to selectively bind mast cells and basophils. It was obvious from early experiments that binding of IgE to its receptor was likely to involve high-affinity interactions, much higher than those observed for IgG binding to IgG receptors. The high-affinity IgE binding was also restricted to a much smaller variety of cells than IgG receptors.

After the discovery of this high-affinity receptor, another IgE receptor was identified that exhibited a lower binding affinity for IgE than FcεRI. The high-affinity receptor was called FcεRI and the low-affinity receptor was called FcεRII [7]. The low-affinity receptor is unlikely to be involved in mast cell/basophil degranulation, but may be an important element in B-cell function and in isotype-specific regulation of IgE. Therefore, both the high- and low-affinity receptors for IgE play important, although very different, roles in the development of allergic disease. In this chapter, these receptors are discussed separately in order to cover not only their pathologic significance but also their recently characterized potential roles in normal physiology.

IMMUNOGLOBULIN E AS PRIMARY HOMOCYTOTROPIC ANTIBODY IN MAN
Genetic control of Immunoglobulin E production

Genetic predisposition for allergic disease appears, in part, to center on genetic polymorphisms related to IgE production. The human 5q31-33 cytokine gene cluster contains polymorphisms in the promoters of the *IL4* and *IL10* genes [8]. For IgE class switching to occur, interleukin (IL)-4 activates the IgE germline promoter by inducing interaction of the signal transducer and activator transcription factor 6 (STAT6) with a responsive DNA element in the proximal region of the promoter. In 1995, a polymorphism in the human IL-4 receptor-coding region was demonstrated to be linked to IgE-mediated allergic inflammatory disorders [9]. Mice with genetically disrupted STAT6 genes are deficient in IL-4–mediated functions, including Ig class switching to IgE [10•,11•]. Interestingly, the human IL-4R polymorphism linked to allergic disease is located within a receptor domain known to control STAT6 activation [12••].

Synthesis of IgE is strictly regulated by cytokines and cell surface molecules. The required cytokines are IL-4 or IL-13, and the second signal is provided by the CD40-CD40 ligand interaction. As with other Ig classes, switching to IgE is preceded by transcription of a germline epsilon transcript. Analysis of this promoter demonstrates several transcription-factor binding motifs, and Delphin and Stavnezer [13] suggested that three transcription factors, STAT6, nuclear factor-κB (NF-κB) and CCAAT/enhancer binding protein are important in enhancing transcription of the germline epsilon transcript (Figure 4-1). We have shown a similar synergistic action for the induction of FcεRII (discussed later in this chapter) [14]. In this model, the inactive transcription factors are activated by interaction of either IL-4 or CD40L with its respective receptor. The activated transcription factors then move to the nucleus and synergistically activate either the germline epsilon transcript or FcεRII promoters, presumably by interacting with RNA polymerase.

Interleukin-4 signaling

Interleukin-4 is a cytokine that has been shown to play a major role in B- and T-cell immune responses [15,16]. The IL-4 receptor is a member of the hematopoietin-receptor superfamily and is composed of two chains, IL-4Rα and IL-2Rγ$_C$ [17–19] as shown in Figure 4-2, a model based on the study by Keegan *et al.* [19]). The receptor chain termed γ$_c$ stands for "common γ" because this same chain is shared by the IL-2, IL-4, IL-7, IL-9, and IL-15 receptors [20, 21]. Two general signaling pathways for the IL-4 receptor have been described. The first involves insulin receptor substrate 1/2 [22,23] and the second involves Janus protein tyrosine kinase (JAK) and STAT [24,25]. Separate sites on the cytoplasmic domain of the IL-4Rα chain interact with members of the JAK and STAT families as well as with insulin receptor substrate 1/2 [12••, 26]. IL-4 induction of IgE involves the activation of STAT6 [24]. It has now been demonstrated that an IL-4–induced protein termed "IL-4–STAT" [27], another termed "signal transducing factor—IL-4" [28], and STAT6 are identical [24]. This protein binds to a consensus DNA sequence composed of an inverted GAA repeat, TTC N4 GAA [29]. Three separate groups have generated STAT6$^{-/-}$ mice and demonstrated the requirement for IgE production, CD23 induction, and lymphocyte proliferative responses [10•,11•,30].

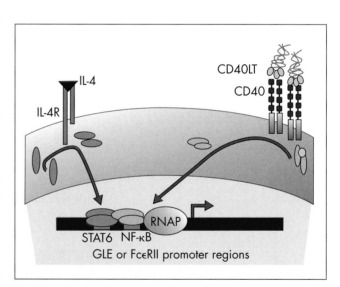

FIGURE 4-1.

Model for germline epsilon transcript (GLE) and FcεRII synergistic induction. STAT6 and nuclear factor (NF)-κB are involved in the induction of both IgE and FcεRII. These transcription factors exist in an inactive form in the cytoplasm and are induced by the combined action of interleukin (IL)-4 and CD40L interacting with the B cell. Once in the nucleus, these transcription factors are believed to interact with each other as well as with the respective DNA motif, an interaction resulting in the synergistic induction observed. The model is based on research by Delphin and Stavnezer [13] as well as on that of Tinnell *et al.* [14]; note that a CCAT enhancer binding protein (CEBP) family member has also been reported to be involved in GLE, but not in CD23 induction. RNAP—RNA polymerase.

Interleukin-13 signaling

Interleukin-13 is a cytokine that shares many biological functions with IL-4. It is secreted by activated T cells and mast cells. Human IL-13 induces FcεRII expression on B cells, enhances B-cell proliferation, and stimulates IgE and IgG4 production [31]. However, IL-13 does not induce IgE switching in mice, presumably because this receptor is not expressed on mouse B cells. Four types of IL-13 receptors exist [32].

CD40-CD40L

CD40 is a 45-kDa membrane glycoprotein that is a member of the tumor necrosis factor (TNF) receptor superfamily [33,34•]. CD40 contains four homologous cysteine-rich extracellular domains and is expressed on B cells, monocytes, dendritic cells, and several other cell types. Its ligand, CD40L, is also known as gp39, is related to TNF, and is expressed on activated CD4+ T lymphocytes, basophils, and activated B cells in humans and mice. CD40L forms a noncovalent trimer that is critical for initiation of CD40 signaling. The CD40-CD40L interaction stimulates B-cell proliferation, Ig secretion, and the upregulation of several other cell sur-

face molecules. This triggering signal is now generally recognized to be the physiologically relevant signal that explains cognate B-cell activation by T-helper cells.

Proteins called TNF receptor–associated factor have been identified that interact with the intracellular domain of CD40 and are involved in CD40 signaling. These signaling events include the modulation of nonreceptor tyrosine kinases, such as Lyn, Fyn, and PI-3 kinase. CD40 also has been shown to stimulate the activation of several transcription factors, such as NF-κB, activator protein-1 (Fos/Jun), NF-activated T cells [35], activating transcription factor 2 [36], and STATs [37•,38].

Biologic functions

Immunoglobulin E does not remain long in serum or other biologic fluid because of its high catabolic rate (2.5 day half life for IgE versus 21 days for IgG). Although IgE is a rare serum antibody, it is a major isotype of plasma cells at many local sites of ongoing immune response. Elevated IgE levels are observed during parasite infections in man and animal models. Mice with a targeted deletion of the IgE gene were shown to have increased worm burdens and reduced granulomatous inflammation following primary infection with *Schistosoma mansoni* [39]. In addition, the finding that mast cells respond to IgE immune complexes by making and releasing many cytokines (discussed later in this chapter) supports a positive role for IgE in immunity. In spite of this, IgE is commonly associated with immunologic problems rather than with protective immunity. IgE is clearly the primary antibody responsible for type I allergic disease, although some controversy remains regarding the anaphylactic role of IgG4. Because of the central role of IgE in the development of immediate hypersensitivity, a concerted effort has been made by research investigators to inhibit IgE responses without affecting other isotypes.

Structure

The IgE molecule is composed of two identical light chains, either λ or κ, which each contain a variable and constant domain, and two identical heavy chains (termed ε *chains*) with one variable domain and four constant region domains. The variable regions give the molecule antigen-binding specificity. The heavy chain constant region gives the molecule its isotype specificity and effector function. At the molecular level, IgE is produced through two processes called variable/diversity/joining recombination and heavy-chain class switching. Variable, diversity, and joining regions comprise the variable region of the heavy chain. Switch recombination to the ε-chain locus occurs only after germline epsilon transcript expression. IgE (molecular weight = 188,000) is slightly larger than IgG (molecular weight =155,000) because it has a fifth domain on the C terminus and it is more heavily glycosylated (12% for IgE versus 3% for IgG).

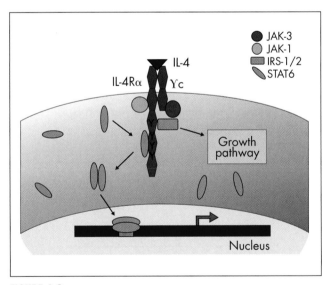

FIGURE 4-2.
A model for the signal transducer and activator of transcription (STAT)6 activation through the interleukin (IL)-4 receptor. The cytokine IL-4 binds to the type I cytokine receptor [21], which is composed of the IL-4 receptor α chain and the γ$_C$ chain. The α chain is composed of five domains, the third of which contains a tyrosine residue and a region termed the *I4R motif*. The phosphorylated tyrosine in this motif interacts with the insulin receptor substrate (IRS)1/2 and is involved in proliferation responses. The fourth domain of the α chain contains three tyrosines that, on phosphorylation, interact with STAT6 to enable its phosphorylation and hence dimerization. The STAT6 homodimer may then enter the nucleus, interact with its DNA binding site, and enhance transcription. IL4Rα—interleukin-4 receptor α; JAK-Janus protein tyrosine kinase.

FcεRI AS HIGH-AFFINITY Fc RECEPTOR FOR IMMUNOGLOBULIN E

Discovery

The two major categories of Fc receptors for IgE are based on their relative affinities for IgE. Although initially thought to be related, molecular cloning has demonstrated that the only similarity between the FcεRI and FcεRII is the sharing of a common ligand. The FcεRI was discovered when it was demonstrated that radiolabeled human IgE is preferentially bound to human basophils and, subsequently, monkey mast cells. Much of the research has been in rodents because of the availability of the rat basophilic cell line as well as of cultured mouse mast cells.

Affinity

FcεRI has the highest affinity for Ig of the known Fc receptors. Affinity measurements have been performed in both the human and rodent systems, and the affinity is in the range of 10^{10} to 10^{12} M^{-1}. Reflected in this high affinity is an extremely low dissociation rate (k_1 below 10^{-5} seconds^{-1}), resulting in retention of monomeric IgE on the mast cell/basophil surface for long periods of time. This interaction has recently been studied using biosensor technology, and this measurement, although consistent with a high affinity, has indicated that the interaction occurs in a biphasic rather than monophasic manner [40]. Early studies on the fate of IgE bound to FcεRI indicated that, although turnover and endocytosis of IgE dimers, trimers, and larger oligomers exist, significant residual IgE could be detected 3 days after loading, particularly if the IgE was not cross-linked.

Structure and interaction with Immunoglobulin E

The FcεRI is composed of three different protein subunits, illustrated in Figure 4-3. The FcεRI is composed of peptides designated α, β, and γ, respectively, and its stoichiometry is known to be $\alpha\beta\gamma_2$. The α-chain was discovered first; it is a 55 to 60 kDa glycoprotein that can be easily radiolabeled by surface iodination procedures. The cDNA for the rat α-chain was the first to be isolated [41] and the subsequent analysis of the human α-chain indicated that the two chains were highly homologous. Early biochemical studies suggested that the α-chain was highly surface-exposed, and no evidence for a cytoplasmic tail was seen. However, the predicted amino acid sequence clearly indicated a single transmembrane sequence followed by a short cytoplasmic tail containing charged amino acids. The extracellular region contains two domains with inter-chain disulfide bonds and amino acid homology so as to place the α-chain in the *Ig* gene superfamily. The extracellular portion of the α-chain is both necessary and sufficient for IgE binding [42]. Indeed, molecularly engineered soluble α-chain, in which the transmembrane and cyto-

plasmic regions have been deleted, will bind IgE with high affinity and thus block IgE binding to the mast cell/basophil [42]. These soluble α-chain constructs may provide a new avenue for blocking allergic reactions, analogous to the monoclonal antibody anti-IgE mentioned above. However, the short serum half life of the recombinant FcεRIα may preclude this use.

The other two components of FcεRI, termed the β and γ chains, are hydrophobic membrane proteins. The β chain is predicted to traverse the membrane four times, meaning that both the amino and carboxyl termini are cytoplasmic [43]. This chain was initially identified as part of the FcεRI on rat basophilic leukemia cells. Recent studies indicate that the primary role of the β-chain is to amplify the signal from the γ-chain [44].

The γ-chain is a 9-kDa disulfide–linked dimer; its cloning allows expression of the complete FcεRI [45]. The predicted sequence is highly homologous to the ζ-chain of the T-cell receptor, which is a similar disulfide-linked dimer [46]. Intriguingly, the γ-chain and ζ-chain are interchangeable—the γ-chain can be used in place of the ζ in the T-cell receptor and the ζ can be used in place of the γ-chain in the FcεRI [47].

Reth [48] was the first to note that the cytoplasmic region of the γ-chain and ζ-chain are similar in structure to various other receptor-associated proteins. Like γ- and ζ-chains, these other proteins are required for efficient expression of the "ligand-binding" subunit. These proteins include the FcεRI, FcγRIII, the T-cell antigen receptor, and the B-cell antigen receptor. These receptors require aggregation to transduce an activation signal,

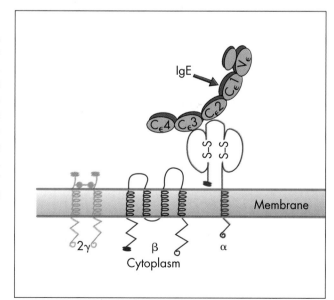

FIGURE 4-3.

The structure of FcεRI. The three different protein components of this receptor. The external portion of the α-chain consists of two immunoglobulin (Ig)-like domains that are shown involved in interaction with IgE at the $C_\epsilon 2$ -$C_\epsilon 3$ domain region.

and the concept of multichain immune recognition receptors (MIRR) is a general term used to designate these receptors [49]. A minimal consensus motif in the cytoplasmic domain required for signaling is YxxLxxxY. This motif is now known as the immunoreceptor tyrosine-based activation motif (ITAM) [50•]. A partial listing of proteins that contain an ITAM is shown in Figure 4-4, as well as the alignment of the sequences to demonstrate homology with the consensus sequence. During receptor subunit aggregation, the tyrosine residues in the ITAM motifs become phosphorylated. This process initiates the activation cascade discussed later in this chapter. FcεRI expression appears to be most effectively upregulated by IgE itself. The binding of IgE to FcεRI expressed on the surface of mouse mast cells is a stimulus for cytokine production by these cells. Furthermore, baseline levels of FcεRI expression on peritoneal mast cells from genetically IgE-deficient mice are reduced by approximately 83% compared with those on cells from corresponding normal mice [51]. FcεRI expression on basophils is similarly regulated by IgE, because the administration of IgE in vivo can significantly upregulate FcεRI expression on mouse basophils, and genetically IgE-deficient mice exhibit a dramatic reduction of basophil FcεRI expression compared with the corresponding normal mice [52]. Therapeutic implications in the findings suggest down-regulation of FcεRI expression on human basophils during in vivo treatment of atopic patients with anti-IgE antibody [53••]. A possible explanation for these results is that FcεRI density is directly or indirectly regulated by plasma-free IgE levels.

IL-4 appears to upregulate FcεRI expression in the human [54,55], although murine mast cells may not respond directly to IL-4 by up-regulation of FcεRI.

The site on IgE that interacts with FcεR is of some interest in view of the possible development of inhibitors of the IgE-FcεR interaction and an extensive review is available [2]. Several approaches have been taken to map the site of IgE-FcεR interaction, including limited proteolysis, energy transfer, and inhibition of IgE binding with a monoclonal antibody with specificity for IgE itself [56]. These reports indicate that the most likely site of interaction is in the $C_\epsilon 2$-$C_\epsilon 3$ domains, because energy transfer studies indicate that IgE adopts a "bent" configuration when bound to the FcεRI. Regarding monoclonal antibody blocking, considerable progress has been made; antibodies that block IgE binding to the FcεRI in both murine and human samples have been identified and have been shown to represent a potential therapy option [57–60]. Because they interact with IgE at the site of interaction with the FcεRI, these monoclonal antibodies cannot interact with FcεRI-bound IgE and therefore do not induce allergic mediator release. Indeed, injection of monoclonal antibodies into mice and humans results in very low IgE levels and amelioration of allergic symptoms [57,61]. In addition, the anti-IgE monoclonal antibodies being tested in humans have been "humanized" to reduce the possibility of immune complex problems [61]. The mechanism through which anti-IgE lowers IgE levels is not known; however, clearance of IgE immune complexes is certainly operative, and suppression of ongoing IgE synthesis may also occur.

CONSENSUS   DXXXXXXXDXXYXXLXXXXXXXYXXL
               E   E   I

FCεRIγ   RLKIQVRKAAIASREKADAVYTGLNTRSQETYETLKHEKPPQ

FCεRIβ   RIGQELE – SKKVPDDRLYEEL–NVYSPIYSELEDKGETSSPVDS

Ig–β   DKDDGKAGMEEDHTYEGLNIDQTATYEDIVTLRTGEVKWSVGEHPGQE

Ig–α   RKRWQNEKFGVDMPDDYEDENLYEGLNLDDCSMYEDISRGLQGTYQDVGNLGIGDAQLEK

CD3γ   GQDGVRQSRASDKQTLLQNEQLYQPLKDREDDQYSHLQGNQLRRN

CD3δ   GHETGRPSGAAEVQALLKNEQLYQPLRKREDTQYSSLGGNWPRNNKS

CD3ζ   ADAYSDIGTKGERRRGKGHDGLYQGLSTATKDTYDALHMQTLAPR

FIGURE 4-4.
Immunoreceptor tyrosine-based activation motifs (ITAMs). The cytoplasmic tails of several receptor-associated molecules share a consensus motif. Tyrosine residues in ITAM motifs are phosphorylated on receptor subunit aggregation–induced activation. The identity of the molecules: Ig-β and Ig-α are associated with B-cell surface Ig; clusters of differentiation (CD)3K, CD3L, and CD3N are associated with the T-cell antigen receptor. The consensus sequence is shown at the top with amino acid residues matching the consensus indicated in brown. (*Adapted from* Reth [48]; with permission.)

FcεRI function

Early studies demonstrated that FcεRI was intimately involved in the allergic mediator–release process, and that cross-linking of FcεRI, even in the absence of IgE, resulted in mast cell triggering. Evidence for the importance of all three proteins (α, β, and γ) has been shown through mutagenesis studies. Transfection of α-, β-, and γ-chains into P815, a mast cell–derived line which does not naturally express the FcεRI, resulted in expression of a functional FcεRI, as measured by calcium intracellular translocation studies [62]. Although the primary function of the α-chain appears to be IgE binding, specific mutations in either the β- or γ-chains resulted in defective signaling, suggesting that all three proteins play a role in the signaling process [62,63]. Interestingly, transfection of COS cells (monkey kidney origin) with the three chains results in the expression of the FcεRI, as evidenced by ligand binding; however, the COS-expressed receptor does not cause calcium translocation subsequent to aggregation, indicating that signaling is defective [62]. Thus, these studies emphasize the importance of all three proteins of FcεRI for both expression and function and indicate that other, as yet unknown, mast cell–specific proteins are required for the signaling process.

Characterization of events between FcεRI aggregation and mediator or cytokine release continues to be an area of active investigation. As previously discussed, the observation that signaling is seen only when the FcεRI is transfected into a mast cell line indicates the importance of other mast cell/basophil-specific components. Various pathways have been implicated in the FcεRI signaling system. An induced increase in cytoplasmic calcium and inositol phosphate metabolites has been known for some time [3], although the exact role that these agents play in the mediator release cascade remains unknown. Additionally, interest has focused on the increased tyrosine kinase phosphorylation that is seen upon FcεRI aggregation. The γ- and β-chains have been shown to be specifically phosphorylated as a result of FcεRI aggregation [64]. In addition, other proteins are also phosphorylated by a tyrosine-specific kinase. One of the most prominent is a 72-kDa protein, which has been identified as a protein tyrosine kinase related to the Syk family [65]. The importance of Syk was first indicated by the preparation of a chimeric cell surface molecule in which the cytoplasmic domain was the Syk kinase [66]. In addition, a Syk-negative rat basophilic leukemia cell line was identified and FcεRI release capacity was restored by transfection with Syk [67•]. The protooncogene *vav* has been implicated in MIRR-induced signaling [68,69]; another component frequently implicated in cell-triggering phenomena is phospholipase C, which has several isoforms [70]. Phospholipase C-γ_1 has recently been shown to be phosphorylated

upon FcεRI aggregation [69,70]. Regarding FcεRI, the Src-related kinases Lyn or Yes were shown to be associated with FcεRI on rat basophilic leukemia cells or the mouse mast cell line PT-18, respectively [71,72]. When Lyn-deficient mice were examined, mast cell triggering through FcεRI was shown to be deficient, confirming the importance of Lyn in IgE-mediated mast cell activation. Association of Lyn with Syk after aggregation has been reported [67•]; thus, this kinase is presumably responsible for phosphorylation of both the ITAMs and Syk during mast cell activation.

Regulation of FcεRI-mediated activation

For obvious reasons, a great deal of interest centers on the mechanisms by which IgE-mediated mast cell activation could be controlled. Recent interest in how ITAM activation might be controlled and dampened has centered on the control motif termed immunoreceptor tyrosine-based inhibitory motif (ITIM). The consensus sequence for this motif is I/VxYxxL/V. Although initially recognized and studied as part of the cytoplasmic domain of the FcγRII, this motif is now recognized to be part of a large number of regulatory molecules [49,73,74]. Mechanistically, the tyrosine in the ITIM is phosphorylated, presumably by the same kinase that phosphorylates the ITAM (Lyn with mast cells), and the phosphotyrosine then recruits other molecules to the vicinity of the cross-linked complex. Note that this mechanism requires that the ITIM-bearing molecule be co–cross-linked to the ITAM-bearing activation complex. Two molecules, the Src homology 2 domain (SH2) containing protein tyrosine phosphatase 1 (SHP-1) and the SH2 domain containing inositol-polyphosphate 5-phosphatase (SHIP), have been recently identified as binding to the ITIM [74,75,76]. Binding in both cases is through an SH_2 domain on the respective molecule. Once recruited, these molecules then act to shut down the triggering signal by dephosphorylating downstream effector molecules (yet to be identified) in the case of SHP-1; with SHIP, this occurs presumably by interfering with the calcium signal [76]. Using appropriately transfected cell lines, Daeron *et al.* [77] demonstrated that the ITIM down-regulation mechanism was operative for FcεRI, B-cell sIg, and T-cell receptor–mediated triggering [77]. Current work indicates that SHIP is important for FcεRI down-regulation, whereas SHP-1 is more important for B-cell receptor and T-cell receptor regulation [78••]. Lack of FcγRIIB expression by human mast cells and basophils indicates that ITIM-mediated regulation of human FcεRI requires other molecules. Two potential candidates have been identified. The first is gp49, which contains two ITIMs in its cytoplasmic domain, and the second is mast cell function–associated antigen, which is a member of the C-type animal lectin family [79,80]. Its cytoplasmic domain has a sequence, YSTL, that closely resembles the YSLL motif of the ITIM sequence. In addition, co–cross-linking with appropriate monoclonal antibodies results in inhibition of FcεRI-mediated activation [81]. Obviously, the natural ligands for both gp49 and mast cell function–associated antigen are being actively sought, and, when found, may offer new avenues for control of mast cell–basophil IgE-mediated activation.

LOW-AFFINITY IMMUNOGLOBULIN E RECEPTOR (FcεRII/CD23)

Discovery and structure

The low-affinity receptor for IgE (FcεRII) is the most unusual of the Fc receptors because it has no Ig-like domains. It is a member of the calcium-dependent animal lectin family, and can be cleaved from the membrane to form a soluble fragment (sCD23). FcεRII is reviewed further by Conrad [4] and Delespesse et al [5]. The FcεRII was initially discovered in 1975 by Lawrence et al. [82] using aggregated IgE on human peripheral blood mononuclear cells. A 45-kDa B-cell activation antigen was designated CD23 at the Second International Workshop on Human Leukocyte Differentiation Antigen in 1984. CD23 was identified using several monoclonal antibodies prepared by immunization of Epstein-Barr virus–transformed human B cells. CD23 was not detected on resting B cells isolated from peripheral blood, lymphoid tissues, or mantle zone B cells, but on activated B cells and germinal center B cells. Subsequently, it was shown that CD23 and FcεRII are the same protein. Cloning studies demonstrated that CD23 is a type II integral membrane glycoprotein [4]. Human CD23 consists of a 23-amino acid N-terminal intracytoplasmic domain, a 21-amino acid transmembrane domain, and a 277-amino acid C-terminal extracellular domain, resulting in a 321-amino acid protein. The gene for human CD23 is found on chromosome 19 and is a single copy gene consisting of 11 exons [83]. In humans, this gene encodes two transcripts, FcεRIIa (CD23a) and FcεRIIb (CD23b), which differ in their 5′ untranslated region and in the first 6 amino acids, which are found in the intracytoplasmic region [84]. The cellular distribution of each transcript is also different. CD23a is present only on B cells and possibly follicular dendritic cells, but CD23b is expressed on a much wider number of hematopoietic cell types, such as CD5+ B cells, T cells, eosinophils, bone marrow–derived mast cells, platelets, monocytes, and Langerhan's cells.

Interaction with Immunoglobulin E

The site of interaction of FcεRII has been mapped by similar techniques, and the results indicate that the interaction site is in the $C_\varepsilon 3$ domain, which is close, but not identical to, the FcεRI interaction site [56,85]. IgE-

CD23 binding is Ca^{2+}-dependent but does not require carbohydrate because deglycosylation of IgE does not significantly influence the binding [85,86]. Mutations in the lectin domain change IgE binding, indicating that the interaction site of CD23 with IgE is in the lectin cassette [87,88]. The stalk region of the molecule has homology with tropomyosin and other similar molecules that exhibit α-helical coiled-coil motifs [89,90]. These molecules are anticipated to form trimers and even higher oligomers, and situations have been reported for both the asialoglycoprotein receptor and mannose binding protein, two members of the C-lectin family. Dierks et al. [91], using chemical cross-linkers, demonstrated that the intact form of CD23 is oligomerized to at least a trimeric form and also showed that the stalk repeat region mediated this oligomerization. This finding has led to a new model for CD23 (Figure 4-5). Unlike human CD23, mouse sCD23 does not exhibit this oligomerization capacity and only interacts with IgE with a single low affinity $10^6 M^{-1}$) [92]. Beavil et al. [93] found that sCD23 could be cross-linked to trimers and higher oligomers, suggesting that the multimeric structure was more stable in human CD23. This may explain the increased biologic activity reported for human sCD23. In recent studies, a modified leucine zipper has been attached to the extracellular portion of CD23 just after the transmembrane region. The transmembrane and cytoplasmic domains are deleted in this

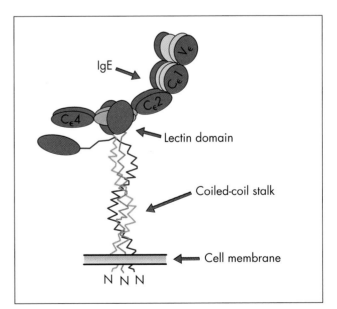

FIGURE 4-5.

CD23 binds IgE as a trimer. This model shows CD23 resulting from the coiled-coil interaction within the stalk region. This interaction frees the lectin heads to interact with IgE. It is hypothesized that two lectin heads can bind an IgE molecule, leaving the third lectin head to interact with another CD23 molecule, cross-linking a second IgE molecule. (*Adapted from* Dierkes et al. [91] and Beavil et al., unpublished data; with permission.)

chimera [94]. This soluble molecule efficiently inhibits IgE binding to the FcεRI, presumably because the increased avidity that is seen for the oligomeric CD23 results in efficient competition even for the FcεRI [95,96]. A schematic of this molecule is shown in Figure 4-6. The above data, taken together, implicate oligomerization in mediating a strong interaction with IgE.

Function of CD23—membrane CD23

CD23 has several potential functions that are related to B-cell proliferation and differentiation, regulation of IgE production, antigen presentation, and cell adhesion. Other reviews should be consulted for discussion of the functions of soluble CD23 [4,5]. Because CD23 was initially discovered as a receptor for IgE, many functional studies were performed to determine its role in IgE regulation. Addition of anti-CD23 monoclonal antibodies to mononuclear cells from either tonsils or peripheral blood cells results in the inhibition of IL-4–induced IgE secretion; the ability of anti-CD23 monoclonal antibodies to inhibit IgE secretion was restricted to those that are identical or close to the IgE binding site on CD23, thus indicating that anti-CD23 monoclonal antibodies have their effect through either steric hindrance or by binding to the same site [97]. In in vivo studies, injection of polyclonal antibodies specific to the lectin homology region of CD23 inhibits IgE synthesis

in a rat model [98]. Recent studies have demonstrated that transgenic mice that overexpress CD23 have a drastic decrease in IgE production to both antigen and parasite infections [99] and this inhibition occurs subsequent to isotype switching because germline-M transcripts were not affected [100•]. In addition, culture of B cells in vitro with cells overexpressing CD23 also resulted in an inhibition of IgE production [100•]; these findings have renewed interest in the use of CD23 as a controlling agent for type I allergy [101]. Data with CD23 knockout animals has been more controversial. In one study, an enhancement of IgE production was reported [102], but this was not supported by other studies [103,104].

When IgE is bound to antigen and CD23, CD23 mediates endocytosis of the antigen-IgE complex and causes an increase in an antigen-specific IgE production [105]; this phenomena is not seen in CD23 knockout animals [104]. Antigen-targeting through CD23 has also been shown to greatly enhance antigen processing and presentation in both the human and the mouse systems [104–107]. This IgE- and CD23-mediated antigen presentation is considered to increase allergen presentation to specific T cells and exacerbate allergy in atopic patients. In addition to endocytosis, CD23 on the monocyte/macrophage can mediate phagocytosis and IgE-dependent cytotoxicity. This function was observed by the killing of IgE-coated schistosomes by eosinophils, macrophages, and platelets. IgE depletion inhibited this killing function, whereas addition of IgE antischistosome antibody increased the killing function. The phagocytic aspect of CD23 is more evident with the CD23b isoform [108]. Additional investigation of CD23's role in monocyte function revealed that ligation of CD23 with IgE–anti-IgE complexes caused monocytes to produce nitric oxide and also enabled monocytes to kill tumor cells and cells infected with *Leishmania* [109,110].

CONCLUSIONS

Progress in this area has continued to be rapid. The recent exciting developments using humanized anti-IgE with FcεRI shows promise in the clinical arena. Development of a chimeric CD23 that blocks binding of IgE to the FcεRI is another promising area for control of IgE-mediated allergic disease. Characterization and isolation of the FcεRI and FcεRII in large amounts will potentially allow crystallization of the receptors or receptor-IgE complexes. This information will ultimately pave the way for more sophisticated inhibitor design. Clearly, much work remains to be done, but as we look forward to the 21st century, the goal of a general control of allergic disease appears ever more attainable.

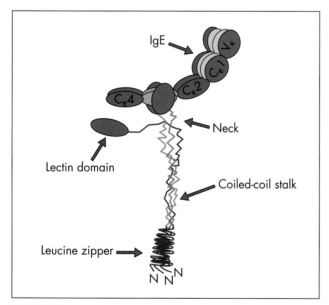

FIGURE 4-6.
Model for stable soluble CD23. The addition of an isoleucine zipper motif to the amino terminus of the extracellular region of CD23 results in the formation of a stable trimer that interacts with IgE in a manner similar to membrane CD23. The trimeric isoleucine zipper presumably stabilizes the native α-helical coiled-coil stalk in a manner similar to the cell membrane with intact CD23 [95]. (*Adapted from* Kelly *et al.* [96]; with permission.)

REFERENCES AND RECOMMENDED READING

Recently published papers of particular interest have been highlighted as:

- • Of interest
- •• Of outstanding interest

1. Sutton BJ, Gould HJ: The human IgE network. *Nature* 1993, 366:421–428.

2. Hulett MD, Hogarth PM: Molecular basis of Fc receptor function. *Adv Immunol* 1994, 57:1–128.

3. Adamczewski M, Kinet J-P: The high-affinity receptor for immunoglobulin E. *Chem Immunol* 1994, 59:173–190.

4. Conrad DH: FcεRI, e-BP and FcεRII: structure and involvement in allergic disease. In *Immunopharmacology of Allergic Diseases*. Edited by Townley RG, Agrawal DK. New York: Marcel Dekker; 1996; 79–98.

5. Delespesse GM, Sarfati CY, Wu S, et al.: The low-affinity receptor for IgE. *Immunol Rev* 1992, 125:77–97.

6. Prausnitz D, Kustner H: Studien über die Überempfindlichkeit. *Zentrabl Bakteriol [A]* 1921, 86:160–175.

7. Ravetch JV, Kinet J-P: Fc receptors. *Annu Rev Immunol* 1990, 9:457–492.

8. Rosenwasser LJ, Borish L: Genetics of atopy and asthma: the rationale behind promoter-based candidate gene studies (IL-4 and IL-10). *Am J Respir Crit Care Med* 1997, 156:S152–S155.

9. Duschl A: An antagonistic mutant of interleukin-4 fails to recruit γ into the receptor complex. Characterization by specific crosslinking. *Eur J Biochem* 1995, 228:305–310.

10.• Kaplan MH, Schindler U, Smiley ST, Grusby MJ: STAT6 is required for mediating responses to IL-4 and for development of T_H2 cells. *Immunity* 1996, 4:313–319.
This source demonstrates the crucial necessity of STAT6 for IgE production.

11.• Shimoda K, van Deursen J, Sangster MY, et al.: Lack of IL-4-induced T_H2 response and IgE class switching in mice with disrupted STAT6 gene. *Nature* 1996, 380:630–633.
Another demonstration of the crucial necessity of STAT6 for IgE production.

12.•• Ryan JJ, McReynolds LJ, Keegan A, et al.: Growth and gene expression are predominantly controlled by distinct regions of the human IL-4 receptor. *Immunity* 1996, 4:123–132.
This study discusses dissection of the majority of tyrosine residues in the cytoplasmic domain of the IL-4 receptor and demonstrates their function thereof.

13. Delphin S, Stavnezer J: Characterization of an interleukin 4 (IL-4) responsive region in the immunoglobulin heavy chain germline ε promoter: regulation by NF–IL-4, a C/EBP family member and NF-kappaB/p50. *J Exp Med* 1995, 181:181–192.

14. Tinnell SB, Jacobs-Helber SM, Sterneck E, et al.: STAT6, NF-κβ and C/EBPb in CD23 expression: STAT6 enhances CD40 induced expression, but is not required for CD40/IL-4 induced superinduction. *Int Immunol* 1998: in press.

15. Keegan A, Nelms K, Paul WE:. The IL-4 receptor-signaling mechanisms. *Adv Exp Med Biol* 1994, 365:211–215.

16. Paul WE: Interleukin-4: a prototypic immunoregulatory lymphokine. *Leuk Lymphoma* 1991, 77:1859–1870.

17. Kondo M, Takeshita T, Ishii N, et al.: Sharing of the interleukin-2 (IL-2) receptor gamma chain between receptors for IL-2 and IL-4. *Science* 1993, 262:1874–1877.

18. Russell SM, Keegan AD, Harada N, et al.: Interleukin-2 receptor gamma chain: a functional component of the interleukin-4 receptor. *Science* 1993, 262:1880–1883.

19. Keegan AD, Ryan JJ, Paul WE: IL-4 regulates growth and differentiation by distinct mechanisms. *Immunologist* 1996, 4:194–198.

20. Ihle JN: Signaling by the cytokine receptor family in normal and transformed hematopoietic cells. *Adv Cancer Res* 1996, 68:24–61.

21. Witthuhn BA, Silvennoinen O, Miura O, et al.: Involvement of the JAK-3 Janus kinase in signalling by interleukins 2 and 4 in lymphoid and myeloid cells. *Nature* 1994, 370:153–157.

22. Keegan AD, Nelms K, White M, et al.: An IL-4 receptor region containing an insulin receptor motif is important for IL-4–mediated IRS-1 phosphorylation and cell growth. *Cell* 1994, 76:811–820.

23. Pernis AB, Witthuhn B, Keegan AD, et al.: Interleukin 4 signals through two related pathways. *Proc Natl Acad Sci USA* 1995, 92:7971–7975.

24. Quelle FW, Shimoda K, Thierfelder W, et al.: Cloning of murine STAT6 and human STAT6, STAT proteins that are tyrosine phosphorylated in responses to IL-4 and IL-3 but are not required for mitogenesis. *Mol Cell Biol* 1995, 15:3336–3343.

25. Malabarba MG, Kirken RA, Rui H, et al.: Activation of JAK3, but not JAK1, is critical to interleukin-4 (IL4)–stimulated proliferation and requires a membrane-proximal region of IL4 receptor α. *J Biol Chem* 1995, 270:9630–9637.

26. Ihle JN, Kerr IM: JAKs and STATs in signaling by the cytokine receptor superfamily. *Trends Genet* 1995, 11:69–74.

27. Hou J, Schindler U, Henzel WJ, et al.: An interleukin-4–induced transcription factor: IL-4. *Stat Science* 1994, 265:1701–1706.

28. Schindler C, Kashleva H, Pernis A, et al.: STF–IL-4: a novel IL-4-induced signal transducing factor. *EMBO J* 1994, 13:1350–1356.

29. Seidel HM, Milocco LH, Lamb P, et al.: Spacing of palindromic half sites as a determinant of selective STAT (signal transducers and activators of transcription) DNA binding and transcriptional activity. *Proc Natl Acad Sci USA* 1995, 92:3041–3045.

30. Takeda K, Tanaka T, Shi W, et al.: Essential role of STAT6 in IL-4 signaling. *Nature* 1996, 380:627–630.

31. Punnonen J, Aversa G, Cocks BG, et al.: Interleukin 13 induces interleukin 4-independent IgG4 and IgE synthesis and CD23 expression by human B cells. *Proc Natl Acad Sci USA* 1993, 90:3730–3734.

32. Murata T, Obiri NI, Debinski W, and Puri RK: Structure of IL-13 receptor: analysis of subunit composition in cancer and immune cells. *Biochem Biophys Res Communi* 1997, 238:90–94.

33. Van Kooten C, Banchereau J: Functional role of CD40 and its ligand. *Int Arch Allergy Immunol* 1997, 113:393–399.

34.• Van Kooten C, Banchereau J: CD40-CD40 ligand: a multifunctional receptor-ligand pair. *Adv Immunol* 1996, 61:1–77.
This is a good review of the important CD40-CD40 system.

35. Francis DA, Karras JG, Ke XY, et al.: Induction of the transcription factors NF-kappa B, AP-1 and NF-AT during B cell stimulation through the CD40 receptor. *Int Immunol* 1995, 7:151–161.

36. Berberich I, Shu G, Siebelt F, et al.: Cross-linking CD40 on B cells preferentially induces stress-activated protein kinases rather than mitogen-activated protein kinases. *EMBO J* 1996, 15:92–101.

37.• Hanissian SH, Geha RS: JAK3 is associated with CD40 and is critical for CD40 induction of gene expression in B cells. *Immunity* 1997, 6:379–387.
This is a demonstration of the importance of JAK3 in allergy and other CD40-mediated actions.

37. Mohapatra SS, Mohapatra S, Yang M, *et al.*: Molecular basis of cross-reactivity among allergen-specific human T cells: T cell receptor gene usage and epitope structure. *Immunology* 1994, 81:15.

38. Sparholt SH, Larsen JN, Ipsen H, *et al.*: Cross-reactivity and T cell epitope specificity of Bet v 1-specific T cells suggest the involvement of multiple isoallergens in sensitization to birch pollen. *Clin Exp Allergy* 1997, 27:932–941.

39. King TP, Lu G: Hornet venom allergen antigen 5, Dol m 5: its T cell epitopes in mice and its antigenic crossreactivity with a mammalian testis protein. *J Allergy Clin immunol* 1997, 99:630–639.

40. Olsen E, Mohapatra SS: Recombinant allergens and diagnosis of specific allergies. *Ann Allergy* 1994, 72:499

41. Valenta R, Vrtala S, Ebner C, *et al.*: Diagnosis of grass pollen allergy with recombinant timothy grass pollen allergens. *Int Arch Allergy Immunol* 1992, 97:287.

42. Mohapatra SS: Recombinant allergens and allergen standardization. *J Allergy Clin Immunol* 1992, 89:921.

43. Cao Y, Luo Z, Yang M, *et al.*: Vaccination with a multi-epitopic recombinant allergen (MERA) vaccine induces specific immune deviation via T cell anergy. *Immunology* 1997, 90:46.

44. Barres MP, Einarsson R, Bjorksten B: Serum levels of interleukin-4, soluble CD23, and IFN-α in relation to the development of allergic disease during the first 18 months of life. *Clin Exp Allergy* 1995, 25:543.

45. Holt PG: A potential vaccine strategy for asthma and allied atopic diseases during early childhood. *Lancet* 1994, 344:456.

46.•• Mohapatra SS: An integrated approach to immune deviation and prevention of allergies and asthma. *Allergy Clin Immunol Int* 1996, 8:164.
This is an excellent review on the potential of a prophylactic allergy vaccine.

47. Des Roches, Paradis L, Menardo J-L, *et al.*: Immunotherapy with a standardized *D. pteronyssnus* extract: specific therapy prevents the onset of new sensitizations in children. *J Allergy Clin Immunol* 1997, 99:450–453.

48. Jacobsen L, Dreborg S, Moller C, *et al.*: Immunotherapy as preventive allergy treatment (PAT). *J Allergy Clin Immunol* 1996, 97:232.

49. Vrtala S, Grote M, Ferreira F, *et al.*: Humoral immune responses to recombinant tree pollen allergens (Bet v 1 and Bet v 2) in mice: construction of a live oral allergy vaccine. *Int Arch Allergy Immunol* 1995, 107:290.

50. Kumar M, Behera A, Matsuse H, *et al.*: Development of a BCG+ based allergen vaccine. *J Allergy Clin Immunol* 1998, 101:333.

51.•• Raz E, Tighe H, Sato Y, *et al.*: Inhibition of specific IgE antibody formation by naked plasmid DNA immunization. *Proc Natl Acad Sci USA* 1996, 93:5141.
This is an excellent article that presents evidence for naked DNA plasmids expressing allergens as potential immunotherapeutic agent.

52.•• Hsu C-H, Chua K-Y, Tao M-H, *et al.*: Immunoprophylaxis of allergen induced immunoglobulin E synthesis and airway hyperresponsiveness in vivo by genetic immunization. *Nature Med* 1996, 2:540.
This is an excellent article that presents evidence for naked DNA plasmids expressing allergens as potential ingredients of a prophylactic vaccine against allergies.

53. Mohapatra SS, Cao Y, Ni H, *et al.*: In pursuit of "Holy Grail": recombinant allergens as catalysts for the allergen specific immunotherapy. *Allergy* 1995, 50(suppl):37–44.

54. Arora N, Gangal SV: Efficacy of liposome entrapped allergen in down-regulation of IgE response in mice. *Clin Exp Allergy* 1992, 22:35.

55. Wheeler AW, Henderson DC, Youlten LJ, *et al.*: Immunogenicity of in guine pig and tolerance in grass pollen sensitive volunteers of enteric coated grass pollen allergens. *Int Arch Allergy Immunol* 1987, 83:354.

56. Maasch HJ, Marsh DG: Standardized extracts modified allergens-allergoids. *Clin Rev Allergy* 1987, 5:89.

57. Wheeler AW, Whittall N, Cook RM, *et al.*: T cell reactivity of conjugates of N-formyl-methionyl-lencyl-phenylalanine and rye grass pollen allergens. *Int Arch Allergy Immunol* 84:69, 1987.

58. Afonso LCC, Scharton TM, Vieira LQ, *et al.*: The adjuvant effect of IL-12 in a vaccine against Leishmania major. *Science* 1994, 263:235.

59.•• Parronchi P, Mohapatra S, Manett R, *et al.*: Modulation by IFN-α of cytokine profile and epitope specificity of allergen-specific T cells. *Eur J Immunology* 1996, 26:697.
This report illustrates the potential of IFN-α as an agent for immune deviation in an in-vitro model.

60.•• Kim TS, De Kryff RH, Rupper R, *et al.*: An ovalbumin-Il-12 fusion protein is more effective than ovalbumin plus free recombinant IL-12 in inducing a helper T cell type 1 dominated immune response and inhibiting antigen-specific IgE production. *J Immunol* 1997, 158:4137–4144.
This is an excellent article showing the potential use of IL-12 as an adjuvant in allergen specific therapy.

61. Mohapatra SS: IL-12 possibilities. *Science* 1995, 269:1499.

62. Briner T, Kuo M-C, Keating KM, *et al.*: Periperal T cell tolerance induced in naive and primed mice by subcutaneous injection of peptides from the major cat AL Fel d I. *Proc Natl Acad Sci USA* 1993, 90:7608.

63. Rogers BL, Bond JF, Craig SJ, *et al.*: Potential therapeutic recombinant proteins comprised of peptides containing recombined T cell epitopes. *Mol Immunol* 1994, 31:955.

64. Hoyne GF, O'Hehir RE, Wraith DC, *et al.*: Inhibition of T cell and antibody responses to house dust mite allergens by inhalations of the dominant T cell epitopes in naive and sensitized mice. *J Exp Med* 1993, 178:1783.

65. Nicodemus C, Phillip G, Jones N, *et al.*: Integrated clinical experience with tolerogenic peptides. *Int Arch Allergy Immunol* 1997, 113:326–328.

66. Van Neerven RJ, Ebner C, Yssel H, *et al.*: T cell responses to allergens. *Immunol Today* 1996, 17:526–532.

67. Litwin A, Pesce AJ, Fischer T, *et al.*: Regulation of the human immune responses to ragweed pollen by immunotherapy: a control trial comparing the effect of immunosuppressive peptidic fragments of short ragweed with standard treatment. *Clin Exp Allergy* 1991, 21:457.

68. Michael JG, Litwin A, Hassert V, *et al.*: Modulation of the immune response to ragweed allergens by peptidic fragments. *Clin Exp Allergy* 1990, 20:669.

69. Muller UR, Dudler T, Schneider T, *et al.*: Type-1 skin reactivity to native and recombinant phospholipase A_2 from honeybee venom is similiar *J Allergy Clin Immunol* 1995, 96:395–402.

70. Adkis CA, Adkis M, Blesken T, *et al.*: Epitope-specific T cell tolerance to phospholipase A_2 in bee venom immunotherapy and recovery by Il-2 and IL-15 in vitro. *J Clin Invest* 1996, 98:1676–1683.

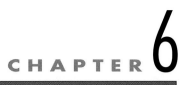

CHAPTER 6

Pathophysiology of Asthma

Martha V. White

Asthma is a chronic inflammatory disease of the airways affecting 14 to 15 million persons in the United States alone. The disease, manifest as variable airflow obstruction, occurs because of mucous plugging, airway edema, inflammation, and smooth muscle contraction, and is responsive to bronchodilators and corticosteroids. The symptoms of coughing, wheezing, shortness of breath, and chest tightness may be triggered by various stimuli, including allergen exposure, respiratory tract infections, exercise, emotional stress, cold air, strong smells, aspirin, fatigue, and others. Asthma frequently begins during the first decade in atopic individuals; however, it may present at any time during life, particularly in nonatopic persons. Disease severity, which is highly variable, ranges from a single mild episode to daily debilitating dyspnea and wheeze.

INHERITANCE OF ASTHMA

Although the tendency to develop asthma seems to be hereditary, the heterogeneous phenotypic expression suggests a complex interaction between multiple genetic factors and environmental exposure. Evidence for an at least partially genetic etiology includes the higher concordance of asthma in monozygotic twins compared with dizygotic twins. Linkage with the high-affinity IgE receptor on chromosome 11q13 has been found for asthma, atopy, and total serum IgE. Asthma has also been linked with the genes for interleukin (IL)-3, IL-4, IL-5, IL-9, IL-13, and granulocyte-macrophage colony-stimulating factor (GM-CSF) on chromosome 5q31; the β2-adrenergic receptor gene on chromosome 5q32; the human leukocyte antigen (HLA) complex on chromosome 6p; and numerous other pro-inflammatory genes on chromosomes 6p21 to 23, 12q, 13q, and 14q [1••].

The importance of environmental factors in asthma expression is apparent from studies revealing deficient peripheral mononuclear cell production of interferon (IFN)-γ in infants who later develop asthma [2,3]. This defect may lead to the up-regulation of cytokines associated with the T-helper 2 (T$_H$2) response. Indeed, a T$_H$2-mediated inflammatory response develops early, with increased mast cell and eosinophil concentrations seen in virally infected asthmatic children as young as 5 years of age compared with a primarily neutrophilic response in children who wheeze only when they are afflicted with virus infections. It has been suggested that environmental exposures during the first 3 years of life are particularly important in providing the stimulus for local sensitization of the airways and for the development of the asthma phenotype. Thus, exposure to measles and other frequent viral pathogens during the first year of life may decrease the risk of asthma by production of large amounts of IL-12, IL-18, and IFN-γ, leading to up-regulation of the T_H1 response [4]. This would partially explain the association between asthma and socioeconomic status, and also the lower incidence of asthma in rural, compared with urban, areas. In contrast, infection with respiratory syncytial virus early in life augments the T_H2 phenotype in susceptible individuals and is positively associated with asthma.

GROSS PATHOLOGY

Pathologic features of asthma leading to airways obstruction include smooth muscle contraction, airway edema, increased mucous secretion, and inflammation. Postmortem studies have revealed large and small airway plugs containing mucous, cellular debris, serum proteins, and inflammatory cells. An inflammatory infiltrate consisting of eosinophils, mast cells, lymphocytes, macrophages, and plasma cells is seen in association with vasodilation and evidence of microvascular leakage, although neutrophils may predominate in patients who die of sudden asphyxic asthma.

Biopsy studies of patients with mild to moderate asthma show similar inflammatory changes and airway epithelial desquamation. The airways of these patients contain increased numbers of macrophages and T lymphocytes, whereas the lamina propria holds increased numbers of eosinophils, lymphocytes, and mast cells [5]. Elevated numbers of resting as well as degranulating mucosal mast cells are found in airway epithelia of patients with mild asthma. Following subsegmental antigen challenge, bronchial biopsy specimens reveal increased numbers of eosinophils, mast cells, lymphocytes, and neutrophils in the airway mucosa. The adhesion molecules, intercellular adhesion molecule type 1 (ICAM-1) and E-selectin, are up-regulated in submucosal and epithelial leukocytes. Elevation in the numbers of these inflammatory cells and adhesion molecules correlate positively with asthma severity and bronchial hyper-responsiveness [6•].

ASTHMATIC INFLAMMATION

In contrast to infectious inflammation, asthmatic inflammation is characterized by elaboration of cytokines that promote IgE production as well as eosinophil recruitment and activation. The process is orchestrated through a complex series of cell-to-cell interactions beginning with the antigen-presenting dendritic cell. These cells, which are abundant in the airway epithelium and submucosa, differentiate in the asthmatic lung under the influence of GM-CSF and stem-cell factor (SCF) to express major his-

tocompatibility complex (MHC) class II with gradual loss of their ability to secrete IL-12. In the presence of IL-4 and tumor necrosis factor (TNF)-α, the high- and low-affinity receptors for IgE are expressed on the dendritic cell's surface, increasing its ability to capture, process, and present antigen. After processing antigen, dendritic cells migrate to local lymph nodes where they present the antigen, in association with their MHC II molecules, to the T-cell receptor [7–9]. In genetically susceptible individuals, antigen presentation by IL-12–deficient dendritic cells leads to the transformation of naive (T_H0) cells into committed T_H2-like cells with the capacity to secrete a series of cytokines encoded on chromosome 5q31, known as the IL-4 gene cluster (IL-3, IL-4, IL-5, IL-9, IL-13, GM-CSF) [10]. These cytokines up-regulate IgE production as well as mast cell, basophil, and eosinophil function. Infectious inflammation leads to an alternative pathway of T cell maturation in which microorganisms, presented to T cells by IL-12–producing dendritic cells, cause production of T_H1 cells capable of secreting IL-2, IFN-γ, and TNF-β. These two T-cell populations are under reciprocal control; IL-12 drives a T_H1 response while IL-4 drives the T_H2 response. T_H1 cells are inhibited by T_H2-derived IL-10, whereas T_H2 cells are inhibited by IFNs [11]. Further direction to T-cell differentiation is supplied by dendritic cell B7.1 and B7.2 molecules interacting with CD28 on T cells. If either molecule interacts with cytotoxic lymphocyte antigen 4 (CTLA-4) on T cells, apoptosis, rather than differentiation, is initiated [7, 11]. The B7.2 molecules are also expressed on B cells, and expression, regulated by T_H2-type cytokines, is increased in allergic asthmatics after antigen exposure [12]. Asthma is characterized by a disproportionate maturation of T lymphocytes along the T_H2 lineage.

CELLS MEDIATING ASTHMATIC INFLAMMATION

The cells that primarily mediate asthmatic inflammation are eosinophils and mast cells. Both cells derive from CD34-bearing bone marrow precursors. These precursors differentiate into mast cells under the influence of epithelial and mesenchymal-cell–derived SCF, and further develop into mucosal mast cells in the presence of T-cell–derived IL-4 and IL-6 [13,14]. IL-3 induces the CD34+ precursors to commit toward eosinophil development, and further maturation and priming are stimulated by IL-5 and GM-CSF [15]. Mast cells, eosinophils, and basophils contain on their cell surfaces both the high-affinity (FcϵRI) and the low-affinity (FcϵRII) receptors for the C3 domain of IgE. Both IgE production by B cells and expression of the IgE receptor are up-regulated by IL-4 and its homologue IL-13 [16]. All three inflammatory cells are abundant in the asthmatic airway submucosa, although mucosal type mast cells are also prominent in the epithelium. Cross-linking of the IgE receptor provides the stimulus for a tyrosine kinase– and protein kinase C–mediated cascade leading to noncytotoxic degranulation and production of leukotrienes and the cytokines IL-4, IL-5, IL-6, IL-8, IL-13, GM-CSF, and TNF-α [17]. Mast cell degranulation leads to rapid release of histamine, prostaglandin D_2, and leukotriene (LT) D_4, which mediate increased microvascular permeability, airway smooth muscle contraction, and initiation of neutrophil and eosinophil recruitment.

INFLAMMATORY CELL RECRUITMENT

Inflammatory cell recruitment is initiated by histamine and LTD_4, which promote transport of P selectin from Weibel-Palade bodies located in the endothelial cell cytoplasm to the endothelial cell surface. The adhesion molecule, P selectin, interacts with sialyl-Lewis lectins and similar types on cell surfaces of leukocytes, initiating rolling of the cells along the endothelium [18]. Over the next 2 to 3 hours, TNF-α released from mast cells induces up-regulation of more specific cell adhesion molecules on the endothelium, including E selectin, intercellular adhesion molecule 1 (ICAM-1), and vascular cell adhesion molecule 1 (VCAM-1), which mediate firm leukocyte adhesion, cell priming, and eventual transendothelial migration of leukocytes [19]. VCAM-1 is particularly important in asthma, selectively binding very late antigen 4 (VLA-4), expressed on eosinophils, basophils, and T cells, but not neutrophils, thus mediating selective recruitment of eosinophils, basophils, and T cells characteristic of asthmatic inflammation. VCAM-1 is under dual regulation by TNF-α and combined IL-4/IL-13 (Table 6-1) [20].

Directed migration of leukocytes through the endothelial wall toward the site of asthmatic inflammation is regulated by various chemoattractant cytokines: monocytes chemotactic protein 3 (MCP3); eotaxin; reg-

ulated upon activation, normal T-cell expressed and secreted (RANTES); and IL-8. Eosinophil migration, priming, and prolonged survival are specifically regulated by IL-5 and GM-CSF [21]. These two groups of cytokines are secreted by mast cells and T cells, as well as certain structural components of the airway, including epithelial cells, endothelial cells, smooth muscle cells, and fibroblasts. Thus, initiation and propagation of asthmatic inflammation require complex interactions between resident and recruited inflammatory cells as well as structural cells.

AIRWAY REMODELING

In chronic, inadequately treated asthma, irreversible airway remodeling is observed, with hypertrophy and increased microvascularization of smooth muscle, increased numbers of goblet cells, and subepithelial collagen deposition. Bronchial epithelium transforms into a repair phenotype, expressing cytokines, inducible nitric oxide synthetase, cyclo-oxygenase 2, and phospholipase A_2. Mast cell and eosinophil-mediated tissue injury causes epithelial disruption with desquamation into the airway lumen, thus leading to loss of barrier function [22, 23]. In addition to the arginine-rich eosinophil granule proteins mediating epithelial injury, metalloendoproteases (MMP) from eosinophils (MMP-9), mast cells (MMP-3 and MMP-9), and from the epithelium (MMP-2 and MMP-9) disrupt epithelial cell adhesion molecules responsible for the integrity of the epithelium [24]. Epithelial disruption, coupled with secretion of growth factors for epithelial cells, fibroblasts, and smooth muscle cells, results in tissue regeneration and remodeling and deposition of collagen type III and V fibers [25]. Smooth muscle hypertrophy and microvascular proliferation further contribute to structural alterations and asthma chronicity [26]. Allergen-independent T-cell expansion of both CD4+ and CD8+ cells occurs. In the presence of increased nitric oxide, which inhibits T_H1 cells and their elaboration of IFN-γ [27], and increased IL-4, which enhances T_H2 differentiation, both of these cell types secrete the T_H2 profile of cytokines encoded on the IL-4 gene cluster [28]. Upregulation of viral receptors, such as ICAM-1, may lead to increased susceptibility to viral infections, which is a prominent trigger of asthma exacerbations [29,30].

CLINICAL CORRELATIVES

Although the inflammatory response observed in asthma supports an allergic etiology, similar inflammatory pathology is seen in nonatopic, or intrinsic, asthma. Indeed, asthma severity correlates with the degree of airway inflammation. Thus, in poorly controlled atopic as well as nonatopic asthmatics, increased bronchial mucosal expression of IL-4 and IL-5 mRNA is observed.

Table 6-1. ASTHMATIC INFLAMMATION: STEPS IN CELL RECRUITMENT

Histamine and LTD_4 cause transportation of P selectin to endothelium

P selectin interacts with Sialyl-Lewis and other lectins on leukocytes, thus initiating rolling

TNF-α up-regulates endothelial expression of E-selectin, ICAM-1, and VCAM-1, allowing for firm adhesion, cell priming, and transendothelial migration

VCAM-1 interacts with VLA-4 on eosinophils, basophils, and T cells, and is regulated by IL-4, IL-13, and TNF-α

ICAM—intercellular adhesion molecule; IL—interleukin; LTD— leukotriene D; TNF—tumor necrosis factor; VCAM—vascular cellular adhesion molecule; VLA—vascular lymphocyte antigen.

Approximately 70% of the mRNA+ cells are CD3+ T cells (75% CD4+, 25% CD8+), whereas the remaining cells expressing increased message for IL-4 and IL-5 are mast cells and eosinophils. In contrast, immunohisto-chemical analysis reveals most cells staining positively for the IL-4 and IL-5 gene product to be mast cells and eosinophils, probably because T cells do not possess granules containing preformed cytokines [31]. Available data suggest that increased expression of the IL-4 gene cluster is not limited to the airways. For example, increased expression of IL-3, IL-4, IL-5, and GM-CSF mRNA and gene product have been found in peripheral blood mononuclear cells of asthmatics [32–35]. The intestinal mucosa has also been observed to have increased expression of mRNA for IL-3, IL-5, and GM-CSF in asthmatics and atopic controls, but not in nonatopic controls or patients with chronic obstructive pulmonary disease (COPD), suggesting that the increased expression of the IL-4 gene cluster predisposes to asthma, rather than the asthma, which is phenotypi-cally similar to COPD, predisposing to overexpression of the IL-4 gene cluster [36].

Medical therapy of asthma needs to include both anti-inflammatory agents and bronchodilators to relieve the symptoms of asthma. Under use of anti-inflammatory medications is associated with irreversible tissue damage and increased risk of asthma death. Thus, the *Guidelines for the Diagnosis and Management of Asthma*, published by the National Institutes of Health's National Heart, Lung, and Blood Institute [37••], recommend early ther-apy with anti-inflammatory agents as primary treatment for all but the mildest cases of asthma.

The most effective anti-inflammatory agents are the corticosteroids (Table 6-2), which are available both for oral and inhaled use. Treatment with these agents results in decreased airway reactivity and symptomatic improve-ment correlating with reductions in markers of inflam-mation. Following corticosteroid treatment, bronchial

mucosal anti-inflammatory effects include a decrease in IL-4 and IL-5 mRNA expressing cells, CD3+ T cells, mucosal mast cells, and activated (EG2+) eosinophils. The number of cells expressing mRNA for IFN-γ increas-es, suggesting a shift towards the T_H1 phenotype [38]. Concomitantly, mRNA for IL-5, IL-3, and GM-CSF decreases in circulating CD4+ T cells [32,33], and serum eosinophilic cationic protein falls, suggesting a decrease in eosinophil activation [34]. The decrease in activated eosinophils seems to be cytokine rather than migration related, because the corticosteroid, dexamethasone, has no effect on expression of adhesion molecules [39].

Inhaled corticosteroids also reduce some of the struc-tural changes associated with airway remodeling. For instance, asthmatic patients treated with inhaled corti-costeroids had less collagen deposition beneath the air-way basement membrane than placebo-treated controls [40,41]. Likewise, treatment with the inhaled corticos-teroid budesonide resulted in reduced numbers of gob-let cells in the airways [42] as well as a reduction in exhaled nitric oxide [43]. The reduction in nitric oxide exhalation can be observed before onset of clinical effects of inhaled corticosteroids [44], suggesting that reduction in airway remodeling may contribute to the clinical improvement observed with inhaled corticos-teroids. The effects of glucocorticosteroid inhalation on reversal of airway function abnormalities associated with existing airway remodeling are short lived, lasting only a week after discontinuation of the inhaled corti-costeroids [45,46]. Inhaled corticosteroids are more effective in preventing than reversing airway remodel-ing. Thus, maximal achievable forced expiratory vol-ume in 1 second (FEV_1) is obtained when inhaled corti-costeroids are given within the first 2 years after asthma diagnosis in children, with lesser results obtained if treatment is delayed for 5 or more years postdiagnosis [47]. Maximal results in adults are attained if inhaled corticosteroid treatment is begun at the time of diagno-

---

Table 6-2. ANTI-INFLAMMATORY EFFECTS OF CORTICOSTEROIDS

Decreased airway reactivity

Decreases in IL-5, IL-3, and GM-CSF mRNA in circulating CD4+ T cells as well as in serum ECP

Bronchial effects: Increase in IFN-γ mRNA+ cells, decrease in IL-4 and IL-5 mRNA+ cells, CD3+ cells, mucosal mast cells, and activated eosinophils

No effect on adhesion molecules

ECP—eosinophil cationic protein; GM-CSF—granulocyte-macrophage colony-stimulating factor; IFN—interferon; IL—interleukin.

Table 6-3. CELLULAR EFFECTS OF GLUCOCORTICOIDS

Inflammatory cells
  Eosinophil apoptosis (T-cell mediated)
  Decreased T-cell cytokines
  Decreased numbers of mast cells and dendritic cells
  Decreased macrophage cytokines
Structural cells
  Decreased cytokines and other epithelial cell mediators
  Decreased endothelial cell leakage
  Increased B_2 receptors on airway smooth muscle
  Decreased mucus-gland secretion of mucus

sis, but the results are reduced if treatment is delayed as little as 2 years [48]. These data suggest that airway remodeling, with irreversible effects on lung function, begins early in the course of asthma.

Although corticosteroids are the most effective anti-inflammatory agents used in the treatment of asthma, their exact mechanism of action is uncertain. Inhaled corticosteroids, because of their lipophilic properties, are able to rapidly enter target cells of the epithelium, endothelium, and other cells where they bind to cytosolic glucocorticoid receptors [49]. The glucocorticoid-receptor complex then translocates to the nucleus, where the glucocorticoid receptor binds to DNA at specific consensus sites, termed *glucocorticoid response elements* on the upstream promoter sequence of steroid-responsive genes. This results in altered transcription of genes involved in asthmatic inflammation [50,51]. Another mechanism whereby glucocorticoids may influence inflammatory cytokine transcription is by direct binding of the translocated glucocorticoid receptor to the transcription factors, nuclear factor-κB and activator protein-1. These factors, when activated in the nucleus by inflammatory cytokines, regulate gene transcription by binding to response elements on the promoter sequence of genes. Thus, binding of these factors within the nucleus by the glucocorticoid receptor may inhibit cellular effects of inflammatory cytokines (Table 6-3) [51,52].

Allergen exposure has been shown to decrease glucocorticoid receptor-binding affinity and steroid responsiveness of peripheral blood mononuclear cells of atopic asthmatics. This effect is mediated both by IL-2 and IL-4, and is limited to atopic asthmatics because the effect was not observed in atopic nonasthmatics [53]. These findings may help explain the relative resistance to therapy of asthmatic patients constantly bombarded with allergen stimulation and also demonstrates the importance of a comprehensive approach to the treatment of asthma, including environmental control of allergens. Asthma is phenotypically heterogeneous; however, the inflammatory pathology underlying asthma is not only systemic but considerably more homogeneous than the phenotypic expression would suggest. The recent explosion in research into the inflammatory pathogenesis of asthma opens the door to many novel therapies of the future.

REFERENCES AND RECOMMENDED READING

Recently published papers of particular interest have been highlighted as:
•   Of interest
••   Of outstanding interest

1.•• Holgate ST: The cellular and mediator basis of asthma in relation to natural history. *Science* 1997, 350(suppl):5–9.
This is a good review of genetic and inflammatory contributions to asthma pathophysiology. It is located in a special asthma supplement to the *Lancet*.

2.   Warner JA, Miles EA, Jones AC, *et al.*: Is deficiency of interferon gamma production by allergen triggered cord blood T cells a predictor of atopic eczema? *Clin Exp Allergy* 1994, 24:223–230.

3.   Tang MLK, Kemp AS, Thornburn J, Hill DJ: Reduced interferon-gamma and subsequent atopy. *Lancet* 1994, 344:983–985.

4.   Shaheen SO, Asby P, Hall AJ, *et al.*: Measles and atopy in Guinea Bissau. *Lancet* 1996, 347:1792–1796.

5.   Dunhill MS. The pathophysiology of asthma, with special reference to changes in the bronchial mucosa. *J Clin Pathol* 1960, 13:27–33.

6.• Fischer TJ: Allergy and clinical immunology: asthma. In *Allergy Immunology Medical Knowledge Self Assessment Program* 2nd edn. Edited by Condemi JJ, Dykewicz MS. Philadelphia: American College of Physicians; 1997:37–55.
This is a general review of asthma pathophysiology and treatment.

7.   Semper AE, Hartley JA: Dendritic cells in the lung: what is their relevance to asthma? *Clin Exp Allergy* 1996, 26:485–490.

8.   Hartley JA, Semper AE, Holgate ST. In vivo and in vitro expression of FcεR1 in human peripheral blood (PB) *Immunology* 1996, 89(suppl):41.

9.   Igarashi Y, Goldrich MS, Kaliner MA, *et al.*: Quantification of inflammatory cells in the nasal mucosa of allergic rhinitis and normals. *J Allergy Clin Immunol* 1995, 95:716–725.

10. Robinson DS, Hamid Q, Ying S, *et al.*: Predominant T$_H$2-type bronchoalveolar lavage T-lymphocyte population in atopic asthma. *N Engl J Med* 1992, 326:298–304.

11. Drazen JM, Arm JP, Austen KJ: Sorting out the cytokines of asthma. *J Exp Med* 1996, 183:1–5.

12. Hofer MF, Jirapongsananuruk O, Trumble AE, *et al.*: Up-regulation of B7.2 but not B7.1 on B cells from patients with allergic asthma. *J Allergy Clin Immunol* 1998, 101:96–102.

13. Yanagida M, Fukamachi H, Ohgami K, *et al.*: Effects of T helper 2-type cytokines, interleukin-3 (IL-3), IL-4, IL-5 and IL-6 on the survival of cultured human mast cells. *Blood* 1995, 86:3705–3714.

14. Denburg JA: Microenvironmental influences on inflammatory cell differentiation. *Allergy* 1995, 50(suppl):25–28.

15. Abbas AK, Murphy KM, Sher A: Functional diversity of helper T lymphocytes. *Nature* 1996, 383:787–793.

16. Church MK, Levi-Schaffer F: The human mast cell. *J Allergy Clin Immunol* 1997, 997:155–160.

17. Springer TS: Adhesion receptors of the immune system. *Nature* 1990, 346:425–34.

18. Casale TB, Costa JJ Galli SJ: TNF-α is important in human lung allergic reactions. *Am J Respir Cell Mol Biol* 1966, 15:35–44.

19. Abraham WM, Sielczar MW, Ahmed A, *et al.*: α$_4$-Integrins mediate antigen-induced late bronchial responses and prolonged airway hyperresponsiveness in sheep. *J Clin Invest* 1994, 93:776–87.

20. Baggiolini M, Dahinden CA: CC chemokines in allergic inflammation. *Immunol Today* 1994, 15:127–133.

21. Lackie PM, Baker JE, Gunther U, *et al.*: Expression of CD44 isoforms is increased in the airway epithelium of asthmatic subjects. *Am J Respir Cell Mol Biol* 1967, 16:14–22.

22. Raeburn D, Webber SE: Proinflammatory potential of the airway epithelium in bronchial asthma. *Eur Respir J* 1994, 7:266–233.

23. Robinson C: The airway epithelium: the origin and target of inflammatory airways disease and injury. In *Immunopharmacology of the Respiratory System*. Edited by Holgate ST. London: Academic Press; 1995:187–207.

24. Roche WR, Beasley R, Williams JH, *et al.*: Subepithelial fibrosis in the bronchi of asthmatics. *Lancet* 1989, 1:520–523.

25. Holgate ST, Djukanovic R, Howarth PH, *et al.*: The T-cell and the airways fibrotic response in asthma. *Chest* 1993, 103:125S–28S.

26. Stanciu LA, Shute J, Promwong C, *et al.*: Increased levels of IL-4 in CD8+T cells in atopic asthma. *J Allergy Clin Immunol* 1997,100:373–378.

27. Barnes PJ, Liew FY: Nitric oxide and asthmatic inflammation. *Immunology Today* 1995, 16:128–130.

28. Tomassini JE, Graham D, DeWill CM, *et al.*: CDNA cloning reveals that the major group rhinovirus receptor on HeLa cells is intercellular adhesion molecule 1. *Proc Natl Acad Sci USA* 1989, 86:4907–4911.

29. Johnston SL, Pattermore PK, Sanderson G, *et al.*: Community study of the role of viral infections in exacerbations of asthma in school children in the community. *BMJ* 1995, 310:1225–1229.

30. Fraenkel DJ, Bardin PG, Sanderson G, *et al.*: Lower airway inflammatory response during rhinovirus colds in normal and asthmatic subjects. *Am J Respir Crit Care Med* 1995, 151:879–886.

31. Ying S, Humbert M, Barkans J, *et al.*: Expression of IL–4 and IL–5 mRNA and protein product by CD4+ and CD8+ T cells, eosinophils, and mast cells in bronchial biopsies obtained from atopic and nonatopic (intrinsic) asthmatics. *J Immunol* 1997, 158:3539–3544.

32. Doi S, Gemou-Engasaeth V, Kay AB, *et al.*: Polymerase chain reaction quantification of cytokine messenger RNA expression in peripheral blood mononuclear cells of patients with acute exacerbations of asthma: effect of glucocorticoid therapy. *Clin Exp Allergy* 1994, 24:854–867.

33. Corrigan CJ, Hamid Q, North J, *et al.*: Peripheral blood CD4 but not CD8 T-lymphocytes in patients with exacerbation of asthma transcribe and translate messenger RNA encoding cytokines which prolong eosinophil survival in the context of a T_H2-type pattern: effect of glucocorticoid therapy. *Am J Resp Cell Mol Biol* 1995, 12:567–578.

34. Lai CK, Ho AS, Chan CH, *et al.*: Interleukin-5 messenger RNA expression in peripheral blood CD4+ cells in asthma. *J Allergy Clin Immunol* 1996, 97:1320–1328.

35. Till S, Dickason R, Huston D, *et al.*: IL-5 secretion by allergen-stimulated CD4+ T cells in primary culture: relationship to expression of allergic disease. *J Allergy Clin Immunol* 1997, 99:563–569.

36. Wallaert B, Desreumaux P, Copin MC: Immunoreactivity for interleukin 3 and 5 and granulocyte/macrophage colony-stimulating factor of intestinal mucosa in bronchial asthma. *J Exp Med* 1995, 182:1897–1904.

37.•• National Institutes of Health: *Guidelines for the Diagnosis and Management of Asthma*. Bethesda: National Institute of Health publication no. 97-4051. 1997:1–86.
This is an expert panel report outlining pathophysiology and treatment of asthma. It gives state of the art information, and includes patient information hand outs.

38. Bentley AM, Hamid Q, Robinson DS, *et al.*: Prednisolone treatment in asthma: reduction in the numbers of eosinophils, T cells, tryptase-only positive mast cells, and modulation of IL-4, IL-5, and interferon-gamma cytokine gene expression within the bronchial mucosa. *Am J Resp Crit Care Med* 1996, 153:551–556.

39. Hughes JM, Sewell WA, Black JL, *et al.*: Effect of dexamethasone on expression of adhesion molecules on CD4+ lymphocytes. *Am J Physiol* 1996, 271:L79–L84.

40. Trigg CJ, Manolitssas ND, Wang J, *et al.*: Placebo-controlled immunopathologic study of four months of inhaled corticosteroids in asthma. *Am J Respir Crit Care Med* 1994, 150:17–22.

41. Oliveri D, Chetta A, Del Donno A, *et al.*: Effect of short-term treatment with low dose inhaled fluticasone propionate on airway inflammation and remodeling in mild asthma: a placebo-controlled study. *Am J Respir Crit Care Med* 1997, 155:1864–1871.

42. Laitinen L, Laitinen A, Haahtela T: A comparative study of the effects of an inhaled corticosteroid, budesonide, and a β2-agonist, terbutaline, on airway inflammation in newly diagnosed asthma: a randomized double-blind, parallel-group controlled trial. *J Allergy Clin Immunol* 1992, 90:32–42.

43. Kharitonov SA, Yates DH, Barnes PJ: Regular inhaled budesonide decreases nitric oxide concentrations in the exhaled air of asthmatic patients. *Am J Respir Crit Care Med* 1996, 153:454–457.

44. Kharitonov SA, Yates DH, Chung KF, *et al.*: Changes in the dose of inhaled steroid affect exhaled nitric oxide levels in asthmatic patients. *Eur J Respir Dis* 1966, 9:196–201.

45. Vathenen AS, Knox AJ, Wisniewski A, *et al.*: Time course of change in bronchial reactivity with an inhaled corticosteroid in asthma. *Am Rev Respir Dis* 1991, 143:1317–1321.

46. Gershman NH, Wong HH, Liu J, *et al.*: Comparison of high versus low dose fluticasone propionate (FP) on clinical outcomes and markers of inflammation in asthmatic subjects. *Am J Respir Crit Care Med* 1997, 155:A288.

47. Agertoft L, Pedersen S: Effects of long-term treatment with an inhaled corticosteroid on growth and pulmonary function in asthmatic children. *Respir Med* 1994; 88:373–381.

48. Haahtela T, Jarvinen M, Kava T, *et al.*: Effects of reducing or discontinuing inhaled budesonide in patients with mild asthma. *N Engl J Med* 1994, 331:700–705.

49. Adcock IM, Gilbey T, Gelder CM, *et al.*: Glucocorticoid receptor localization in normal human lung and asthmatic lung. *Am J Respir Crit Care Med* 1996, 154:771–782.

50. Barnes PJ: Current issues for establishing inhaled corticosteroids as the antiinflammatory agents of choice in asthma. *J Allergy Clin Immunol* 1998, 10(suppl):427–433.

51. Barnes PJ, Adcock IM: Anti-inflammatory actions of steroids: molecular mechanisms. *Trends Pharmacol Sci* 1993, 14:436–41.

52. Barnes PJ, Adcock IM. Transcription factors in asthma. *Clin Exp Allergy* 1995, 27(suppl):46–49.

53. Nimmagadda SR, Szefler SJ, Spahn JD, *et al.*: Allergen exposure decreases glucocorticoid receptor binding affinity and steroid responsiveness in atopic asthmatics. *Am J Resp Crit Care Med* 1997, 155:87–93.

CHAPTER 7

Anti-leukotriene Agents in the Treatment of Asthma

Noreen R. Henig
William R. Henderson Jr.

Over the last decade, the medical community has changed its thinking about asthma. Once thought to be a disease primarily of airway smooth-muscle dysfunction, asthma is now recognized to be a chronic inflammatory disease of the airways. With this new understanding, our approach to the treatment of asthma has changed. Early institution of anti-inflammatory drugs, *eg*, corticosteroids, has become the mainstay of asthma therapy. Prolonged treatment with corticosteroids, however, has potentially serious complications, making both physicians and their patients uneasy. Thus, there has been considerable effort to develop new anti-inflammatory agents to treat asthma.

Leukotrienes belong to a family of inflammatory mediators known as eicosanoids [1–3]. Leukotrienes and their family members, prostaglandins, thromboxanes, and lipoxins, are derived from the common precursor arachidonic acid. In response to injury, inflammatory cells synthesize eicosanoids de novo rather than releasing them from preformed repositories. Leukotrienes are involved in the pathogenesis of a wide range of inflammatory diseases, including asthma, psoriasis, rheumatoid arthritis, and inflammatory bowel disease. Novel anti-leukotriene agents that block either the synthesis or actions of leukotrienes are now available for clinical use in the treatment of asthma.

LEUKOTRIENE SYNTHESIS
Arachidonic acid release

The first step in the synthesis of leukotrienes is the mobilization of arachidonic acid from cell membrane phospholipid. Release of arachidonic acid is the rate-limiting step in a multistep, enzymatic cascade. A receptor-mediated process at the cell surface (*eg*, mast cell binding of IgE) causes an intracellular influx of calcium. This influx of calcium ions initiates translocation of cytoplasmic phospholipase A_2 ($cPLA_2$) from the cytosol to the nuclear or plasma membrane [4,5]. The $cPLA_2$ then catalyzes the hydrolysis of arachidonic acid at the phospholipid sn-2 position [6,7]. $cPLA_2$ is found in cells mediating airway inflammation, such as alveolar macrophages, eosinophils, and mast cells. A secretory phospholipase A_2, which is also involved in the liberation of arachidonic acid, is found on the surface of inflammatory cells, including mast cells [8,9].

5-Lipoxygenase and 5-lipoxygenase-activating protein

Leukotriene synthesis begins when the cytosolic enzyme 5-lipoxygenase (5-LO) translocates from the cytosol to the nuclear or plasma

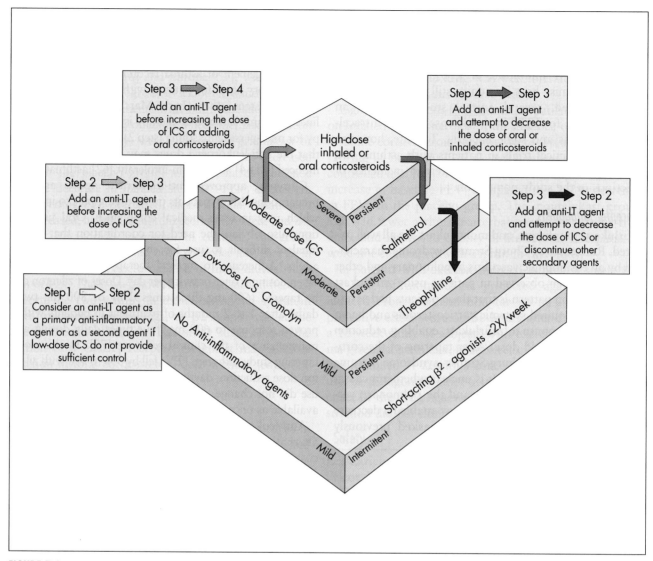

FIGURE 7-6.
Stepwise approach to asthma management according to National Institutes of Health guidelines [69]. The National Asthma Education and Prevention Program outlines a stepwise approach to the management of asthma. Steps one through four are illustrated. The medications on each step are added to the individual asthma patient's regime. Uses for anti-leukotriene agents are only suggestions, as their role in therapy is not fully established. Anti-LT—antileukotriene; ICS—inhaled corticosteroids.

now underway to examine the use of these agents in patients with acute severe asthmatic exacerbations and in patients with emphysema or chronic bronchitis. Other potential therapeutic targets include patients with cystic fibrosis, ulcerative colitis, psoriasis, and rheumatoid arthritis.

Laboratory evidence showing the role of leukotrienes in asthma is strong. Clinical studies examining the efficacy and safety of the anti-leukotriene drugs in asthma are encouraging, but many questions remain. For example, whether these drugs will prevent airway remodeling in asthma is not known. The role of these novel anti-inflammatory drugs in asthma management should be clarified in the near future with completion of current clinical research studies.

REFERENCES AND RECOMMENDED READING

Recently published papers of particular interest have been highlighted as:
- •   Of interest
- ••   Of outstanding interest

1. Samuelsson B, Dahlén S-E, Lindgren JÅ, *et al.*: Leukotrienes and lipoxins: structures, biosynthesis, and biological effects. *Science* 1987, 237:1171–1176.

2. Henderson WR Jr: Eicosanoids and platelet-activating factor in allergic respiratory diseases. *Am Rev Respir Dis* 1991, 143:S86–S90.

3. Henderson WR Jr: The role of leukotrienes in inflammation. *Ann Intern Med* 1994, 121:684–697.

4. Sharp JD, White DL, Chiou XG, *et al.*: Molecular cloning and expression of human Ca^{2+}–sensitive cytosolic phospholipase A_2. *J Biol Chem* 1991, 266:14850–14853.

5. Clark JD, Lin L-L, Kriz RW, et al.: A novel arachidonic acid-selective cytosolic PLA$_2$ contains a Ca^{2+}–dependent translocation domain with homology to PKC and GAP. Cell 1991, 65:1043–1051.

6. Mayer RJ, Marshall LA: New insights on mammalian phospholipase A$_2$(s): comparison of arachidonyl-selective and -nonselective enzymes. FASEB J 1993, 7:339–348.

7. Glaser KB, Mobilio D, Chang JY, et al.: Phospholipase A$_2$ enzymes: regulation and inhibition. Trends Pharmacol Sci 1993, 14:92–98.

8. Murakami M, Kudo I, Umeda M, et al.: Detection of three distinct phospholipases A$_2$ in cultured mast cells. J Biochem (Tokyo) 1992, 111:175–181.

9. Kramer RM, Hession C, Johansen B, et al.: Structure and properties of a human nonpancreatic phospholipase A$_2$. J Biol Chem 1989, 264:5768–5775.

10. Matsumoto T, Funk CD, Ridmark O, et al.: Molecular cloning and amino acid sequence of human 5-lipoxygenase. Proc Natl Acad Sci USA 1988, 85:26–30.

11. Miller DK, Gillard JW, Vickers PJ, et al.: Identification and isolation of a membrane protein necessary for leukotriene production. Nature 1990, 343:278–281.

12. Reid GK, Kargman S, Vickers PJ, et al.: Correlation between expression of 5-lipoxygenase-activating protein, 5-lipoxygenase, and cellular leukotriene synthesis. J Biol Chem 1990, 265:19818–19823.

13. Wong A, Cook MN, Foley JJ, et al.: Influx of extracellular calcium is required for the membrane translocation of 5-lipoxygenase and leukotriene synthesis. Biochemistry 1991, 30:9346–9354.

14. Penrose JF, Gagnon L, Goppelt-Struebe M, et al.: Purification of human leukotriene C$_4$ synthase. Proc Natl Acad Sci USA 1992, 89:11603–11606.

15. Nicholson DW, Klemba MW, Rasper DM, et al.: Purification of human leukotriene C$_4$ synthase from dimethylsulfoxide -differentiated U937 cells. Eur J Biochem 1992, 209:725–734.

16. Penrose JF, Spector J, Baldasaro M, et al.: Molecular cloning of the gene for human leukotriene C$_4$ synthase. J Biochem 1996, 271:11356–11361.

17. Claesson H-E, Haeggström J: Human endothelial cells stimulate leukotriene synthesis and convert granulocyte released leukotriene A$_4$ into leukotrienes B$_4$, C$_4$, D$_4$ and E$_4$. Eur J Biochem 1988, 173:93–100.

18. Maclouf JA, Murphy RC: Transcellular metabolism of neutrophil-derived leukotriene A$_4$ by human platelets: a potential cellular source of leukotriene C$_4$. J Biol Chem 1988, 263:174–181.

19. Buckner CK, Krell RD, Laravuso RB, et al.: Pharmacological evidence that human intralobar airways do not contain different receptors that mediate contractions to leukotriene C$_4$ and leukotriene D$_4$. J Pharmacol Exp Ther 1986, 237:558–562.

20. Martin TR, Pistorese BP, Chi EY, et al.: Effects of leukotriene B$_4$ in the human lung. Recruitment of neutrophils into the alveolar spaces without a change in protein permeability. J Clin Invest 1989, 84:1609–1619.

21. Sampson SE, Costello JF, Sampson AP: The effect of inhaled leukotriene B$_4$ in normal and in asthmatic subjects. Am J Respir Crit Care Med 1997, 155:1789–1792.

22. Palmblad JE, Lerner R: Leukotriene B$_4$-induced hyperadhesiveness of endothelial cells for neutrophils: relation to CD54. Clin Exp Immunol 1992, 90:300–304.

23. Rola-Pleszczynski M, Chavaillaz PA, Lemaire I: Stimulation of interleukin 2 and interferon gamma production by leukotriene B$_4$ in human lymphocyte cultures. Prostaglandins Leukot Med 1986, 23:207–210.

24. Claesson H-E, Dahlberg N, Gahrton G: Stimulation of human myelopoiesis by leukotriene B$_4$. Biochem Biophys Res Commun 1985, 131:579–585.

25. Rola-Pleszczynski M, Staňková J: Leukotriene B$_4$ enhances interleukin-6 (IL-6) production and IL-6 messenger RNA accumulation in human monocytes in vitro: transcriptional and posttranscriptional mechanisms. Blood 1992, 80:1004–1011.

26. Brach MA, deVos S, Arnold C, et al.: Leukotriene B$_4$ transcriptionally activates interleukin-6 expression involving NK-K B and NF-IL6. Eur J Immunol 1992, 22:2705–2711.

27. Turner CR, Breslow R, Conklyn MJ, et al.: In-vitro and in-vivo effects of leukotriene B$_4$ antagonism in a primate model of asthma. J Clin Invest 1996, 97:381–387.

28. Yong EC, Chi EY, Henderson WR Jr: Toxoplasma gondii alters eicosanoid release by human mononuclear phagocytes: role of leukotrienes in interferon-gamma–induced antitoxoplasma activity. J Exp Med 1994, 180:1637–1648.

29. Henderson WR, Chi E: The importance of leukotrienes in mast cell-mediated Toxoplasma gondii cytotoxicity. J Infect Dis 1998, 177:1437–1443.

30. Bailie MB, Standiford TJ, Laichalk LL, et al.: Leukotriene-deficient mice manifest enhanced lethality from Klebsiella pneumonia in association with decreased alveolar macrophage phagocytic and bactericidal activities. J Immunol 1996, 157:5221–5224.

31.•• Henderson WR Jr, Lewis DB, Albert RK, et al.: The importance of leukotrienes in airway inflammation in a mouse model of asthma. J Exp Med 1996, 184:1483–1494.
This study demonstrates that leukotrienes play an important role in asthma pathogenesis. It shows that anti-leukotriene agents effectively block lung inflammation by inhibiting airway eosinophil influx and mucus release.

32. Becker AB, Black MK, Lilley K, et al.: Antiasthmatic effects of a leukotriene biosynthesis inhibitor (MK-0591) in allergic dogs. J Appl Physiol 1995, 78:615–622.

33. Muñoz NM, Douglas I, Mayer D, et al.: Eosinophil chemotaxis inhibited by 5-lipoxygenase blockade and leukotriene receptor antagonism. Am J Respir Crit Care Med 1997, 155:1398–1403.

34. Laitinen LA, Laitinen A, Haahtela T, et al.: Leukotriene E$_4$ and granulocytic infiltration into asthmatic airways. Lancet 1993, 341:989–990.

35. Diamant Z, Hiltermann JT, van Rensen EL, et al.: The effect of inhaled leukotriene D$_4$ and methacholine on sputum cell differentials in asthma. Am J Respir Crit Care Med 1997, 155:1247–1253.

36. Wenzel SE, Westcott JY, Larsen GL: Bronchoalveolar lavage fluid mediator levels 5 minutes after allergen challenge in atopic subjects with asthma: relationship to the development of late asthmatic responses. J Allergy Clin Immunol 1991, 87:540–548.

37. Wenzel SE, Larsen GL, Johnston K, et al.: Elevated levels of leukotriene C$_4$ in bronchoalveolar lavage fluid from atopic asthmatics after endobronchial allergen challenge. Am Rev Respir Dis 1990, 142:112–119.

38. Sladek K, Dworski R, Fitzgerald GA, et al.: Allergen-stimulated release of thromboxane A$_2$ and leukotriene E$_4$ in humans: effect of indomethacin. Am Rev Respir Dis 1990, 141:1441–1445.

39. Drazen JM, O'Brien J, Sparrow D, et al.: Recovery of leukotriene E$_4$ from the urine of patients with airway obstruction. Am Rev Respir Dis 1992, 146:104–108.

40. Ferreri NR, Howland WC, Stevenson DD, et al.: Release of leukotrienes, prostaglandins, and histamine into nasal secretions of aspirin-sensitive asthmatics during reaction to aspirin. Am Rev Respir Dis 1988, 137:847–854.

41. Christie PE, Tagari P, Ford-Hutchinson AW, et al.: Urinary leukotriene E$_4$ concentrations increase after aspirin challenge in aspirin-sensitive asthmatic subjects. Am Rev Respir Dis 1991, 143:1025–1029.

42. Naclerio RM, Proud D, Togias AG, et al.: Inflammatory mediators in late antigen-induced rhinitis. N Engl J Med 1985, 313:65–70.

43. Henderson WR Jr: New modalities for the pharmacotherapy of asthma: leukotriene inhibitors and antagonists. *Immunol Allergy Clin North Am* 1996, 16:797–808.

44.• Israel E, Cohn J, Dubé L, *et al.*: Effect of treatment with zileuton, a 5-lipoxygenase inhibitor, in patients with asthma: a randomized controlled trial. *JAMA* 1996, 275:931–936.
This study demonstrates the clinically beneficial effects of chronic treatment with zileuton, a 5-LO inhibitor, in patients with mild to moderate asthma.

45. Liu MC, Dubé L, Lancaster J, *et al.*: Clinical aspects of allergic disease: acute and chronic effects of a 5-lipoxygenase inhibitor in asthma, a 6-month randomized multicenter trial. *J Allergy Clin Immunol* 1996, 98:859–871.

46. Bellia V, Cuttitta G, Mirabella M, *et al.*: Urinary leukotriene E_4 as a marker of nocturnal asthma. *Am Rev Respir Dis* 1992, 145:A16.

47. Wenzel SE, Trudeau JB, Kaminsky DA, *et al.*: Effect of 5-lipoxygenase inhibition on bronchoconstriction and airway inflammation in nocturnal asthma. *Am J Respir Crit Care Med* 1995, 152:897–905.

48. Meltzer SS, Hasday JD, Cohn J, *et al.*: Inhibition of exercise induced bronchospasm by zileuton: a 5-lipoxygenase inhibitor. *Am J Respir Crit Care Med* 1996, 153:931–935.

49. In KH, Asano K, Beier D, *et al.*: Naturally occurring mutations in the human 5-lipoxygenase gene promoter that modify transcription factor binding and reporter gene transcription. *J Clin Invest* 1997, 99:1130–1137.

50. Evans DJ, Barnes PJ, Spaethe SM, *et al.*: Effect of a leukotriene B_4 receptor antagonist, LY293111, on allergen-induced responses in asthma. *Thorax* 1996, 51:1178–1184.

51. Taylor IK, O'Shaughnessy KM, Fuller RW, *et al.*: Effect of cysteinyl-leukotriene receptor antagonist ICI 204,219 on allergen-induced bronchoconstriction and airway hyperreactivity in atopic subjects. *Lancet* 1991, 337:690–694.

52. Finnerty JP, Wood-Baker R, Thomson H, *et al.*: Role of leukotrienes in exercise-induced asthma: inhibitory effect of ICI 204,219, a potent leukotriene D_4 receptor antagonist. *Am Rev Respir Dis* 1992, 145:746–749.

53. Spector SL, Smith LJ, Glass M, *et al.*: Effects of 6 weeks of therapy with oral doses of ICI 204,219, a leukotriene D_4 receptor antagonist, in subjects with bronchial asthma. *Am J Respir Crit Care Med* 1994, 150:618–623.

54. Zeneca Pharmaceuticals: A multicenter, double-blind, placebo-controlled trial of Accolate in mild to moderate asthmatic patients needing chronic treatment: trial number 9188IL/0029. Wilmington, DE; 1992.

55. Suissa S, Dennis R, Ernst P, *et al.*: Effectiveness of the leukotriene receptor antagonist zafirlukast for mild-to-moderate asthma: a randomized, double-blind, placebo-controlled trial. *Ann Intern Med* 1997, 126:177–183.

56. Grossman J, Faiferman I, Dubb JW, *et al.*: Results of the first US double-blind, placebo-controlled, multicenter clinical study in asthma with pranlukast, a novel leukotriene receptor antagonist. *J Asthma* 1997, 34:321–328.

57. Barnes NC, Pujit JC: Pranlukast, a novel leukotriene receptor antagonist: results of the first European, placebo controlled, multicenter clinical study in asthma. *Thorax* 1997, 52:523–527.

58.• Tamaoki J, Kondo M, Sakai N, *et al.*: Leukotriene antagonist prevents exacerbation of asthma during reduction of high-dose inhaled corticosteroid. *Am J Respir Crit Care Med* 1997, 155:1235–1240.
This study demonstrates that the dose of inhaled corticosteroids can be reduced in the presence of pranlukast, a $CysLT_1$ receptor antagonist.

59. Leff JA, Israel E, Noonan MJ, *et al.*: Montelukast (MK-0476) allows tapering of inhaled corticosteroids (ICS) in asthmatic patients while maintaining clinical stability. *Am J Respir Crit Care Med* 1997, 155:A976.

60. Reiss TF, Chervinsky P, Edwards T, *et al.*: Montelukast (MK-0476), a $CysLT_1$ receptor antagonist, improves asthma outcomes over a 3-month treatment period. *Am J Respir Crit Care Med* 1997, 155:A622.

61. Knorr BA, Matz J, Bernstein JA, *et al.*: Montelukast for chronic asthma in 6- to 14-year old children: a randomized, double-blind trial. *JAMA* 1998, 279:1181–1186.

62. Kuna P, Malmstrom K, Dahlen S-E, *et al.*: Montelukast (MK-0476), a $CysLT_1$ receptor antagonist, improves asthma control in aspirin-intolerant asthmatic patients. *Am J Respir Crit Care Med* 1997, 155:A975–A975.

63. Bronsky EA, Kemp JP, Zhang J, *et al.*: Dose-related protection of exercise bronchoconstriction by montelukast, a cysteinyl leukotriene-receptor antagonist, at the end of a once-daily dosing interval. *Clin Pharmacol Ther* 1997, 62:556–561.

64. Leff JA, Busse WW, Pearlman D, *et al.*: Montelukast, a leukotriene–receptor antagonist, for the treatment of mild asthma and exercise–induced bronchoconstriction. *N Engl J Med* 1998, 339:147–152.

65. Chen X-S, Sheller JR, Johnson EN, *et al.*: Role of leukotrienes revealed by targeted disruption of the 5-lipoxygenase gene. *Nature* 1994, 372:179–182.

66. Goulet JL, Snouwaert JN, Latour AM, *et al.*: Altered inflammatory responses in leukotriene-deficient mice. *Proc Natl Acad Sci USA* 1994, 91:12852–12856.

67. Lazarus SC, Lee TM, Wright S, *et al.*: Secondary outcomes analysis of zileuton plus usual care vs usual care alone in the treatment of patients with asthma. In *Proceedings.* Boston, MA: American College of Allergy, Asthma, and Immunology meeting; November 1996.

68. Wechsler ME, Garpestad E, Flier SR, *et al.*: Pulmonary infiltrates, eosinophilia, and cardiomyopathy following corticosteroid withdrawal in patients with asthma receiving zafirlukast. *JAMA* 1998, 279:455–457.

69. National Heart, Lung, and Blood Institute: *Guidelines for the Diagnosis and Management of Asthma: National Institutes of Health Publ. No. 97-4051.* Bethesda, MD: National Institutes of Health, 1997.

70. DuBuske LM, Grossman J, Dube LM, *et al.*: Randomized trial of zileuton inpatients with moderate asthma: effect of reduced dosing frequency and amounts on pulmonary function and asthma symptoms. *Am J Managed Care* 1997, 3:633–640.

71. Cumming RG, Mitchell P, Leeder SA: Use of inhaled corticosteroids and the risk of cataracts. *N Engl J Med* 1997, 337:8–14.

72. Garbe E, LeLorier J, Boivin J, *et al.*: Inhaled and nasal glucocorticoids and the risks of ocular hypertension on open-angle glaucoma. *JAMA* 1997, 277:722–727.

73. Oral and inhaled corticosteroids reduce bone formation as shown by plasma osteocalcin levels. *Am J Respir Crit Care Med* 1995, 151:333–336.

74. Ip M, Lam K, Yam L, *et al.*: Decreased bone mineral density in premenopausal asthma patients receiving long-term inhaled steroids. *Chest* 1994, 105:1722–1727.

75. Herrala J, Puolyoki H, Impivaara O, *et al.*: Bone mineral density in asthmatic women on high dose inhaled beclomethasone dipropionate. *Bone* 1994, 15:621–623.

76. Hopp RJ, Degan JA, Biven RE, *et al.*: Longitudinal assessment of bone mineral density in children with chronic asthma. *Ann Allergy Asthma Immunol* 1995, 75:143–148.

CHAPTER 8

Bronchodilators

William F. Schoenwetter
Richard J. Sveum

There are four classes of bronchodilator drugs: β-adrenergic agonists, methylxanthines, anticholinergics, and leukotriene modifiers. Each drug has specific characteristics, indications, and shortcomings. β-agonists are used as first-line therapy for asthma because of the rapid onset of action and their effectiveness as bronchodilators.

In 1997, the National Heart, Lung, and Blood Institute [1] released the National Asthma Education and Prevention Program Expert Panel Report 2, which furthers our understanding of asthma management. Medications are now categorized into two classes: long-term control drugs, used to achieve and maintain control of persistent asthma, and quick-relief agents, used to treat acute symptoms and exacerbations. Bronchodilators fall into both classifications. The report reemphasizes that drugs that have anti-inflammatory effects are the most effective for long-term control. A stepped therapy approach suggests initiating more intense therapy at the onset in order to establish prompt control, and then reducing treatment as tolerated.

Patients with asthma can expect the β-agonists to deliver the greatest bronchodilatation. β-agonists are effective for relief of acute and exercise-induced bronchospasm and are generally well tolerated. The recent availability of the long-acting β-agonists salmeterol and formoterol increases their usefulness in asthma management for long-term control.

β–AGONIST SAFETY

There is a definite association between high dose and excessive use of inhaled β-agonists and the risk of death from asthma. What is not understood is whether this association is a result of a causal effect of the drugs or simply reflects the greater severity of asthma.

The issue of β-agonist safety was raised by a report from New Zealand suggesting that inhaled fenoterol use was associated with an increased risk of death from asthma [2]. Then Sears et al. [3] reported that the regular rather than as-needed use of aerosolized fenoterol resulted in less asthma control. This was followed shortly by a large case-control study from Saskatchewan by Spitzer et al. [4] showing an association between the excessive use of β-agonists and the risk of near death or death from asthma. The publication of these papers within a 2-year period initiated a controversy, summarized by Fahy and Boushey [5], over the appropriate use of β-agonists in asthma. Some experts recommended limited β-agonist use whereas others questioned the data. Conflicting opinions led to numerous articles and debates featured at various medical meetings. Studies by Wong et al. [6] compared

CHAPTER 9

The New Antihistamines

Robert A. Nathan

Antihistamines are an integral part of pharmacologic therapy for patients with allergic rhinitis, chronic urticaria, atopic dermatitis, and other allergic disorders. For years, the customary first-line pharmacotherapeutic approach for the treatment of patients with allergic rhinitis and pruritus consisted of antihistamines despite their pronounced unwanted side effects. New or second-generation antihistamines are now the focus of therapy, largely because these agents are nonsedating or less sedating than their predecessors.

Although various inflammatory mediators play a role in producing clinical signs and symptoms of allergic rhinitis, histamine still is recognized as the primary mediator in this disorder. Histamine is released within minutes after contact between an allergen and specific IgE molecules on the surface of mast cells. Once released from mast cells and basophils, histamine produces vascular permeability and vasodilation in the skin (Table 9-1) [1••]. In the nose, histamine stimulates sensory nerves, causing itching and sneezing. Histamine also increases mucosal blood flow, resulting in nasal congestion, and increases goblet cell secretion and vascular permeability, evoking symptoms of rhinorrhea (Table 9-1) [1••].

Antihistamines act in the skin to suppress the wheal and flare response by inhibiting histamine binding at its receptors on nerves, vascular smooth muscle, endothelium, and mast cells. In the nose, antihistamines competitively inhibit histamine receptors on nasal mucosa cells, diminishing the early phase reaction.

PHARMACOKINETICS

Collectively, the second-generation antihistamines are similar in their ability to competitively antagonize histamine at its receptors. Individually, these agents differ considerably in their pharmacokinetic and pharmacodynamic profiles (Table 9-2) [2••,3]. Second-generation antihistamines possess a similar core moiety, but the side chains adjoining the core determine their pharmacokinetic properties.

Pharmacokinetic profiles of second-generation antihistamines allow for once- or twice-daily treatment. All new agents are well absorbed after oral administration, with peak plasma concentrations generally occurring within 1 to 2 hours. Terfenadine, astemizole, and loratadine are metabolized extensively in the liver, each with active metabolites. Cetirizine (the carboxylated metabolite of hydroxyzine), fexofenadine (the active metabolite of terfenadine), and acrivastine are poorly metabolized and excreted largely unchanged.

Table 9-1. PHYSIOLOGIC RESPONSES TO HISTAMINE CHALLENGE AND MECHANISMS UNDERLYING THESE RESPONSES IN THE SKIN AND NASAL MUCOSA

	Response	Mechanism
Skin		
Wheal	Increased vascular permeability	H_1-receptor–mediated endothelial cell contraction (via EDRF (NO)/PGI$_2$)
Flare	Vasodilation	H_1/H_2-receptor–mediated axonal reflex (substance P/CGRP/NKA-mediated)
Nasal mucosa		
Itch	Sensory nerve activation	H_1-receptor–mediated trigeminal nerve activation
Congestion	Increased mucosal blood flow (vasodilation)	H_1/H_2-receptor–mediated stimulation of sympathetic nerves; VIP release from parasympathetic (?) nerves
Rhinorrhea	Increased goblet cell secretion, increased vascular permeability	H_1-receptor interaction with parasympathetic nerves (goblet cells); H_1-receptor–mediated increase in engorgement (sympathetic) of highly fenestrated capacitance vessels.

EDRF—endothelium-derived relaxing factor; NO—nitric oxide; PGI$_2$—prostaglandin I$_2$; P/CGRP—substance P/calcitonin gene-related peptide; NKA—neurokinin A; VIP—vasoactive intestinal peptide.
From Monroe et al. [1••]; with permission.

Table 9-2. PHARMACOKINETIC PROPERTIES OF SELECTED ORAL SECOND-GENERATION ANTIHISTAMINES

Antihistamine	Dosage*	Elimination half-life	Active metabolite	Onset of action	Duration of action, h	Metabolized in liver	Protein binding, %
Astemizole	10 mg qd	20 h 7 to 10 d †	Yes	2 to 4 d	>24	Yes	~97
Cetirizine	5 or 10 mg qd	7 to 10.6 h	No	<1 h	12 to 24	Minimally	93
Fexofenadine	60 mg bid	14.4 h	No	1 h	12	Minimally	60 to 70
Loratadine	10 mg qd	8 to 11 h	Yes	1 to 3 h	>24	Yes	~97
Terfenadine	60 mg bid	20 h	Yes	1 to 2 h	12	Yes	97

*Adult
† Biphasic half-life: 20 h for distribution, 7 to 10 days for elimination.
bid—twice daily; qd—once daily

Most new antihistamines have a rapid onset of action—defined as a significant therapeutic effect within 1 to 2 hours—and duration of action 12 to 24 hours after a single dose. One exception is the second-generation antihistamine astemizole. This drug has an onset of action within 2 days and a prolonged duration of action. Steady-state plasma levels of astemizole are reached in as long as 4 weeks, with the wheal response taking as long as 8 weeks to recover to normal [4••].

Typically, the onset of action of antihistamines is determined by suppression of histamine-induced wheal and flare in the skin. However, Day et al. [5•] at Kingston General Hospital (Kingston, Ontario) recently used the environmental exposure unit (EEU) to investigate the onset of action of terfenadine, astemizole, cetirizine, and loratadine in patients with seasonal allergic rhinitis. The EEU is designed to eliminate confounding

factors (eg, seasonal and geographic variations in pollen counts) encountered during evaluation of antihistamines by exposing individuals to a predetermined, controlled, constant level of airborne pollen. Essentially, the unit is a modified classroom with a feeder system that delivers controlled levels of commercially available ragweed pollen into a study area (Fig. 9-1). A modified laser counter measures the grains emitted and records concentrations using a computer. Fans circulate room air continuously, while six impact-type particle samplers determine pollen levels in the patients' seating area. Patients are moved every 30 minutes, ensuring that they spend an equal amount of time in each section of the chamber. Day's group [5•] found no significant ($P = 0.119$) difference among antihistamines in the time to onset of clinically important relief (mean range, 1:45 to 2:28 h), with the quickest to slowest agents being cetirizine, terfenadine, astemizole, and loratadine, respectively. They also used the EEU to study fexofenadine, the newest antihistamine available in the United States. Using a "relaxed" criteria of clinically important relief (slight to complete relief rather than marked or complete relief), they showed that fexofenadine (60- and 120-mg doses) had a median time to onset of clinically important relief of 60 minutes [6•].

EFFICACY

The clinical effects of antihistamines result primarily from competitive inhibition of H_1 receptors in the skin and nasal mucosa during an allergic response. Antihistamines are most effective when occupying the H_1 receptor site before histamine is released. Hence, maximum therapeutic benefits are gained through prophylactic treatment before allergen exposure.

Several methods are used to assess the potency and activity of antihistamines. The most popular method is the suppression of epicutaneous histamine-induced wheal and flare. All H_1 antihistamines inhibit wheal and flare response but differ in the strength of their effect, time to peak effect, and duration of action. Investigators

previously have suggested that the inhibition of wheal and flare by antihistamines correlates with relief of allergic rhinitis symptoms [7,8].

Recently, however, Monroe et al. [1••] challenged the reliability of antihistamine suppression of histamine-induced wheal and flare as a predictor of clinical effect. The authors concluded, based on a comprehensive literature review, that the method is useful in determining dose-response relationships for individual drugs, but correlates poorly with the ability of various antihistamines to modify clinical responses (Tables 9-3 and 9-4). Histamine, although an important mediator of allergic response in the skin, is just one of a number of significant mediators and cells involved in an allergic reaction. Structural, functional, and inflammatory responses differ between the skin and nasal mucosa and, as such, a cutaneous histamine-antihistamine interaction may not accurately predict the potency of antihistamines in other tissues and organs or their effect on clinical symptoms of allergic disease.

Epicutaneous histamine injection produces a rapid wheal and flare response that lasts approximately 1 hour [1••]. However, this response mimics only a portion of the early phase reaction—before mast cell degranulation and multiple mediator release—and does not reflect late-phase

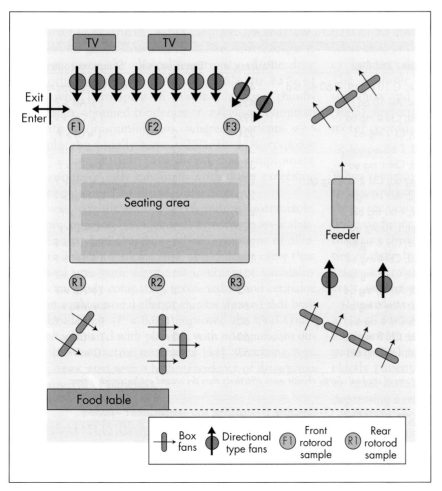

FIGURE 9-1.

Representation of the environmental exposure unit. *Adapted from* from Day JH, *et al.* [5•]; with permission.

as 78% of patients with asthma report nasal symptoms, and as many as 38% of patients with allergic rhinitis have asthma [57•].

Histamine is recognized as an important mediator in the pathogenesis of asthma; however, first-generation antihistamines were not considered as a treatment for asthma because the high doses required produced intolerable side effects. Moreover, product labels for antihistamines contraindicated their use in patients with asthma, warning that these agents may thicken mucous and cause bronchoconstriction. Later investigations would prove that antihistamines do not cause bronchoconstriction but instead have bronchodilating effects [58].

Concerns about side effects with second-generation antihistamines are less troublesome and not substantiated by studies investigating their effects in patients with asthma. In fact, some nonsedating antihistamines demonstrate mild anti-asthmatic effects. Terfenadine [59,60], loratadine [4], and astemizole [61,62] have exhibited modest bronchodilating effects, reduced bronchial hyperreactivity to histamine, and protected against exercise- and antigen-induced bronchospasm, although most treatment benefits were reported with doses higher than currently recommended. Cetirizine demonstrated some protective effects against bronchial hyperreactivity to methacholine at 6 hours [63], and when used concomitantly with salbutamol provided prolonged relief (over 7 to 8 hours) of lower airway obstruction [64]. In patients with allergic rhinitis and perennial asthma, cetirizine (20 mg) significantly reduced baseline severity of both rhinitis (itchy nose, nasal congestion, watery eyes) and asthma symptoms (chest tightness, wheezing, shortness of breath, and nocturnal asthma) [65].

Some antihistamines also demonstrate treatment effects when used at recommended dosages. In one study, cetirizine (10 mg daily) reduced the severity of seasonal rhinitis and asthma but had no effect on pulmonary function [66]. Combination treatment with loratadine (5 mg twice daily) and pseudoephedrine (120 mg twice daily) improved asthma symptoms, peak expiratory flow rates, spirometry, and quality-of-life measurements for patients with seasonal rhinitis and asthma [57•]. It is interesting to speculate about the potential effects of fexofenadine in patients with asthma. Unlike other second-generation antihistamines, the dosage of fexofenadine can be increased to maximize anti-inflammatory effects without the risk of sedation and cardiovascular events.

One study also has shown that combination therapy with loratadine (10 mg twice daily) and the leukotriene receptor antagonist zafirlukast (80 mg twice daily) reduced ($P < 0.05$) early and late asthmatic reactions in patients with allergic asthma more than either agent alone, suggesting that combination therapy may present a new strategy for treating asthma [67••]. What remains to be seen is whether the improvement in chest symptoms was the direct effect of two antimediator drugs on the lower airway or the result of appropriate treatment of allergic rhinitis in the upper airway.

GUIDELINES FOR THE USE OF ANTIHISTAMINES

When prescribing antihistamines for patients, physicians should consider drug action and efficacy as well as safety profile. First- and second-generation antihistamines may show equivalent efficacy but differ in terms of side effects. From a patient's perspective, one of the most important considerations when choosing an appropriate therapy is its impact on quality of life.

Because of the sedation and psychomotor impairment associated with first-generation antihistamines, some physicians recommend the use of these agents only at bedtime so that the sedative effects occur during sleep. Other physicians recommend a combination regimen as a cost-saving measure, prescribing a nonsedating antihistamine in the morning and a sedating antihistamine in the evening. However, until studies confirm the safety of a mixed morning/evening regimen, caution is advised. The side effects of sedating antihistamines can persist into the morning hours, contributing to potential adverse consequences during the day (eg, traffic accidents, work-related injuries, and impaired performance).

Kay et al. [68••] investigated the carryover effects of a morning/evening treatment regimen with terfenadine (mornings) and the over-the-counter sedating antihistamine chlorpheniramine (evenings). Results of the Multiple Sleep Latency test and Stanford Sleepiness Scale test showed that the morning/evening regimen increased daytime sleepiness, decreased alertness, and caused a carryover sedation effect (ie, patients fell asleep more quickly and were less able to concentrate the following day). In an editorial, Simons [69••] summarized the safety concerns of first-generation antihistamines and cautioned that cost containment should not impel health-care providers to prescribe a first-generation antihistamine over a second-generation agent. Moreover, studies have shown that patients may not recognize when performance is impaired [70,71]. CNS impairment can exist even when drowsiness is not reported by patients, as demonstrated by discrepancies between subjective reporting and objective measures of sedation [25,72,73].

Compliance may be another issue to consider when prescribing an antihistamine. A number of anecdotal and subjective reports describe tolerance to first-generation antihistamines over time; however, this decrease in clinical response may be related to a gradual decrease in compliance rather than drug tolerance. In one study, the decrease in clinical response to chlorpheniramine over 3 weeks was associated with a decrease in patient compliance [74]. Noncompliance was attributed to side effects, such as drowsiness, lightheadedness, and anticholinergic effects (dry mouth and urinary hesitancy). Hence, the adverse effects of first-generation antihistamines may interfere with their value as long-term treatment.

Second-generation antihistamines, therefore, play a prominent role in the international consensus report on the diagnosis and management of rhinitis (Fig. 9-4) [75]. The first step in the medical management of patients with mild allergic rhinitis begins with a nonsedating antihistamine. Patients with moderate disease fall into two categories: those with predominantly nasal symptoms and those with predominantly ocular symptoms. Moderate disease patients with eye symptoms should begin therapy with a nonsedating antihistamine daily. However, if symptoms are not controlled with antihistamines alone or if patients have more prominent nasal blockage, a topical anti-inflammatory medication should also be prescribed.

CONCLUSIONS

The new, nonsedating antihistamines are the recommended first-line pharmacotherapeutic approach for the management of mild-to-moderate allergic rhinitis, especially when ocular symptoms predominate. Advantages of the new antihistamines include oral or topical administration; a once- or twice-daily treatment regimen (which should improve compliance); specific H_1 receptor antagonism; inhibition of other inflammatory mediators involved in the allergic response; and mild anti-asthmatic effects. Aside from their lack of sedative effects, perhaps the most compelling reason to prescribe second-generation antihistamines is that they do not interfere with performance and learning. Factors that will most likely dictate drug choice among the newer agents are cost, convenience, compliance, and patient preference.

REFERENCES AND RECOMMENDED READING

Recently published papers of particular interest have been highlighted as:
- •   Of interest
- •• Of outstanding interest

1.•• Monroe EW, Daly AF, Shalhoub RF: Appraisal of the validity of histamine induced wheal and flare to predict the clinical efficacy of antihistamines. *J Allergy Clin Immunol* 1997, 99:S798–S806.
This is a review of comparative studies of antihistamines in the treatment of chronic idiopathic urticaria and seasonal allergic rhinitis, and the lack of predictive value of antihistamine suppression of cutaneous histamine-induced wheal and flare reaction.

2.•• Garbus SB, Moulton BW, Meltzer EO, *et al.*: Considerations in pharmaceutical conversion: focus on antihistamines. *Am J Man Care* 1997, 3:617–630.
This paper discusses issues related to and implications of pharmaceutical conversion using the antihistamine class of drugs as the case situation.

3.   Kastrup EK, ed.: *Drug Facts and Comparisons.* St. Louis: Facts and Comparisons; 1997:188–194a.

4.•• Du Buske LM: Clinical comparison of histamine H_1 receptor antagonist drugs. *J Allergy Clin Immunol* 1996, 98:S307–S318.
This is a comprehensive review of the second-generation antihistamines, focusing on their pharmacokinetics, adverse effect profiles, antiallergic activities, and antiasthmatic effects.

5.• Day JH, Briscoe MP, Clark RH, *et al.*: Onset of action and efficacy of terfenadine, astemizole, cetirizine, and loratadine for the relief of symptoms of allergic rhinitis. *Ann Allergy Asthma Immunol* 1997, 79:163–172.
This study employs an environmental exposure unit as a model to differentiate the onset of action and efficacy of second-generation antihistamines.

6.• Day JH, Briscoe MP, Welsh A, *et al.*: Onset of action, efficacy, and safety of a single dose of fexofenadine hydrochloride for ragweed allergy using an environmental exposure unit. *Ann Allergy Asthma Immunol* 1997, 79:533–540.
This paper extends findings by Day et al. [5] to include the onset of action and efficacy of fexofenadine hydrochloride without a direct comparison to other antihistamines.

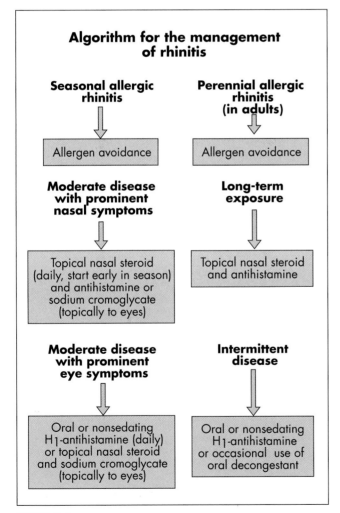

FIGURE 9-4.
Guidelines for the stepwise approach to the treatment of patients with rhinitis. *Adapted from* International Rhinitis Management Working Group [75]; with permission.

7. Watson WTA, Simons KJ, Chen XY, *et al*.: Cetirizine: a pharmacokinetic and pharmacodynamic evaluation in children with seasonal allergic rhinitis. *J Allergy Clin Immunol* 1989, 84:457–464.

8. Howarth PH, Emmanual MB, Holgate ST, *et al*.: Astemizole, a potent histamine H_1 receptor antagonist: effect in allergic rhinoconjunctivitis, on antigen and histamine induced skin wheal responses and relationship to serum levels. *Br J Clin Pharmacol* 1984, 18:1–8.

9.• Klein GL, Littlejohn T III, Lockhart EA, *et al*.: Brompheniramine, terfenadine, and placebo in allergic rhinitis. *Ann Allergy Asthma Immunol* 1996, 77:365–370.
This is a thought-provoking study comparing a first-generation antihistamine with a second-generation antihistamine.

10. Meltzer EO, Schatz M: Pharmacotherapy of asthma: 1987 and beyond. *Immunol Allergy Clin North Am* 1987, 7:57–91.

11. Data presented at the annual meeting of British Society of Allergy and Clinical Immunology [abstract 05]; September 1996; Manchester, UK.

12. Simons FER, Simons KJ: Second-generation H_1 receptor antagonists. *Ann Allergy* 1991, 66:5–19.

13. Drouin MA: H_1 antihistamines: perspective on the use of the conventional and new agents. *Ann Allergy* 1985, 55:747–752.

14. Kaliner MA, Check WA: Nonsedating antihistamines. *Allergy Proc* 1988, 9:649–661.

15.•• Adelsburg BR: Sedation and performance issues in the treatment of allergic conditions. *Arch Intern Med* 1997, 157:494–500.
This is an excellent review article on CNS effects with particular emphasis on psychomotor and cognitive effects of second-generation antihistamines.

16.• Nolan TM: Sedative effects of antihistamines: safety, performance, learning, and quality of life. *Clin Ther* 1997, 19:39–55.
This is another review article on the side-effect profile of the sedating and nonsedating antihistamines with emphasis on patient satisfaction and quality-of-life parameters.

17. Simons FER, Simons KJ: H_1 receptor antagonist treatment of chronic rhinitis. *J Allergy Clin Immunol* 1988, 81:975–980.

18.•• Simons FER, Fraser TG, Reggin JD, *et al*.: Comparison of the central nervous system effects produced by six H_1 receptor antagonists. *Clin Exp Allergy* 1996, 26:1092–1097.
This is a comprehensive comparative study of the newer antihistamines and their effects on cognitive functioning and somnolence.

19. Spencer CM, Faulds D, Peters DH: Cetirizine. *Drugs* 1993, 46:1055–1080.

20. Falliers CJ, Brandon ML, Buchman E, *et al*.: Double-blind comparison of cetirizine and placebo in the treatment of seasonal rhinitis. *Ann Allergy* 1991, 66:257–262.

21.• Davies RJ, Bagnall AC, McCabe RN, *et al*.: Antihistamines: topical vs oral administration. *Clin Exp Allergy* 1996, 26(suppl):11–17.
This paper gives supporting evidence that it is logical to administer antihistamines directly to the target organ, the nose.

22. Cimbura G, Lucas DM, Bennett RC, *et al*.: Incidence and toxicological aspects of drugs detected in 484 fatally injured drivers and pedestrians in Ontario. *Forensic Sci* 1982, 27:855–867.

23. Warren R, Simpson H, Hilchie J, *et al*.: Drugs detected in fatally injured drivers in the province of Ontario. In: *Alcohol, Drugs and Traffic Safety*, vol 1. Edited by Goldburg L. Stockholm: Almquist & Wiskell, 1981:203–217

24. US Department of Transportation: *Digest of the State Alcohol-Highway Safety Related Legislation*, edn 14. Washington, DC: United States Department of Transportation, 1996.

25. O'Hanlon JF: Antihistamines and driving performance: the Netherlands. *J Respir Dis* 1988, 9:12–17.

26. Van Cauwenberge PB: New data on the safety of loratadine. *Drug Invest* 1992, 4:283–291.

27. Ramaekers JG, Uiterwijk MM, O'Hanlon JF: Effects of loratadine and cetirizine on actual driving and psychometric test performance, and EEG during driving. *Eur J Clin Pharmacol* 1992, 42:363–369.

28. Offenloch K, Zahner G: Rated performance, cardiovascular and quantitative EEG parameters during stimulated instrument flight under the effect of terfenadine. *Arzeimittelforschung* 1992, 42:864–868.

29. Neves-Pinto RM, Lima GM, da Mota Teixeira R: A double-blind study of the effects of loratadine versus placebo on the performance of pilots. *Am J Rhinology* 1992, 6:23.

30. Gilmore TM, Alexander BH, Mueller BA, *et al*.: Occupational injuries and medication use. *Am J Ind Med* 1996, 30:234–239.

31. Walsh JK, Muehlbach MJ, Schweitzer PK: Simulated assembly line performance following ingestion of ceterizine or hydroxyzine. *Ann Allergy* 1992, 69:195–200.

32. Vuurman EF, van Veggel L, Uiterwijk MM, *et al*.: Seasonal allergic rhinitis and antihistamine effects on children's learning. *Ann Allergy* 1993, 71:121–126.

33. Vuurman EF, van Veggel L, Sanders RL, *et al*.: Effects of Semprex-D and diphenhydramine on learning in young adults with seasonal allergic rhinitis. *Ann Allergy Asthma Immunol* 1996, 76:247–252.

34. Tatro DS, Olin BR, Hebel SK: *Drug Interaction Facts*. St. Louis: JB Lippincott, 1997.

35. Pratt C, Mason J, Russel T, Ahlbrandt R: Effect of fexofenadine HCl on corrected QT interval (QT_c) [abstract]. *Allergy* 1997, 52:67.

36.• Hey JA, del Prado M, Sherwood J, *et al*.: Comparative analysis of the cardiotoxicity proclivities of second generation antihistamines in an experimental model predictive of adverse clinical ECG effects. *Arneimittelforschung* 1996, 46:153–158.
This is an interesting article using a guinea pig model to predict the arrhythmogenic potential of second-generation antihistamines in humans.

37. Bahmer FA, Ruprecht KW: Safety and efficacy of topical levocabastine compared with oral terfenadine. *Ann Allergy* 1994, 72:429–434.

38. Gastpar H, Nolte D, Aurich R, *et al*.: Comparative efficacy of azelastine nasal spray and terfenadine in seasonal and perennial rhinitis. *Allergy* 1994, 49:152–158.

39. Janssens MM-L: Levocabastine: A new topical approach for the treatment of paediatric allergic rhinoconjunctivitis. *Rhinology* 1992, 13(suppl):39–49.

40. Janssens MM-L, Vanden Bussche G: Levocabastine: an effective topical treatment of allergic rhinoconjunctivitis. *Clin Exp Allergy* 1991, 21(suppl):29–36.

41. Thomas KE, Ollier S, Ferguson H, *et al*.: The effect of intranasal azelastine, Rhinolast, on nasal airways obstruction and sneezing following provocation testing with histamine and allergen. *Clin Exp Allergy* 1992, 22:642–647.

42. Falconieri P, Monteleone AM, Mancuso T, *et al*.: Effectiveness of levocabastine eye drops in children with allergic conjunctivitis: a double-blind study. *Pediatr Asthma Allergy Immunol* 1994, 8:111–115.

43. Dechant KL, Goa KL: Levocabastine: a review of its pharmacological properties and therapeutic potential as a topical antihistamine in allergic rhinitis and conjunctivitis. *Drugs* 1991, 41:202–224.

44. Grossman J, Halverson PC, Meltzer EO, *et al*.: Double-blind assessment of azelastine in the treatment of perennial allergic rhinitis. *Ann Allergy* 1994, 73:141–146.

45. Canonica GW, Ciprandi G, Buscaglia S, et al.: Adhesion molecules of allergic inflammation: recent insights into their functional roles. Allergy 1994, 49:135–141.

46. Ciprandi G, Pronzato C, Ricca V, et al.: Evidence of intracellular adhesion molecule-1 expression on nasal epithelial cells in acute rhinoconjunctivitis caused by pollen exposure. J Allergy Clin Immunol 1994, 94:738–746.

47.• Campbell A, Chanal I, Czarlewski W, et al.: Reduction of soluble ICAM-1 levels in nasal secretion by H₁ blockers in seasonal allergic rhinitis. Allergy 1997, 52:1022–1025.
This study examines the ability of both loratadine and cetirizine to reduce the release of soluble ICAM-1 in nasal secretions supporting an anti-inflammatory effect of second-generation antihistamines.

48. Ciprandi G, Pronzato C, Ricca V, et al.: Loratadine treatment of rhinitis due to pollen allergy reduces epithelial ICAM-1 expression. Clin Exp Allergy 1997, 27:1175–1183.

49. Ciprandi G, Tosca M, Ricca V, et al.: Cetirizine treatment of rhinitis in children with pollen allergy: evidence of its anti-allergic activity. Clin Exp Allergy 1997, 27:1160–1166.

50. Devalia JL, Abdelaziz MM, Baytam H, et al.: Effect of fexofenadine on eosinophil-induced changes in epithelial permeability and mediator release from nasal epithelial cells of seasonal allergic rhinitics [abstract 2015]. J Allergy Clin Immunol 1997, 99:S497.

51. Naclerio RM, Porud D, Kagey-Sobotka A, et al.: The effect of cetirizine on early allergic response. Laryngoscope 1989, 99:596–599.

52. Charlesworth EN, Massey WA, Kagey-Sobotka A, et al.: Effect of H₁ receptor blockade on the early and late response to cutaneous allergen challenge. J Pharmacol Exp Ther 1992, 262:964–970.

53. Pazdrak K, Gorski P, Ruta U: Inhibitory effect of levocabastine on allergen-induced increase of nasal reactivity to histamine and cell influx. Allergy 1993, 48:598–601.

54. Buscaglia S, Catrullo A, Ciprandi G, et al.: Levocabastine eye drops reduce ICAM-1 expression both in vitro and in vivo [abstract]. Allergy 1995, 50(suppl):79.

55. Pronzato G, Ricca V, Varese P, et al.: Evaluation of anti-allergic activity of azelastine nasal spray [abstract]. Allergy 1995, 50(suppl):69.

56.• Grossman J: One airway, one disease. Chest 1997, 111:11S–16S.
This paper suggests that allergic rhinitis and asthma are not separate diseases but a continuum of inflammation in a common airway.

57.• Corren J, Harris AG, Aaronson D, et al.: Efficacy and safety of loratadine plus pseudoephedrine in patients with seasonal allergic rhinitis. J Allergy Clin Immunol 1997, 100:781–788.
This study demonstrates that treating allergic rhinitis with an antihistamine and decongestant can also improve symptoms of asthma, pulmonary function, and quality of life.

58. Popa VT: Bronchodilating activity of an H₁ blocker, chlorpheniramine. J Allergy Clin Immunol 1977, 59:54–63.

59. Taytard A, Beaumont D, Pujet JC, et al.: Treatment of bronchial asthma with terfenadine: a randomized controlled trial. Br J Clin Pharmacol 1987, 24:743–746.

60. Raffety P, Jackson L, Smith R, et al.: Terfenadine, a potent H₁ receptor antagonist in the treatment of grass pollen sensitive asthma. Br J Clin Pharmacol 1990, 30:229–235.

61. Clee MD, Ingram CG, Reid PC, et al.: The effect of astemizole on exercise-induced asthma. Br J Dis Chest 1984, 78:180–183.

62. Cistero A, Abadias M, Lieonaart R: Effect of astemizole on allergic asthma. Ann Allergy 1992, 69:123–127.

63. Aubier M, Neukirch C, Melac M: Effect of cetirizine on bronchial hyperresponsiveness in patients with allergic rhinitis [abstract]. J Allergy Clin Immunol 1996, 97:316.

64. Spector SL, Nicodemus CF, Corren J, et al.: Comparison of the bronchodilatory effects of cetirizine, salbuterol, and both together versus placebo in patients with mild to moderate asthma. J Allergy Clin Immunol 1995, 96:174–181.

65. Aaronson DW: Evaluation of cetirizine in patients with allergic rhinitis and perennial asthma. Ann Allergy Asthma Immunol 1996, 76:440–446.

66. Grant JA, Nicodemus CF, Findlay SR, et al.: Cetirizine in patients with seasonal allergic rhinitis and concomitant asthma: prospective, randomized, placebo-controlled trial. J Allergy Clin Immunol 1995, 95:923–932.

67.•• Roquet A, Dahlen B, Kumlin M, et al.: Combined antagonism of leukotrienes and histamine produces predominant inhibition of allergen-induced early and late phase airway obstruction in asthmatics. Am J Resp Crit Care Med 1997, 155:185–186.
This study examines the effects of a second-generation antihistamine, loratadine, alone and in combination with a leukotriene receptor antagonist, zafirlukast, on allergic asthma.

68.•• Kay GG, Plotkin KE, Quig MB, et al.: Sedating effects of AM/PM antihistamine dosing with evening chlorpheniramine and morning terfenadine. Am J Man Care 1997, 3:1843–1848.
This study investigates and clearly demonstrates the carryover sedative effects of giving a sedating antihistamine at bedtime.

69.•• Simons FER: The eternal triangle: benefit, risk, and cost of therapeutic agents. Ann Allergy Asthma Immunol 1996, 77:337–338.
This editorial criticizes employing a sedating antihistamine only for the purpose of cost containment.

70. Goetz DW, Jacobson JM, Murnane JE, et al.: Prolongation of simple and choice reaction times in a double-blind comparison of twice daily hydroxyzine versus terfenadine. J Allergy Clin Immunol 1989, 84:316–322.

71. Seidel WF, Cohem S, Bliwise NG, et al.: Direct measurement of daytime sleepiness after administration of cetirizine and hydroxyzine with a standardized electroencephalographic assessment. J Allergy Clin Immunol 1990, 86:1029–1033.

72. Seidel WF, Cohen S, Bliwise NG, et al.: Cetirizine effects on objective measures of daytime sleepiness and performance. Ann Allergy 1987, 59:58–62.

73. Goetz DW, Jacobson JM, Apaliski SJ, et al.: Objective antihistamine side effects are mitigated by evening dosing of hydroxyzine. Ann Allergy 1991, 67:448–454.

74. Bantz EW, Dolan WK, Chadwick EW, et al.: Chronic chlorpheniramine therapy: subsensitivity, drug metabolism and compliance. Ann Allergy 1987, 59:341–346.

75. International Rhinitis Management Working Group: International Consensus Report on the Diagnosis and Management of Rhinitis. Allergy 1994, 49(suppl):1–34.

CHAPTER 10

Nonallergic rhinitis

Russell A. Settipane

Guy A. Settipane

Nonallergic rhinitis represents a broad classification of nasal diseases that share the occurrence of nasal symptoms without an allergic etiology. As many as half the patients presenting to physicians with chronic nasal symptoms (obstruction/congestion, rhinorrhea, and hyperirritability) may have this disorder [1]. Nasal symptoms may be indistinguishable from those in allergic rhinitis; therefore, negative testing for IgE sensitivity to relevant aeroallergens is necessary to confirm this diagnosis. Nonallergic rhinitis may be subclassified on the basis of various characteristics. These include immunologic/cytologic features [2] (Table 10-1), etiology/systemic disease association (Table 10-2), and frequency of occurrence (Table 10-3). This chapter focuses on frequency of occurrence as it pertains to chronic rhinitis conditions, excluding acute infectious etiologies, such as viral upper respiratory infections and acute bacterial sinusitis. The epidemiology of nonallergic rhinitis is discussed first, followed by a review of the clinical presentation, diagnosis, pathophysiology, and treatment of individual nonallergic rhinitis syndromes. Discussion focuses on common nonallergic rhinitis syndromes, and only briefly reviews uncommon or rare forms of rhinitis.

EPIDEMIOLOGY OF NONALLERGIC RHINITIS

The frequency of nonallergic rhinitis and the different syndromes that comprise this disorder are poorly defined. Mullarkey *et al.* [1] determined that 52% of 142 rhinitis patients seen in an allergy clinic could be classified as having nonallergic rhinitis. Togias [3] found that only 17% of 362 rhinitis patients at an academic allergy clinic had nonallergic rhinitis. Rough data from large population surveys indicate the prevalence of chronic sinusitis to be 13.5% [4] and chronic rhinitis to be 20.4% [5]. Presumably, a substantial portion of subjects surveyed would be more precisely labeled as nonallergic rhinitis if skin testing and sinus imaging were performed. In addition, many of the patients labeled as having allergic rhinitis may have a concomitant nonallergic component to their rhinitis, and therefore represent a mixed rhinitis. The prevalence of nonallergic rhinitis can only be estimated due to the lack of hard data. Based on estimates that 10% to 20% of the population has allergic rhinitis [6,7] and 17% to 52% of all rhinitis sufferers are nonallergic, the prevalence of nonallergic rhinitis may well extend into the tens of millions in the United States alone.

We looked at the breakdown of nonallergic rhinitis in 78 patients, and found nonallergic rhinitis with eosinophils syndrome (NARES) in glucose measurements accurately identify the fluid as CSF if it contains > 30 mg/100 mL glucose. A more specific test for CSF rhinorrhea is β2 transferrin, which has come into common use in recent years [79]. In addition, thin coronal CT, radionuclide cisternography, and magnetic resonance cisternography can help to localize the site of CSF leakage [80].

Foreign bodies in the nose may present as unilateral nasal blockage and purulent nasal discharge. This may be seen not only in children with objects, such as pebbles, erasers, buttons, peas, and beans, but also in hospitalized adults with nasal tubes in place.

Systemic autoimmune/vasculitis diseases, such as Churg-Strauss vasculitis [35], systemic lupus erythematosus, relapsing polychondritis, and Sjögrens syndrome, can also result in rhinitis [35,81–83]. Granulomatous diseases such as sarcoidosis and, more commonly, Wegner's can produce nasal manifestations in a large proportion of affected patients [84,85].

Rhinitis sicca can result from Sjögrens syndrome. It also may occur as a normal part of aging. Treatment with the liberal use of nasal saline sprays is appropriate.

FUTURE AREAS OF STUDY

Little is known as to what extent inflammation may play in nonallergic rhinitis. New information on proinflammatory cytokines, chemokines, regulated upon activation normal T cell expressed and secreted (RANTES), macrophage inflammatory protein (MIP), monocyte chemoattractant protein (MCP), and eotaxin will help to better understand the process of the proinflammatory response [86,87,88•]. Current concepts of inflammation begin with T-helper-2 (T_H2) lymphocyte producing IL-4 and IL-5. IL-5 stimulates eosinophil as well as IgE production. IL-4 also stimulates IgE production. IL-12 and interferon-γ induce the differentiation of T_H1 suppressor cells, which antagonizes the differentiation of T_H2 cells. T_H1 cells are associated with cell-mediated inflammation and T_H2 cells are associated with humoral-mediated allergic inflammation. Development of new drugs to inhibit or enhance cytokines and chemokines will play a significant role on controlling proinflammatory responses and treating many diseases, one of which may be nonallergic rhinitis.

CONCLUSIONS

Nonallergic rhinitis is a common disease entity that can occur in about 50% of all patients with rhinitis. These patients have negative allergy skin tests and normal serum IgE. Symptoms are similar to allergic rhinitis but usually are not associated with sneezing episodes and conjunctival complaints. Nonallergic rhinitis is more frequently found in adults (> 20 years of age) than in children. Common causes of nonallergic rhinitis include

vasomotor, chronic sinusitis, NARES/BENARS, drug-induced pregnancy, nasal polyps, and physical/chemical/irritant triggers. Infrequent causes include aspirin sensitivity, hypothyroidism, atrophic mucosa, CSF rhinorrhea, ciliary dyskinesia, and nasal mastocytosis. The frequency of these causes ranges from vasomotor rhinitis (61%) to hypothyroidism (2%). Treatment of nonallergic rhinitis should be individualized according to patient symptoms and should include antihistamines, decongestants, anticholinergic agents, a trial of nasal steroids, and nasal lavage (saline washing). Experimental medical treatment includes capsaicin and silver nitrate applications. Experimental surgical treatment includes vidian nerve section, electrocoagulation of anterior ethmoidal nerve, sphenopalatine ganglion block, and turbinectomy.

Experimental new drug treatments may include future medications that enhance or inhibit proinflammatory proteins, such as cytokines, chemokines, MIP, MCP, RANTES, and eotaxin.

REFERENCES AND RECOMMENDED READING

Recently published papers of particular interest have been highlighted as:
•   Of interest
••   Of outstanding interest

1. Mullarkey MF, Hill JS, Webb DR: Allergic and nonallergic rhinitis: their characterization with attention to the meaning of nasal eosinophilia. *J Allergy Clin Immunol* 1980, 65:122–126.

2. Zeiger RS: Differential diagnosis and classification of rhinosinusitis. In *Nasal Manifestations of Systemic Diseases.* Edited by Schatz M, Zeiger RS, Settipane GA. Providence, RI: OceanSide Publications; 1991:3–20.

3. Togias A: Age relationships and clinical features of nonallergic rhinitis. *J Allergy Clin Immunol* 1990, 85:182.

4. Moss AJ, Parsons VL: Current estimates from the national health interview survey, United States, 1985: DHHS publication number (PHS)86-1588. Hyattsville, MD: National Center for Health Statistics, 1986:66–67.

5. Turkeltaub PC, Gergen PJ: The prevalence of allergic and nonallergic respiratory symptoms in the US population: data from the second national health and nutrition examination survey 1976–1980 (NHANES II). *J Allergy Clin Immunol* 1988, 81:305.

6. Broder I, Higgins MW, Mathews KP, *et al.*: Epidemiology of asthma and allergic rhinitis in a total community: Tecumseh, Michigan. *J Allergy Clin Immunol* 1974, 54:100–110.

7. Hagy GW, Settipane GA: Prognosis of positive allergy skin tests in an asymptomatic population. *J Allergy* 1971, 48:200–211.

8. Settipane GA, Klein DE: Nonallergic rhinitis: dermography of eosinophils in nasal smear, blood total eosinophil counts and IgE levels. *NER Allergy Proc* 1985, 6:363–366.

9. Mygind N: Definition, classification, terminology. In *Allergic and Nonallergic Rhinitis: Clinical Aspects.* Copenhagen: Munksgaard; 1993:11–14.

10. Lindberg S, Malm L: Comparison of allergic rhinitis and vasomotor rhinitis patients on the basis of a computer questionnaire. *Allergy* 1993, 48:602–607.

11. Borum P: Nasal methacholine challenge. *J Allergy Clin Immunol* 1979, 63:253–257.

12. Stjärne P, Lundblad L, Änggard A, *et al.*: Local capsaicin treatment of the nasal mucosa reduces symptoms in patients with nonallergic nasal hyperreactivity. *Am J Rhinol* 1991, 5:145–151.

13. Togias A, Proud D, Kagey-Sobotka A, *et al.*: Cold dry air (CDA) and histamine (HIST) induce more potent responses in perennial rhinitis compared to normal individuals. *J Allergy Clin Immunol* 1991, 87:148.

14. Berger G, Marom Z, Ophir D: Goblet cell density of the inferior turbinates in patients with perennial allergic and nonallergic rhinitis. *Am J Rhinol* 1997, 11:233–236.

15. Berger G, Goldberg A, Ophir D: The inferior turbinate mast cell population of patients with perennial allergic and nonallergic rhinitis. *Am J Rhinol* 1997, 11:63–66.

16.• Grossman J, Banov C, Boggs P, *et al.*: Use of ipratropium bromide in chronic treatment of nonallergic perennial rhinitis, alone and in combination with other perennial rhinitis combinations. *J Allergy Clin Immunol* 1995, 95:1123–1127.
This paper demonstrates that added effectiveness may be obtained by combining ipratropium bromide and corticosteroid nasal spray therapy.

17.• Bronsky EA, Druce H, Findlay SR, Hampel FC: A clinical trial of ipratropium bromide nasal spray in patients with perennial nonallergic rhinitis. *J Allergy Clin Immunol* 1995, 95:1117–1122.
This is one of the primary references demonstrating the effectiveness of ipratropium bromide for treatment of perennial nonallergic rhinitis.

18. Malm L, Wihl J: Intranasal beclomethasone dipropionate in vasomotor rhinitis. *Acta Allergol* 1976, 31:245–253.

19. Wight RG, Jones AS, Beckingham E, *et al.*: A double-blind comparison of intranasal budesonide 400 micrograms and 800 micrograms in perennial rhinitis. *Clin Otolaryngol* 1992, 17:354–358.

20. Small P, Black M, Frenkiel S: Effects of treatment with beclomethasone dipropionate in subpopulations of perennial rhinitis patients. *J Allergy Clin Immunol* 1982, 70:178–182.

21. Bhargava KB, Shirali GN, Abhyankar US, Gadre KC: Treatment of allergic and vasomotor rhinitis by the local application of different concentrations of silver nitrate. *J Laryngol Otol* 1992, 106:699–701.

22. Samarrae SM: Treatment of vasomotor rhinitis by the local application of silver nitrate. *J Laryngol Otol* 1991, 105:285–287.

23. Guindy A: Endoscopic transseptal vidian neurectomy. *Arch Otolaryngol Head Neck Surg* 1994, 120:1347–1351

24. Dong Z: Anterior ethmoidal electrocoagulation in the treatment of vasomotor rhinitis. *Chung Hua Erh Pi Yen Hou Ko Tsa Chih* 1991, 26:358–359.

25. Fernandes CM: Bilateral transnasal vidian neurectomy in the management of chronic rhinitis. *J Laryngol Otol* 1994, 108:569–573.

26. Prasanna A, Murthy PS: Vasomotor rhinitis and sphenopalatine ganglion block. *J Pain Symptom Manage* 1997, 13:332–338.

27. Mladina R, Risavi R, Subaric M: CO_2 laser anterior turbinectomy in the treatment of nonallergic vasomotor rhinopathia. A prospective study upon 78 patients. *Rhinology* 1991, 29:267–271.

28. NIAID Task Force Report: Asthma and the other allergic diseases: National Institutes of Health publication 79-387. Washington, DC: US Department of Health, Education and Welfare; 1979:23–31.

29.• Lund VJ, Kennedy DW: Quantification for staging sinusitis. *Ann Otol Rhinol Laryngol* 1995, 104(suppl):17–21.
This paper proposes definitions for chronic sinusitis in adult and pediatric populations.

30. Gwaltney JM Jr: Microbiology of sinusitis. In *Sinusitis*. Edited by Druce HM. New York: Marcel Dekker; 1994:41–56.

31. Stierna P, Carlsoo B: Histopathological observations in chronic maxillary sinusitis. *Acta Otolaryngol (Stockh)* 1990, 110:450–458.

32. Georgitis JW, Matthews BL, Stone B: Chronic sinusitis: characterization of cellular influx and inflammatory mediators in sinus lavage fluid. *Int Arch Allergy Immunol* 1995, 106:416–421.

33. Jacobs RL, Freedman PM, Boswell RN: Nonallergic rhinitis with nasal eosinophilia (NARES syndrome). *J Allergy Clin Immunol* 1981, 67:253–262.

34. Sobol SM, Love RG, Stutman HR, Pysher TJ: Phaeohyphomycosis of the maxilloethmoid sinus caused by *Drechslera spicifera*: a new fungal pathogen. *Laryngoscope* 1984, 94:620–627.

35. Olsen KD, Neel HB, DeRemee RA, Weiland LH: Nasal manifestations of allergic granulomatosis and angiitis (Churg-Strauss syndrome). *Otolaryngol Head Neck Surg* 1980, 88:85–89.

36. Moneret-Vautrin DA, Hsieh V, Wayoff M, *et al.*: Nonallergic rhinitis with eosinophilia syndrome a precursor of the triad: nasal polyposis, intrinsic asthma, and intolerance to aspirin. *Ann Allergy* 1990, 64:513–518.

37. Bousquet J, Chanez P, Lacoste JY, *et al.*: Eosinophilic inflammation in asthma. *N Engl J Med* 1990, 323:1033–1039.

38. Hastie AT, Loegering DA, Gleich GJ, Kueppers F: The effect of purified human eosinophil major basic protein on mammalian ciliary activity. *Am Rev Respir Dis* 1987, 135:848–853.

39. Flavahan NA, Slifman NR, Gleich GJ, Vanhoutte PM: Human eosinophil major basic protein causes hyperreactivity of respiratory smooth muscle. *Am Rev Respir Dis* 1988, 138:685–688.

40. Venge P, Dahl R, Fredens K, Peteerson CGB: Epithelial injury by human eosinophil. *Am Rev Respir Dis* 1988, 138:S54–S57.

41. Spector SL, English G, Jones L: Clinical and nasal biopsy response to treatment of perennial rhinitis. *J Allergy Clin Immunol* 1980, 66:129–137.

42. Ayars GH, Altman LC, McManus MM, *et al.*: Injurious effect of the eosinophil peroxide-hydrogen peroxide-halide system and major basic protein on human nasal epithelium in vitro. *Am Rev Respir Dis* 1989, 140:125–131.

43. Davidson AE, Miller SD, Settipane RJ, *et al.*: Delayed nasal mucociliary clearance in patients with nonallergic rhinitis and nasal eosinophilia. *Allergy Proc* 1992, 13:81–84.

44. Settipane GA: Nasal manifestations of systemic diseases. In *Rhinitis*, edn 2. Providence, RI: OceanSide Publications; 1991:197–208.

45. Graf P, Hallen H, Juto-Je: The pathophysiology and treatment of rhinitis medicamentosa. *Clin Otolaryngol* 1995, 20:224–229.

46. Incaudo GA, Schatz M: Rhinosinusitis associated with endocrine conditions: hypothyroidism and pregnancy. In *Nasal Manifestations of Systemic Diseases*. Edited by Schatz M, Zeiger RS, Settipane GA. Providence, RI: OceanSide Publications; 1991:53–62.

47. Toppozada H, Michaels L, Toppazada M, *et al.*: The human respiratory nasal mucosa in pregnancy. *J Larynol Otol* 1982, 96:613–626.

most relevant allergens and preservation of allergenicity. Successful immunotherapy requires high-quality allergenic extracts, standardized for lot-to-lot and manufacturer-to-manufacturer consistency [3••].

The naming of allergens is based on a convention using the first three letters of the genus, the first letter of the species, and numeration of distinct allergens. For example, the most important allergen thought to derive from cats is Fel d 1. Similarly, the predominant allergens for sensitivity to the dust mite species growing in humid climates are Der p 1 and 2. Finally, the principle allergen in short ragweed is Amb a 1.

Considerable strides have been made in allergen evaluation through introduction of new molecular techniques. The protein structure of several allergens has been determined and this data can be retrieved from the Allergen Database [5]. In addition, several allergens have been cloned and have become available in large quantities through recombinant technology [6,7]. Monoclonal and polyclonal antibodies to major allergens have improved quantitation of allergens by immunochemical analysis. In vitro evaluations have permitted determination of the antibody-combining sites of allergens, referred to as *B-cell epitopes*. Furthermore, it has been possible in some situations to define major allergen peptides recognized by T cells, ie, the T-cell epitopes [8,9].

Standardization of allergens is a vital requisite for safe and effective immunotherapy. To ensure consistency, the prescribing physician must know the most relevant allergens present and their concentration. Comparisons are often made to standardized preparations, and recombinant sources of several allergens should improve the reliability of standards [3••]. Current methods for standardization include detection of IgE antibodies to allergens both in vivo and in vitro. Skin testing remains a popular technique for comparison of the total allergenic potency of extracts; end point titration is a standard of the United States Food and Drug Administration (FDA) [10,11]. Other biologic techniques include bronchial or nasal inhalation challenge and histamine release from basophils. The most commonly used in vitro techniques are radioallergosorbent test (RAST) inhibition and direct immunoassays. The availability of recombinant allergens has increased the precision of standardization. One major breakthrough in standardization is the ability to measure the concentration of major allergens in an extract. Examples include determining the amounts of Der p 1 in house dust-mite extracts, Fel d 1 in cat dander extracts, and Amb a 1 in ragweed pollen extracts.

MECHANISMS OF IMMUNOTHERAPY

Many investigations have evaluated mechanisms for immunotherapy. Initially, modulation of circulating antibodies and changes in effector cells were thought the most important changes. However, recent studies have emphasized the modulation of cytokines and T-cell response.

Modulation of the humoral response

Effective immunotherapy induces an increase in IgG that may block antibodies, preventing the combination of allergen with IgE [12]. A definite quantitative relationship exists between the dose of allergen administered and the levels of allergen-specific IgG. Golden *et al.* [13•] showed the clinical relevance of the venom-specific IgG antibody levels during immunotherapy. Probably the chief value of measuring total IgG levels is to ensure that a significant dose of allergens has been used for immunotherapy. Absolute levels correlate poorly with the clinical response, however, except perhaps in venom immunotherapy. Specific subclasses of IgG have been monitored during immunotherapy, but the relevance of these investigations remains controversial.

Although a rise in serum allergen-specific IgE is noticed initially, prolonged immunotherapy effects a gradual decline over several years [14,15]. Furthermore, the seasonal rise in IgE is blunted. Despite the elevated IgE level, histamine release from basophils and target organ sensitivity tend to decrease with effective immunotherapy [16]. This finding suggests that the reduced biologic responses are unrelated to antibody levels. Increased levels of soluble CD23, the low-affinity receptor for IgE, have been observed in serum of atopic children and adults with allergic rhinitis and asthma. Based on this observation, it was postulated that some down-regulation of soluble CD23 might occur during immunotherapy. Jung *et al.* [17] reported a reduction in CD23 expression on peripheral B cells correlates with successful immunotherapy in grass pollinosis.

Modulation of the cellular response

One effect of prolonged immunotherapy is reduction in the numbers of mast cells and eosinophils in respiratory tissues [18,19]. Another reduction occurs in the release of mediators from IgE-sensitized mast cells and basophils. The recruitment of inflammatory cells into sites of allergic inflammation is also affected. Changes in lymphocyte response were postulated by Rocklin and Sheffer [20]. They described production of CD8+ suppressor T cells during effective immunotherapy. Increased levels in CD8+ cells have been observed [21].

Cytokines have a fundamental role in regulating the maturation, recruitment, and activation of cells during allergic inflammatory responses. Much attention has been focused on changes in cytokine levels and in the cells producing them through effective immunotherapy [22]. These changes in cytokine responses probably have fundamental effects on the end-organ response to allergens. The first cytokine linked to allergic reactions was histamine-releasing factor (HRF) [23]. Kuna *et al.* [24] showed that immunotherapy suppresses the production of allergen-stimulated HRF in patients experiencing clinical benefits. It is now clear that the principal HRFs synthesized by mononuclear cells are members of the beta (Cys-Cys) family of chemokines. Monocyte chemoattractant peptide-1 (MCP-1) is the most potent chemokine, inducing release of histamine from basophils [25]. Hsieh *et al.* [26] demonstrated reduced synthesis of MCP-1 after immunotherapy.

One fundamental advance in understanding the roles of cytokines was the description of two classes of T-helper (T_H) cells [27]. T_H1 cells synthesize interferon (IFN)-γ, interleukin (IL)-2, tumor necrosis factor (TNF)-β, and other cytokines. In contrast, T_H2 cells produce IL-4, IL-5, IL-9, IL-10, and IL-13. Production of IL-12 by macrophages drives naive cells to differentiate into T_H1 cells, whereas IL-4 stimulates growth of T_H2 cells. T_H2 cells and the cytokines released by these cells are fundamentally linked to development of allergic inflammation through recruitment of inflammatory cells and synthesis of IgE.

A potential goal of immunotherapy is the induction of T_H1 cellular activity with a concomitant reduction in T_H2 cellular activity. Grass pollen immunotherapy inhibits allergen-induced infiltration of CD4+ T lymphocytes and eosinophils into the nasal mucosa and increases the number of cells expressing messenger RNA for IFN-γ, a marker of increase in T_H1 cells [28]. The same results were also manifest in an allergen-induced cutaneous late phase response (LPR) [29]. These changes are accompanied by increased CD4+ cells expressing IFN-γ and a late increase in IFN-γ cells (Fig. 11-1). These immunologic responses were correlated with improvement in clinical responses as assessed by seasonal symptoms and medication requirements (Fig. 11-2). Hamid *et al.* [30•] also showed that the late-phase increase in cells expressed IL-12. Indeed, a reciprocal number of cells expressed IL-12 and IL-4, and a direct correlation was shown between IL-12+ and IFN-γ+ cells (Fig. 11-3). This observation suggests that IL-12 is a driving force for localization of T_H1 cells synthesizing IFN-γ. Other studies have confirmed that immunotherapy reduces T_H2 cells and associated synthesis of cytokines, such as IL-4, made by these cells, along with an increase in synthesis of IFN-γ [22,31].

Modulation of the in vivo response to allergens

Effective immunotherapy is correlated with a reduction in both mucosal and cutaneous responses to allergen challenge [19,28,29,30•]. Both the immediate and late-phase response to allergen skin testing is dramatically reduced (Fig. 11-4). Bronchial late-phase response in asthma with allergen immunotherapy is also reduced.

The hallmark of the late-phase response is the infiltration of eosinophils, which could be a possible cellular target for immunotherapy [19]. It has been shown that immunotherapy can decrease the mast cells in nasal brushing in mite-sensitive children [32]. Conventional immunotherapy inhibits immediate release of mast cell mediators [33] and eosinophil numbers in allergen-stimulated nasal lavage in ragweed sensitive patients [19, 34]. Rak *et al.* [35] demonstrated the inhibitory effects of birch pollen immunotherapy on seasonal increases in bronchial responsiveness to histamine and associated increases in eosinophils and eosinophil cationic protein concentrations in bronchoalveolar lavage fluid during the peak pollen season.

EFFICACY OF IMMUNOTHERAPY

The predominant technique for allergen immunotherapy currently in use is administration of allergens through periodic subcutaneous injections. Controlled evaluations

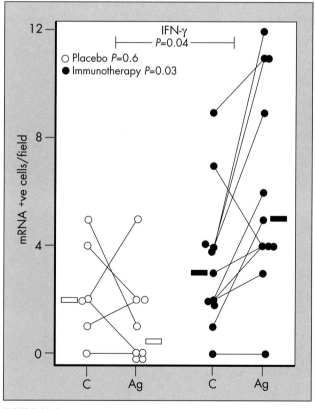

FIGURE 11-1.

In situ hybridization of nasal biopsy specimens with an antisense riboprobe against mRNA for IFN-γ. The difference in mRNA+ cell counts (24 hours after allergen challenge minus counts 24 hours after a control challenge with allergen diluent) for immunotherapy-treated (solid circles) patients were significant using the Mann-Whitney U test. In-group comparisons were performed using the Wilcoxon test. Ag—allergen challenge; C—control challenge. (*Adapted from* Durham *et al.* [28]; with permission.)

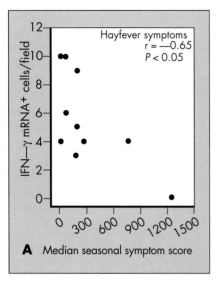

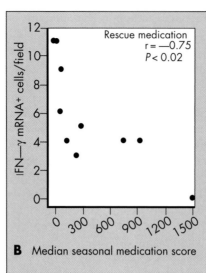

FIGURE 11-2.
Relationship between allergen-induced IFN-γ mRNA+ cells in the nasal mucosa of immunotherapy-treated patients and seasonal hay fever symptoms (area under curve, **A**) and medication (topical cromolyn sodium applied to nose and eyes and oral antihistamine [acrivastine] tablets, **B**) during the 11-week pollen season. (*Adapted from* Durham *et al.* [28]; with permission.)

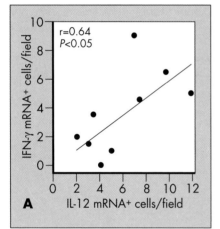

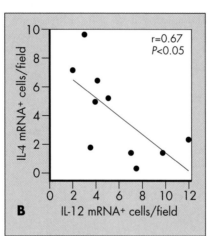

FIGURE 11-3.
Correlations between IL-12 mRNA+ cells and IFN-γ+ (**A**) and IL-4+ (**B**) cells at allergen-challenged sites in patients receiving immunotherapy. (*Adapted from* Hamid *et al.* [30●]; with permission.)

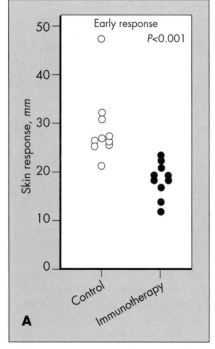

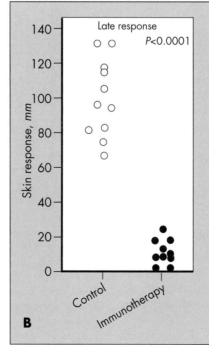

FIGURE 11-4.
Size of early (15 minute, **A**) and late (24 hour, **B**) skin responses after intradermal allergen in control and immunotherapy-treated patients. (*Adapted from* Hamid *et al.* [30●]; with permission.)

showing efficacy of this mode of treatment began appearing after the middle of this century. In the United States, the frequency of injections is usually once or twice weekly during the build-up stage to a maintenance dosage after which injections may be given at longer intervals [2•]. In contrast, the schedule adopted for administration of insect venoms has been referred to as a *clustered rush procedure*. Patients receive several injections of venom at rapidly increasing concentrations at periodic visits and reach maintenance levels within a shorter time. In Europe, it is common for patients to initiate immunotherapy by receiving several injections in 1 to 3 days; this is referred to as *rush immunotherapy* [3••].

Parenteral immunotherapy necessitates frequent visits for injections that may be uncomfortable and associated with other adverse reactions. Thus, other routes have been evaluated. A considerable amount of literature exists regarding topical immunotherapy with allergens delivered intranasally, orally, sublingually, and by inhalation modalities. This subject has been reviewed recently [3••], but because it is not currently practiced to any extent in the United States, it is not considered further in this chapter.

Immunotherapy for respiratory allergic disorders

Most patients receiving immunotherapy suffer from respiratory allergic disorders. The allergens that have been evaluated in controlled studies are outlined in Table 11-1. Also documented are investigations of both allergic rhinitis and asthma. The value of immunotherapy for rhinitis that is not adequately responsive to avoidance and pharmacotherapy is undisputed. Immunotherapy is the only procedure that anticipates significant reduction in target-organ sensitivity over time. Many double-blind controlled trials have shown the efficacy of immunotherapy in allergic rhinitis and conjunctivitis secondary to grass and ragweed [3••,18,28,29,30•,36–39]. A limited number of investigations have been conducted for alleviation of rhinitis due to other pollen, fungal, and mite allergens [3••,40,41].

The use of allergen immunotherapy in asthma is more controversial. There have been a reasonable number of controlled trials with pollen allergens, predominantly the grasses [42•,43,44]. Other trials have been conducted with dust mites [45–50]. When avoidance can not be practiced, as in the home of cat-sensitive patients, the value of immunotherapy has been shown by controlled trials [51–54].

Abramson *et al.* [55••] performed a meta-analysis of randomized placebo-controlled double-blind trials of allergen immunotherapy for asthma that were published between 1966 and 1990. Twenty trials met the rigid standards set by the authors. The parameters evaluated included asthmatic symptoms, medication usage, spirometry, and bronchial hyperreactivity. Improvement

was found for all four parameters. The authors considered whether there were a significant number of unpublished negative trials that might overestimate the benefit of immunotherapy for asthma. They estimated another 33 negative studies would be required to overturn the positive evaluations they calculated from published trials. The authors concluded that "allergen immunotherapy is a treatment option in highly selected patients with extrinsic (allergic) asthma" [55••]. Sigman and Mazer [56] reviewed pediatric literature from 1966 to 1994 to evaluate the clinical efficacy of immunotherapy in childhood asthma and identified twelve purely pediatric studies. Most reports described an improvement in asthmatic symptoms or a decrease in bronchial reactivity.

Two American studies of immunotherapy have been published recently that have attracted considerable attention. Creticos *et al.* [42•] reported a multicenter evaluation of ragweed immunotherapy for asthma. Approximately 1000 individuals were screened initially and 127 started the first year of observation, but only 90 met inclusion criteria to begin the controlled phase of immunotherapy for 2 years. Of this group, 77 completed the first year and 53 the second. A significant improvement in peak flow was seen in both years. Medication use improved in the first, but not the second, year. Clinical symptoms were not significantly different. Our institution participated in a companion trial of allergen immunotherapy with dust mites in asthma, but we suffered even greater attrition of patients during the prolonged protocol. The retained trial group was too small to make an appropriate analysis. These experiences document the difficulties involved in conducting well-controlled trials of immunotherapy in asthma.

Most well-controlled trials of immunotherapy have been conducted with one allergen or a limited panel of allergens, and this is the case of the reports documented in Table 11-1. However, in the United States, the standard of practice is to use a multiplicity of allergens. Adkinson *et al.* [57] conducted a double-blind, placebo-controlled trial of multiple-allergen immunotherapy in 121 children with moderate-to-severe perennial extrinsic asthma. All required daily medication and were assigned to receive subcutaneous injections of placebo or up to seven aeroallergens at maintenance levels for at least 18 months. Children were seen every 2 to 3 weeks for careful management, including adjustment of medications and avoidance measures. Compliance was high. Overall, no differences were found between the two groups. Bousquet *et al.* [36] have also cast doubt on the value of immunotherapy with multiple allergens. The landmark study of Adkinson has received many comments, and perhaps it shows the tremendous power of careful management of asthmatic children by highly competent physicians. In such a situation, the added benefit of immunotherapy may be small. However, in the real

Table 11-1. CONTROLLED STUDIES SHOWING EFFICACY OF ALLERGEN IMMUNOTHERAPY

	Rhinitis	Asthma
Allergen		
Grasses	X	X
Ragweed	X	X
Mountain cedar	X	X
Parietaria	X	
Fungi		
Cladosporium	X	X
Alternaria	X	X
Mites	X	X
Animals		
Dog		X
Cat		X

Adapted from *Bousquet* et al. *[3••] and Weber [4•].*

world, standards for managing patients with asthma rarely reach those achieved by Adkinson, so the precise place of immunotherapy and of multiple-allergen immunotherapy for asthma remains to be adequately evaluated. Clearly, the practitioner should select asthmatic patients carefully for trials of immunotherapy. In all situations, carefully designed avoidance of offending allergens and use of pharmacotherapy is indicated.

Hymenoptera sting immunotherapy

Stings by members of the Hymenoptera family account for a significant number of deaths and life-threatening anaphylactic reactions annually. Hunt *et al.* [58] demonstrated the value of immunotherapy with venoms over the classical formulations prepared from the whole bodies of insects. Commercial venom extracts are available for honeybee, wasp, hornet, and yellowjacket venoms. Several well-controlled trials have demonstrated the efficacy of these venoms for treating IgE-mediated anaphylaxis [59–63,64•,65]. Stings caused by imported fire ants are still treated with whole-body extracts, in which efficacy has been demonstrated [66]. Patients who have experienced significant cardiorespiratory symptoms are candidates for insect immunotherapy. In children, however, reactions involving only cutaneous reactions have been shown to have a low risk of progression with future stings to life-threatening reactions; thus, immunotherapy is not thought necessary under these circumstances [61].

Immunotherapy for food allergy

Anaphylactic reactions to foods are common and may occasionally be fatal. One particularly troublesome sensi-

tivity in the United States is to peanut, because this food is so often used as filler even when not identified in labeling. A significant number of unanticipated deaths from peanut hypersensitivity have been reported, especially in children. For this reason, trials of peanut immunotherapy have been undertaken to achieve protection from the dreadful consequences of peanut hypersensitivity. A controlled study showed decreased skin-prick test reactions to peanut and decreased sensitivity to ingestion of peanut in double-blind, placebo-controlled oral challenge [67]. Another double-blind, placebo-controlled study was designed to evaluate the long-term effects of the peanut immunotherapy [68]. It was concluded that immunotherapy with peanut extract increased the tolerance of patients to oral challenge to peanut; however, it resulted in repeated systemic reactions in most patients even on maintenance injections. Further studies will be required, perhaps using a modified peanut extract, to reduce the frequency of reactions to injections before immunotherapy can be recommended for this and other food allergies.

PRACTICAL ISSUES IN IMMUNOTHERAPY
Selection of patients

Immunotherapy is clearly indicated for patients who have experienced life-threatening reactions to insect stings. The value of this modality for patients with significant upper respiratory symptoms related to aeroallergens is also undisputed. This is the only treatment offering a significant long-term reduction in symptoms as well as the need for time-consuming avoidance procedures and expensive pharmacotherapy. The role for patients with asthma is more complex, but its use in selected patients is indicated by studies outlined earlier [42–56].

Selection of allergenic extracts

The extracts most frequently used in the United States are prepared by aqueous extraction of appropriate source materials. Standardized extracts are highly desirable to ensure reduced variation among lots and manufacturers. Lyophilized extracts can be stored for extended periods before reconstitution. Moreover, commercial extracts are prepared in glycerin to extend potency. Addition of albumin to aqueous solutions also fosters preservation of potency by reducing protein-binding to glass. In all circumstances, extracts should be kept refrigerated to reduce losses. Highly concentrated extracts have increased stability. When highly diluted preparations are made for initiating immunotherapy, strict labeling with short periods before expiration is essential. Finally, care must be taken in mixing certain extracts, because preliminary description of proteases has been found in certain allergens.

A variety of modified extracts has been developed with the anticipation of reducing immediate reactions without reducing the long-term efficacy [3••]. Several of these products are popular in other countries, but the most frequently used extracts in the United States are unmodified aqueous extracts. One technique for modification is the absorption of allergens to carriers such as aluminum and tyrosine [69]. Another procedure involves the cross-linking of allergens with formaldehyde [38,39] or glutaraldehyde [37].

As emphasized previously, most of the controlled trials of immunotherapy have been conducted with only a single or limited number of aeroallergens. In this manner, the therapeutic dose can be optimized. Unfortunately, it is more common in the United States to use a multiplicity of allergens, and this may seriously limit the effectiveness of the dose reached for individual allergens. For this reason, the allergist should carefully select the most critical allergens for inclusion in immunotherapy based on clinical history, knowledge of local allergens, and positive testing for sensitivity.

Risks versus benefits

The chief benefits anticipated from immunotherapy are reductions in the frequency and severity of reactions and the need for avoidance and pharmacotherapy. The most frequent side effect is local reactions at the site of injection, but this does not predict the likelihood of systemic reactions. Most systemic reactions occur within 20 minutes after injection; therefore, patients must be carefully monitored for at least this time period [70,71]. The risk of fatal reactions is low and has been estimated at about one in every two million injections [72,73]. No data suggest the likelihood of immunotherapy inducing autoimmune disorders. Risk factors for systemic reactions include patients with symptomatic asthma, highly sensitive patients, introduction of a new vaccine vial, dosing errors, injections during the pollen season, short stay after injection, and use of concomitant medications such as β-blockers [2•,3••,4•,70–75].

Guidelines for optimal immunotherapy

Recommended guidelines for improving the benefit of immunotherapy and reducing the risk are give in Table 11-2. Although self-administration of allergens has been used in some practices, this procedure is rarely warranted [71]. It is not possible for the prescribing allergist to administer all injections, so a close relationship with the medical facility where injections will be given is essential. The physician supervising the administration of extracts and the office personnel involved must be familiar with the risks of immunotherapy and be able to recognize anaphylaxis and respond appropriately. Patients should be interviewed carefully before each injection for prior systemic symptoms, allergic symptoms, and changes in medications, especially institution of β-blockers. Dosing regimens must be modified when

patients experience systemic reactions. The necessary equipment and drugs have been recommended by the American Academy of Asthma Allergy and Immunology [71]. The waiting time of at least 20 minutes must be carefully monitored. In our practice, all patients receive a routine prescription for injectable epinephrine and antihistamines for self-administration if a systemic reaction occurs after leaving the clinic. All patients with asthma have peak flow monitored before each visit, and the injection is withheld if values fall below 70% of personal best.

Several studies with standardized allergens show the optimal maintenance dose should be between 5 and 20 µg of the major allergen in each injection [3••,19,52,58,59,76–78]. This dose is associated with significant clinical improvement, although systemic reactions would require a lower dose. Lower doses do not improve clinical symptoms or reduce sensitivity to allergen challenge in experimental protocols [19].

The length of time for which patients should receive immunotherapy has been evaluated in several controlled studies. Perhaps the best available data concern venoms. For prevention of anaphylaxis, immunotherapy should

Table 11-2. GUIDELINES FOR OPTIMAL ALLERGEN INJECTION IMMUNOTHERAPY

1. Follow strict criteria for selecting candidates for immunotherapy
2. Obtain written informed consent
3. Maintain close cooperation between the allergist and the physician who is administering injections, with actual administration only under medical supervision
4. Select allergens based on demonstrated sensitivity (usually positive skin tests) and clinical relevance
5. Carefully prepare and store extracts with conservative expiration dates
6. Carefully monitor side effects from immunotherapy, drug usage, and clinical response; ask patients at each visit about reactions to previous injection and use of new drugs since last visit
7. Follow established protocols for adjustment of dosage when systemic reactions occur
8. Make certain that drugs and equipment for treatment of anaphylaxis are available and that personnel know how to treat anaphylaxis
9. Prescribe epinephrine and antihistamines to be carried by patients receiving immunotherapy
10. Measure peak flow routinely before injections in patients with asthma and omit injections if values are less than 70% of personal best
11. Require patients to remain at medical facility for at least 20 minutes
12. Increase dosage to a maintenance dose of 5 to 20 µg of each relevant allergen
13. Obtain commitment of patient to continue maintenance immunotherapy for at least 3 to 5 years

be given for at least 3 to 5 years. Indications are good that it may be safe to discontinue treatment at that point in selected patients [63,64•,65]. However, patients with severe reactions before immunotherapy may be more prone to systemic reactions after discontinuation. Similar studies support the same recommendations for other allergens [19,69,79,80•,81]. Furthermore, indications exist of persistence of protection several years after discontinuation on immunotherapy.

FUTURE TRENDS IN IMMUNOTHERAPY
Modulation of T-cell response and cytokines

Vogel [82••] recently reviewed potential new therapies for asthma involving modulation of the immune system through means other than allergen injection therapy. It appears likely that a change in the profile of the cellular response to allergens from predominantly T_H2 to T_H1 would be useful, and Durham [28] has suggested that this is the major effect of conventional allergen injection therapy. One novel concept proposed by Spiegelberg et al. [83] is the use of plasmid DNA for antigens, rather than proteins, for immunotherapy. They have had preliminary success in achieving a protracted shift to T_H1. Immunization with plasmid DNA encoding for allergens will be a promising approach for treating allergic diseases. Another approach involves injection of modified allergen peptides designed to modify the T-cell response without inducing an IgE response with systemic reactions [84]. Peptides derived from the major cat allergens have been used successfully in initial trials [85]. Finally, allergens can be delivered with new techniques such as liposomes [86] or other microencapsulation devices [87] to reduce the potential for allergic responses.

It is likely that certain cytokines are critical for induction of the allergic response, and that blocking them would achieve clinical benefit. Injection of antibody to IL-5 has been shown to reduce the recruitment of eosinophils following allergen exposure for several weeks [88]. Another approach for antagonism of cytokines is the use of soluble receptors, which has been used with success in initial trials of soluble receptors for IL-1 and IL-4 [89,90]. The main concern is that interference with the function of these cytokines has unanticipated side effects, perhaps by interfering with critical elements of host-defense.

Some cytokines are antagonistic of allergic inflammation. Sur et al. [91] have successfully blocked allergic lung inflammatory responses in rodents by administering IL-12, but it is obvious that the timing of IL-12 administration relative to sensitization and allergen challenge is critical. Furthermore, this cytokine may prove too toxic to administer in doses sufficient to achieve reduction in allergic responses.

A recent report describes use of synthetic CpG oligodeoxynucleotides to shift the response from T_H2 to T_H1 [92]. Trials of this technique to block allergic inflammation will be of great interest.

The critical role of IgE in allergic reactions has served as a stimulus for modulation of this antibody response. Vassella et al. [93] observed that predisposition to atopic diseases is lower in those individuals who have high level of anti-IgE antibodies at birth. Recently, humanized antibodies derived from mouse monoclonal antibodies to human IgE have been developed with specificity for the region binding to FcεRI. The antibody has been shown to bind to free IgE, blocking its binding to FcεRI. Furthermore, the antibody does not bind to IgE-FcεRI complexes on mast cells and basophils, and it does not trigger mediator release. In preliminary trials, this antibody has been beneficial in asthma [94•,95•] and rhinitis [96].

REFERENCES AND RECOMMENDED READING

Recently published papers of particular interest have been highlighted as:
•   Of interest
••   Of outstanding interest

1.   Noon L: Prophylactic inoculation against hay fever. *Lancet* 1911, 1:1572–1573.

2.•   Nicklas RA, Bernstein LI, Blessing-Moore J: Practice parameters for allergen immunotherapy. *J Allergy Clin Immunol* 1996, 98:1–11.
This review gives the consensus of the two American allergy societies for immunotherapy.

3.•• Bousquet J, Lockey R, Malling HJ: Allergen immunotherapy: therapeutic vaccines for allergic diseases: WHO position paper. *Allergy* 1998: in press.
This comprehensive review and update gives the most complete review of current literature and international consensus for management of immunotherapy.

4.•   Weber RW: Immunotherapy with allergens. *JAMA* 1997, 278:1881–1887.
This is an excellent chapter on immunotherapy appearing in the recently revised Primer on Alleric and Immunologic Diseases.

5.   Marsh DG, Freidhoff LR: ALBE: an allergen database. Computerized database, edn 1. Baltimore: International Union of Immunological Societies, 1992.

6.   Chapman MD, Smith AM, Vailes LD, et al.: Recombinant mite allergens: new technologies for the management of patients with asthma. *Allergy* 1997, 52:374–79.

7.   Valenta R, Flicker S, Eibensteiner PB, et al.: Recombinant allergen-specific antibody fragments: tools for diagnosis, prevention and therapy of type-I allergy. *Biol Chem* 1997, 378:745–749.

8.   Schramm G, Bufe A, Petersen A, et al.: Mapping of IgE-binding epitopes on the recombinant major group I allergen of velvet grass pollen, rHol l 1. *J Allergy Clin Immunol* 1997, 99:781–787.

9.   Bousquet J, Des Roches A, Paradis L: Clinical use of recombinant allergens and epitopes. *Adv Exp Med Biol* 1996, 409:463–469.

10. Turkeltaub PC, Campbell G, Mosimann JE: Comparative safety and efficacy of short ragweed extracts differing in potency and composition in the treatment of fall hay fever: use of allergenically bioequivalent doses by parallel line bioassay to evaluate comparative safety and efficacy. *Allergy* 1990, 45:528–546.

11. Van Metre TE Jr, Adkinson NF Jr, Kagey-Sobotka A, *et al.*: How should we use skin testing to quantify IgE sensitivity?. *J Allergy Clin Immunol* 1990, 86:583–586.

12. Leynadier F, Abuaf N, Halpern GM, *et al.*: Blocking IgG antibodies after rush immunotherapy with mites. *Ann Allergy* 1986, 57:325–29.

13.• Golden DB, Meyers DA, Kagey-Sobotka A, *et al.*: Clinical relevance of the venom-specific immunoglobulin G antibody level during immunotherapy. *J Allergy Clin Immunol* 1996, 109:369–375.
This is an excellent evaluation of the use of IgG antibodies in insect venom immunotherapy.

14. Gleich GJ, Zimmermann EM, Henderson LL, Yunginger JW: Effect of immunotherapy on immunoglobulin E and immunoglobulin G antibodies to ragweed antigens: a six-year prospective study. *J Allergy Clin Immunol* 1982, 70:261–271.

15. Peng Z, Naclerio RM, Norman PS, *et al.*: Quantitative IgE- and IgG-subclass responses during and after long-term ragweed immunotherapy. *J Allergy Clin Immunol* 1992, 89:519–529.

16. Malling HJ, Skov PS, Permin H, *et al.*: Basophil histamine release and humoral changes during immunotherapy: dissociation between basophil-bound specific IgE, serum value, and cell sensitivity. *Allergy* 1982, 37:187–190.

17. Jung CM, Prinz JC, Rieber EP, *et al.*: A reduction in allergen-induced FcεRII/CD23 expression on peripheral B cells correlates with successful hyposensitization in grass pollinosis. *J Allergy Clin Immunol* 1995, 25:10–14.

18. Hedlin G, Silber G, Naclerio R, *et al.*: Comparison of the in vivo and in vitro response to ragweed immunotherapy in children and adults with ragweed-induced rhinitis. *Clin Exp Allergy* 1990, 20:491–500.

19. Furin MJ, Norman PS, Creticos PS, *et al.*: Immunotherapy decreases antigen-induced eosinophil migration into the nasal cavity. *J Allergy Clin Immunol* 1991, 88:27–32.

20. Rocklin RE, Sheffer AL: Generation of antigen-specific suppressor cells during allergy desensitization. *N Engl J Med* 1980, 302:1213–1219.

21. Bonno M, Fujisawa T, Iguchi K, *et al.*: Mite-specific induction of interleukin-2 receptor on T lymphocytes from children with mite-sensitive asthma: modified immune response with immunotherapy. *J Allergy Clin Immunol* 1996, 97:680–688.

22. Soderlund A, Gabrielsson S, Paulie S, *et al.*: Allergen-induced cytokine profiles in type I allergic individuals before and after immunotherapy. *Immunol Lett* 1997, 57:177–181.

23. Thueson DO, Speck LS, Lett-Brown MA, Grant JA: Histamine-releasing activity (HRA), I: production by mitogen- or antigen-stimulated human mononuclear cells. *J Immunol* 1979, 123:626–632.

24. Kuna P, Alam R, Kuzminska B, *et al.*: The effect of preseasonal immunotherapy on the production of histamine-releasing factor (HRF) by mononuclear cells from patients with seasonal asthma: result of a double-blind placebo-controlled, randomized study. *J Allergy Clin Immunol* 1989, 83:816–824.

25. Alam R, Grant JA: The chemokines and the histamine-releasing factors: modulation of function of basophils, mast cells and eosinophils. *Chem Immunol* 1995, 61:148–160.

26. Hsieh KH, Chou CC, Chiang BL: Immunotherapy suppresses the production of monocyte chemotactic and activating factor and augments the production of IL-8 in children with asthma. *J Allergy Clin Immunol* 1996, 98:580–587.

27. Huston DP: The biology of the immune system. *JAMA* 1997, 22:1804–1814.

28. Durham SR, Ying S, Veronica A, *et al.*: Grass pollen immunotherapy inhibits allergen-induced infiltration of CD4+ T lymphocytes and eosinophils in the nasal mucosa and increases the number cells expressing messenger RNA for interferon gamma. *J Allergy Clin Immunol* 1996, 97:1356–1365.

29. Varney VA, Hamid QA, Gaga M, *et al.*: Influence of grass pollen immunotherapy on cellular infiltration and cytokine mRNA expression during allergen-induced late-phase cutaneous responses. *J Clin Invest* 1993, 92:644–651.

30.• Hamid QA, Schotman E, Jacobson MR, *et al.*: Increases in IL-12 messenger RNA+ cells accompany inhibition of allergen-induced late skin responses after successful grass pollen immunotherapy. *J Allergy Clin Immunol* 1997, 9:254–260.
This paper reviews the changes in lymphocytes and cytokines with effective immunotherapy.

31. Jutel M, Pichler WJ, Skrbic D, *et al.*: Bee venom immunotherapy results in decrease of IL-4 and IL-5 and increase of IFN-gamma secretion in specific allergen-stimulated T-cells cultures. *J Immunol* 1995, 154:4187–94.

32. Otsuka H, Mezawa A, Ohnishi M, *et al.*: Changes in nasal metachromatic cells during allergen immunotherapy. *Clin Exp Allergy* 1991, 21:115–119.

33. Creticos PS, Adkinson N Jr, Kagey-Sobotka A, *et al.*: Nasal challenge with ragweed pollen in hay fever patients: effect of immunotherapy. *J Clin Invest* 1985, 76:2247–2253.

34. Iliopoulos O, Proud D, Adkinson N Jr, *et al.*: Effects of immunotherapy on the early, late, and rechallenge nasal reaction to provocation with allergen: changes in inflammatory mediators and cells. *J Allergy Clin Immunol* 1991, 87:855–866.

35. Rak S, Lowhagen O, Venge P: The effect of immunotherapy on bronchial hyperresponsiveness and eosinophil cationic protein in pollen-allergic patients. *J Allergy Clin Immunol* 1988, 82:470–480.

36. Bousquet J, Becker WM, Hejjaoui A, *et al.*: Differences in clinical and immunologic reactivity of patients allergic to grass pollens and to multiple-pollen species. II. Efficacy of a double-blind, placebo-controlled, specific immunotherapy with standardized extracts. *J Allergy Clin Immunol* 1991, 88:43–53.

37. Grammer LC, Zeiss CR, Suszko IM, *et al.*: A double-blind, placebo-controlled trial of polymerized whole ragweed for immunotherapy of ragweed allergy. *J Allergy Clin Immunol* 1982, 69:494–499.

38. Meriney DK, Kothari H, Chinoy P, *et al.*: The clinical and immunologic efficacy of immunotherapy with modified ragweed extract (allergoid) for ragweed hay fever. *Ann Allergy* 1986, 56:34–38.

39. Norman PS, Lichtenstein LM, Kagey-Sobotka A, *et al.*: Controlled evaluation of allergoid in the immunotherapy of ragweed hay fever. *J Allergy Clin Immunol* 1982, 70:248–260.

40. Ortolani C, Pastorello EA, Incorvaia C, *et al.*: A double-blind, placebo-controlled study of immunotherapy with an alginate-conjugated extract of Parietaria judaica in patients with Parietaria hay fever. *Allergy* 1994, 49:13–21.

41. McHugh SM, Lavelle B, Kemeny DM, *et al.*: A placebo-controlled trial of immunotherapy with two extracts of *Dermatophagoides pteronyssinus* in allergic rhinitis, comparing clinical outcome with changes in antigen-specific IgE, IgG, and IgG subclasses. *J Allergy Clin Immunol* 1990, 86:521–531.

42.• Creticos PS, Reed CE, Norman PS, *et al.*: Ragweed immunotherapy in adult asthma. *N Engl J Med* 1996, 334:501–506.
This is a recent evaluation of immunotherapy in asthma.

43. Dolz I, Martinez-Cocera C, Bartolome J, *et al.*: A double-blind, placebo-controlled study of immunotherapy with grass-pollen extract Alutard SQ during a 3-year period with initial rush immunotherapy. *Allergy* 1996, 51:489–500.

44. Bousquet J, Norman PS, Robber M, *et al.*: Double-blind, placebo-controlled immunotherapy with mixed grass-pollen allergoids, III: efficacy and safety of unfractionated and high-molecular–weight preparations in rhinoconjunctivitis and asthma. *J Allergy Clin Immunol* 1989, 44:108–115.

45. Pitcher C, Marquardsen A, Sparholt S, *et al.*: Specific immunotherapy with *Dermatophagoides pteronyssinus* and *D. farinae* results in decreased bronchial hyperreactivity. *Allergy* 1997, 2:274–283.

46. Warner JO, Price JF, Soothill JF, *et al.*: Controlled trial of hypsensitization to *Dermatophagoides pteronyssinus* in children with asthma. *Lancet* 1978, 2:912–915.

47. Machiels JJ, Somville MA, Lebrun PM, *et al.*: Allergic bronchial asthma due to *Dermatophagoides pteronyssinus* hypersensitivity can be efficiently treated by inoculation of allergen-antibody complexes. *J Clin Invest* 1990, 85:1024–1035.

48. Oslen O, Larsen K, Jacobsen L, *et al.*: A one year placebo-controlled double-blind house dust mite immunotherapy in asthmatic adults. *Allergy* 1997, 52:853–859.

49. Torres Costa JC, Placido JL, Moreira Silva JP, *et al.*: Effects of immunotherapy on symptoms, PEFR, spirometry, and airway responsiveness in patients with allergic asthma to house-dust mites (*D. pteronyssinus*) on inhaled steroid therapy. *Allergy* 1996, 51:238–244.

50. Dreborg S, Agrell B, Foucard T, *et al.*: A double-blind multi-center immunotherapy trial in children, using a purified and standardized *Cladosporium herbarum* preparation, I: clinical results. *Allergy* 1986, 41:131–140.

51. Sundin B, Lilja G, Graff-Lonnevig V, *et al.*: Immunotherapy with partially purified and standardized animal dander extracts, I: clinical results from a double-blind study on patients with animal dander asthma. *J Allergy Clin Immunol* 1986, 77:478–487.

52. Alvarez-Cuesta E, Cuesta-Herranz J, Puyana-Ruiz J, *et al.*: Monoclonal antibody-standardized cat extract immunotherapy: risk-benefit effects from a double-blind placebo study. *J Allergy Clin Immunol* 1994, 93:556–566.

53. Haugaard L, Dahl R: Immunotherapy in patients allergic to cat and dog dander. I. Clinical results. *Allergy* 1992, 47:249–254.

54. Lilja G, Sundin B, Graff-Lonnevig V, *et al.*: Immunotherapy with cat- and dog- dander extract, IV: effects of 2 years of treatment. *J Allergy Clin Immunol* 1989, 83:37–44

55.•• Abramson MJ, Puy RM, Weiner JM: Is allergen immunotherapy effective in asthma? A meta-anylasis of randomized controlled trials. *Am J Respir Crit Care Med* 1995, 151:969–974.
This is a methodical review of controlled studies of immunotherapy in asthma.

56. Sigman K, Mazer B: Immunotherapy for childhood asthma: is there a rationale for its use? *Ann Allergy Asthma Immunol* 1996, 76:299–305.

57. Adkinson NF, Eggleston PA, Eney D, *et al.*: A controlled trial of immunotherapy for asthma in allergic children. *N Engl J Med* 1997, 336:324–331.

58. Hunt KJ, Valentine MD, Sobotka AK, *et al.*: A controlled trial of immunotherapy in insect hypersensitivity. *N Engl J Med* 1978, 299:157–161.

59. Lockey RF, Turkeltaub PC, *et al.*: The Hymenoptera venom study III: safety of venom immunotherapy. *J Allergy Clin Immunol* 1990, 86:775–780.

60. Laurent J, Smiejan JM, Block-Morot E, *et al.*: Safety of Hymenoptera venom rush immunotherapy. *Allergy* 1997, 52:94–96.

61. Valentine MD, Schuberth KC, Kagey-Sobotka A, *et al.*: The value of immunotherapy with venom in children with allergy to insect stings. *N Engl J Med* 1991, 23:1601–1603.

62. Bernstein JA, Kagen SL, Bernstein DI, Berstein H: Rapid venom immunotherapy is safe for routine use in the treatment of patients with Hymenoptera anaphylaxis. *Ann Allergy* 1994, 73:423–428.

63. Reisman RE, Lantner R: Further observation of stopping venom immunotherapy: comparison of patients stopped because of a fall in serum venom-specific IgE to insignificant levels with patients stopped prematurely by self-choice. *J Allergy Clin Immunol* 1989, 83:1049–1054.

64.• Golden DB, Kwiterovich KA, Kagey-Sobotka A, *et al.*: Discontinuing venom immunotherapy: outcome after 5 years. *J Allergy Clin Immunol* 1996, 997:579–587.
This paper provides useful guides for stopping venom immunotherapy.

65. Bousquet J, Knani J, Velasquez G, *et al.*: Evaluation of sensitivity to Hymenoptera venom in 200 allergic patients followed for up to 3 years. *J Allergy Clin Immunol* 1989, 84:944–950.

66. Freeman TM, Hylander R, Ortiz A, Martin ME: Imported fire ant immunotherapy: effectiveness of whole body extracts. *J Allergy Clin Immunol* 1992, 90:210–215.

67. Oppenheimer JJ, Nelson HS, Bock SA, *et al.*: Treatment of peanut allergy with rush immunotherapy. *J Allergy Clin Immunol* 1992, 90:256–262.

68. Nelson HS, Lahr J, Rule R, *et al.*: Treatment of anaphylactic sensitivity to peanuts by immunotherapy with injections of aqueous peanut extract. *J Allergy Clin Immunol* 1997, 99:744–751.

69. Price JF, Warner JO, Hey EN, *et al.*: A controlled trial of hyposensitization with adsorbed tyrosine *Dermatophagoides pteronyssinus* antigen in childhood asthma: in vivo aspects. *Clin Allergy* 1984, 14:209–219.

70. Stewart GD, Lockey RF: Systemic reactions from allergen immunotherapy. *J Allergy Clin Immunol* 1992, 90:567–578.

71. American Academy of Allergy and Immunology Board of Directors: Guidelines to minimize the risk from systemic reactions caused by immunotherapy with allergenic extracts. *J Allergy Clin Immunol* 1994, 93:811–812.

72. Lockey RF, Benedict LM, Turkeltaub PC, Bukantz SC: Fatalities from immunotherapy (IT) and skin testing (ST). *J Allergy Clin Immunol* 1987, 79:660–677.

73. Reid MJ, Lockey RF, Turkeltaub PC, Platts-Mills TA: Survey of fatalities from skin testing and immunotherapy 1985–1989. *J Allergy Clin Immunol* 1993, 92:6–15.

74. Norman PS: Safety of allergen immunotherapy. *J Allergy Clin Immunol* 1989, 84:438–439.

75. Hepner MJ, Ownby DR, Anderson JA, *et al.*: Risk of systemic reactions in patients taking beta-blocker drugs receiving aller-gen immunotherapy injections. *J Allergy Clin Immunol* 1990, 86:407–411.

76. Creticos PS, Marsh DG, Proud D, *et al.*: Responses to rag-weed-pollen nasal challenge before and after immunotherapy. *J Allergy Clin Immunol* 1989, 84:197–205.

77. Haugaard L, Dahl R, Jacobsen L: A controlled dose-response study of immunotherapy with standardized, partially purified extract of house dust mite: clinical efficacy and side effects. *J Allergy Clin Immunol* 1993, 91:709–722.

78. Bousquet J, Hejjaoui A, Clauzel AM, *et al.*: Specific immunotherapy with a standardized *Dermatophagoides pteronyssinus* extract, II: prediction of efficacy of immunotherapy. *J Allergy Clin Immunol* 1988, 82:971–977.

79. Hedlin G, Heilborn H, Lilja G, *et al.*: Long-term follow-up of patients treated with a three-year course of cat or dog immunotherapy. *J Allergy Clin Immunol* 1995, 96:879–885.

80.• Naclerio RM, Proud D, Moylan B, *et al.*: A double-blind study of the discontinuation of ragweed immunotherapy. *J Allergy Clin Immunol* 1997, 100:293–300.
This is a careful evaluation of the response to stopping pollen immunotherapy.

81. Jacobsen L, Nuchel Petersen B, Wihl JA, *et al.*: Immunotherapy with partially purified and standardized tree pollen extracts, IV: results from long-term (6-year) follow-up. *Allergy* 1997, 52:914–920.

82.•• Vogel G: New clues to asthma therapies. *Science* 1997, 276:1643–1646.
This paper reviews future approaches to immunomodulation for treatment of asthma.

83. Spiegelberg HL, Orozco EM, Roman M, *et al.*: DNA immunization: a novel approach to allergen-specific immunotherapy. *Allergy* 1997, 52:964–970.

84. Ferreira F, Hirtenlehner K, Jilek A, *et al.*: Dissection of immunoglobulin E and T-lymphocyte reactivity of isoforms of the major birch pollen allergen Bet v 1: potential use of hypoallergenic isoforms for immunotherapy. *J Exp Med* 1996, 183:599–609.

85. Norman PS, Ohman JL Jr, Long AA, *et al.*: Treatment of cat allergy with T-cell reactive peptides. *Am J Respir Crit Care Med* 1996, 154:1623–1628.

86. Walls AF: Liposomes for allergy immunotherapy. *Clin Exp Allergy* 1992, 22:1–2.

87. Litwin A, Falanagan M, Entis G, *et al.*: Oral immunotherapy with short ragweed extract in a novel encapsulated preparation: a double-blind study. *J Allergy Clin Immunol* 1997, 100:30–38.

88. Mauser PJ, Pitman AM, Fernandez X, *et al.*: Effects of an antibody to interleukin-5 in a monkey model of asthma. *Am J Respir Crit Care Med* 1995, 152:467–472.

89. Sim TC, Hilsmeier KA, Reece LM, *et al.*: Interleukin-1 receptor antagonist protein inhibits the synthesis of IgE and proinflammatory cytokines by allergen-stimulated mononuclear cells. *Am J Respir Cell Mol Biol* 1994, 11:473–479.

90. Renz H, Bradley K, Enssle K, *et al.* Prevention of the development of immediate hypersensitivity and airway hyperresponsiveness following in vivo treatment with soluble IL-4 receptor. *Int Arch Allergy Immunol* 1996, 109:167–176.

91. Sur S, Lam J, Bouchard P, *et al.*: Immunomodulatory effects of IL-12 on allergic lung inflammation depend on timing of doses. *J Immunol* 1996, 157:4173–4180.

92. Zimmermann S, Egeter O, Hausmann S, *et al.*: CpG oligodeoxynucleotides trigger protective and curative T_H1 responses in lethal muring leishmaniasis. *J Immunol* 1998, 160:3627–3630.

93. Vassella CC, Oderlram H, Laffler S, *et al.*: High anti-IgE levels at birth are associated with a reduced allergy prevalence in infant at risk: a prospective study. *Clin Exp Allergy* 1994, 24:771–777.

94.• Fahy JV, Fleming HE, Wong HH, *et al.*: The effect of an anti-IgE monoclonal antibody on the early and late phase responses to allergen inhalation in asthmatic subjects. *Am J Respir Crit Care Med* 1997, 155:1828–1834.
This paper evaluated the response in asthma to therapy with anti-IgE antibodies.

95.• Boulet LP, Chapman KR, Cote J, *et al.*: Inhibitory effects of an anti-IgE antibody E25 on the allergen-induced early asthmatic response. *Am J Respir Crit Care Med* 1997, 155:1835–1840.
This is another paper on anti-IgE antibody therapy and its response in asthma.

96. Casale TB, Bernstein IL, Busse WW, *et al.*: Use of an anti-IgE humanized monoclonal antibody in ragweed-induced allergic rhinitis. *J Allergy Clin Immunol* 1997, 100:110–121.

to warn them that they may require prolonged use of nasal washings and topical nasal corticosteroids despite surgical resection.

CONCLUSIONS

At this time, there are very few controlled trials of the management of chronic sinusitis, and the only studies of acute sinusitis have focused on the efficacy of various antibiotics. In one trial of 200 consecutive patients with recurrent sinusitis, medical management subjectively and objectively reduced sinusitis in the greatest majority of patients [13••]. However, despite the most appropriate and aggressive medical management, some patients require surgery. Even after surgery, and in the face of continued medical management, some of these patients will continue to experience recurrent episodes of sinusitis. Much more research into the pathophysiology of sinusitis is required before we will understand how to manage these patients or even how to select which patients should undergo surgery and when [2••]. None of these studies will be carried out until the medical and lay communities recognize the importance of sinusitis and urge funding of prospective clinical trials.

REFERENCES AND RECOMMENDED READING

Recently published papers of particular interest have been highlighted as:

- •   of interest
- ••   of outstanding interest

1. Collins JG: Prevalence of selected chronic conditions: United States, 1986–1988. National Center for Health Statistics. *Vital Health Stat* 1993, 10:1–87.

2.•• Kaliner MA, Osguthorpe JD, Fireman P, *et al.*: Sinusitis: bench to bedside. *J Allergy Clin Immunol* 1997, 99:S829–S848.
This manuscript represents a summary of a 2-day meeting held in 1996 involving a select group of allergists and otolaryngologists. The paper summarizes what is known about sinusitis, what is not known, and what needs to be done in order to answer these questions.

3.•• Kaliner MA: Allergy care in the next millennium: guidelines for the specialty. *J Allergy Clin Immunol* 1997, 99:729–734.
This manuscript represents my presidential address to the American Academy of Allergy, Asthma and Immunology's annual meeting in 1996. In this paper, I lay out referral guidelines for primary care physicians for rhinitis, sinusitis, and asthma patients. More importantly, the paper also provides exactly what information should be generated by the specialist and returned to the primary care physician in order to warrant the referral.

4.•• Raphael GD, Baraniuk JN, Kaliner MA: How the nose runs and why. *J Allergy Clin Immunol* 1991, 87:457–467.
This manuscript describes exactly what processes are involved in forming nasal secretions, why these processes are present, and how to control them.

5. McMenamin P: Costs of hay fever in the United States in 1990. *Ann Allergy* 1994, 73:35–39.

6. Ray NF, Thamer M, Rinehart CS, *et al.*: Medical expenditures for the treatment of allergic rhinoconjunctivitis in the United States in 1996. *J Allergy Clin Immunol* 1998: in press.

7. Peynegre R, Rouvier P: Anatomy and anatomical variations of the paranasal sinuses: influence on sinus dysfunction. In *Diseases of the Sinuses*. Edited by Gershwin ME, Incaudo GA. Totowa, NJ: Humana Press; 1996:3–33.

8. Messerklinger W: *Endoscopy of the Nose*. Baltimore: Urban and Schwarzenberg; 1978.

9. Hamilos DL, Leung DYM, Woods R, *et al.*: Chronic hyperplastic sinusitis: association of tissue eosinophilia with mRNA expression of granulocyte-macrophage colony stimulating-factor and interleukin-3. *J Allergy Clin Immunol* 1993, 92:39–48.

10.•• Hamilos DL, Leung DYM, Wood R, *et al.*: Evidence for distinct cytokine expression in allergic versus nonallergic chronic sinusitis. *J Allergy Clin Immunol* 1995, 96:537–544.
This is the second paper in this series, and is of great interest to those who want to understand the pathophysiology of sinusitis.

11. Denburg JA, Gauldie J, Dolovich J, *et al.*: Structural cell-derived cytokines in allergic inflammation. *Int Arch Allergy Appl Immunol* 1991, 94:127–132.

12. Drake-Lee AB, Lowe D, Swanston A, *et al.*: Clinical profile and recurrence of nasal polyps. *J Laryngol Otol* 1984, 98:783–793.

13.•• McNally PA, White MV, Kaliner MA: Sinusitis in an allergist's office: analysis of 200 consecutive cases. *Allergy Asthma Proc* 1997, 18:169–176.
An important article in deciding how to treat sinusitis medically. This is the largest series describing patients with chronic sinusitis, and shows how effective medical management can be.

14. Clerico DM: Rhinopathic headaches: referred pain of nasal and sinus origin. In *Diseases of the Sinuses*. Edited by Gershwin ME, Incaudo GA. Totowa, NJ: Humana Press; 1996:403–424.

15. Zdenek P: The role of allergy in sinus disease. In *Diseases of the Sinuses*. Edited by Gershwin ME, Incaudo GA. Totowa, NJ: Humana Press; 1996:97–166.

16. Stevenson DD: Commentary: the American experience with aspirin desensitization for aspirin-sensitive rhinosinusitis and asthma. *Allerg Proc* 1992, 13:185–192.

17. Mathison DA, Simon RA, Stevenson DD: Aspirin, sulfur dioxide/sulfite, and other chemical sensitivities and challenges in asthmatic patients. In *Provocation Testing in Clinical Practice*. Edited by Spector SL. New York: Marcel Dekker; 1995:599–622.

18. Zinreich SJ: Radiologic diagnosis of the nasal cavity and paranasal sinuses. In *Sinusitis: Pathophysiology and Treatment*. Edited by Druce HD. New York: Marcel Dekker; 1994:57–72.

19. Kaliner MA: Human nasal host defense and sinusitis. In *Diseases of the Sinuses*. Edited by Gershwin ME, Incaudo GA. Totowa, NJ: Humana Press; 1996:53–62.

20. Kowalski ML: Pathophysiology of rhinosinusitis in aspirin-sensitive patients. In *Progress in Allergy and Clinical Immunology*, vol 4. Edited by Oehling AK, Huerta Lopez JG. Seattle: Hogrefe and Huber; 1997:174–178.

CHAPTER 13

Anaphylaxis

Phillip L. Lieberman

The purpose of this chapter to familiarize the reader with recent advances in our knowledge of anaphylaxis and anaphylactoid reactions. It is not intended to be a comprehensive review of the subject, for which the reader is referred to other sources [1••,2–4].

To review these advances within limited space restrictions, six subtopics, in areas where advances are particularly important, have been chosen: clinical profile and epidemiology of anaphylaxis, idiopathic anaphylaxis, the role of nitric oxide, the role of the renin-angiotensin system, diagnosis and treatment, and differential diagnosis. There is also a section on the new and unusual agents of anaphylaxis.

CLINICAL PROFILE AND EPIDEMIOLOGY

Perhaps the most important aspect of dealing with anaphylaxis from the allergist's standpoint is the evaluation of patients presenting to the office after an anaphylactic event in order to identify the cause. There have been several recent series of patients with anaphylaxis who have been evaluated by retrospective chart review [5–9]. The largest series, from the University of Tennessee, describes 380 patients [7,8]. Another series, from Spain, describes 182 patients [6], and a third, from the Mayo Clinic, describes 179 patients [5]. Several salient points arise when these studies are examined as a whole (Table 13-1). In a significant number of patients, no cause could be found, and these patients had to be considered to have recurrent idiopathic anaphylaxis. No cause could be found in 46% of the University of Tennessee patients, 33 % of the patients in the series from Spain, and 21% of the Mayo Clinic patients. Atopy is clearly a risk factor, and in the two series reporting the incidence of atopy, it occurred in 36% [8] and 49% [5] of patients. A rather unexpected finding is the preponderance of females in all three series. The highest percentage of women was in the Mayo Clinic series (61%), followed by the University of Tennessee series (58%) and the Spanish series (55%). In all three series, food and drugs were the most common causative agents. In the two American series, antibiotics and nonsteroidal anti-inflammatory drugs (NSAIDs) were the most common drug offenders. There was a distinct difference, however, between the Mayo Clinic series and the University of Tennessee series with regard to the specific food offenders. Shellfish were, by far, the most common food to cause anaphylaxis in the University of Tennessee series; peanuts were the next most common. Conversely, shellfish were not mentioned in the Mayo Clinic series, and peanuts were the most common food. In both American series,

Table 13-1. CHARACTERISTICS OF PATIENTS WITH ANAPHYLACTIC EPISODES EVALUATED IN ALLERGISTS' OFFICES

Patients	Memphis, TN	Rochester, MN	Albacete, Spain
Number, n	380	182	179
Idiopathic, %	46	21	33
Female, %	61	58	55
Most common cause	Foods	Foods	Drugs
Most common manifestation	Cutaneous	—	Cutaneous
Atopic, %	36	49	—
Study	Kemp et al. [7] Kagy et al. [8]	Yocum and Khan [5]	Perez et al. [6]

foods led drugs as the most common cause of anaphylaxis, whereas in the Spanish series, drugs were the most frequent offenders. As expected, in all three series cutaneous manifestations were the most frequent complaint. In fact, the absence of any cutaneous finding (urticaria, angioedema, flush) speaks strongly against the diagnosis of anaphylaxis, because 90% or more of patients experiencing anaphylactic episodes have one or more of these cutaneous manifestations [6,8].

The data from another large, recent series of anaphylactic episodes was obtained in a different way [9]. The authors identified all residents of a county in Minnesota who had experienced anaphylaxis from 1983 to 1987. A retrospective analysis was done to determine the cause, the incidence of atopy, the mortality rate, the recurrence rate, and the percentage of patients seen by an allergist. Out of 1080 charts reviewed, 125 episodes of anaphylaxis were identified in 110 patients. In keeping with the other studies, cutaneous symptoms were the most common complaint. A suspected allergen was identified in 73% of the episodes. Foods were the most common offenders. One death was reported.

In one of the aforementioned University of Tennessee series [7], an observation pertinent to therapy was made. It was learned that a significant number of patients failed to keep their epinephrine kit with them. Failure to do so was much more frequent in patients in whom a causative agent for the episodes had been identified than in patients with idiopathic anaphylaxis. This implies that the security of knowing the cause lessened the perceived danger of recurrence. Nonetheless, there were several recurrences even when the patient was aware of the causative agent.

Also of note is the fact that, in many instances, there was a gradual remission, and in two series [6,7], an allergy evaluation resulted in a diminished number of episodes for many patients and in a reduction in emergency room visits.

The combined results of these series allow several conclusions. First of all, atopy is far more common in patients who experience anaphylaxis regardless of whether a responsible allergen can be identified. Atopy incidence can be as high as 49% [5]. Second, women seem predisposed to anaphylactic episodes regardless of cause. This incidence can range as high as 61% [5]. When the cause is found, food and drugs head the list, with peanuts and shellfish apparently being the most common offending foods and NSAIDs and antibiotics the most common drug offenders. Cutaneous symptoms are, by far, the most common manifestation. Finally, the prognosis usually is good, with the majority of patients undergoing remission, and deaths are extremely rare.

The importance of drugs as causes of anaphylaxis has recently been reported not only in the retrospective reviews noted above but also in prospective studies. The most recently reported are from Denmark [10] and the Netherlands [11]. In the Netherlands, all adverse drug reactions registered as anaphylaxis between the years 1974 and 1994 were analyzed—a total of 936 reports. The majority of these patients, as in the other studies, were female (65%). Also consistent with the other investigations, the most common agents to cause anaphylaxis in this series were NSAIDs and antibiotics. It is interesting to note that 12 cases of anaphylaxis occurred during allergen immunotherapy [11].

In the Danish study [10], 30 cases of fatal, drug-related anaphylactic reactions occurring between 1968 and 1990 were identified. The most frequent cause of anaphylactic episodes was radiocontrast, and antibiotics were the next most common offender. It is interesting to note that five anaphylactic deaths occurred during allergen immunotherapy. All of these occurred in a family practitioner's office and the allergens involved were molds.

Based on their data, the authors of the Dutch study [11] calculated that there are approximately 50 reports of drug-associated anaphylaxis per year in the

Netherlands, which has a population of 13 to 15 million. However, they believed this incidence to be underestimated because of failure to report all reactions. In fact, in previous studies, only 4% to 8% of anaphylactic reactions were reported to the Dutch Inspectorate for Health Care [12,13].

Another interesting aspect of this study is that 11.9% of the 345 reports classified as "probable anaphylaxis" occurred later than 30 minutes after exposure to the offending agent. The authors interpret these data as support for the policy of observing a patient for 1 hour after the administration of antigen for allergen immunotherapy [11].

Before leaving this discussion of the clinical profile of anaphylactic reactions, it is important to note several unusual manifestations recently reported. One of these was bilateral massive adrenal hemorrhage that occurred as a result of an anaphylactic reaction to a colloid solution (plasmagel) [14]. The importance of this occurrence is that it is extremely difficult to make a diagnosis of adrenal hemorrhage in a patient in acute distress, especially during a hypotensive anaphylactic event. In this case, the diagnosis was made only after computed tomography (CT) of the abdomen.

In another interesting case report, the diagnosis of anaphylaxis was missed because of a failure to consider it as part of the differential diagnosis of recurrent syncope [15]. In this instance, a 36-year-old man had experienced three episodes of syncope and hypotension. Each had required hospitalization, and on each occasion he was evaluated for causes of syncope without the cause having been determined. On the fourth admission, because of a response to antihistamines and corticosteroids, anaphylaxis was considered. This prompted an evaluation that revealed a markedly elevated immunoglobulin (Ig)-E level and positive immediate hypersensitivity testing to banana and latex. Dietary restriction resulted in the prevention of recurrences. The importance of this case is that it represents an exception to the rule, because cutaneous symptoms were not noted.

Finally, it is always important to understand that profound cardiovascular disturbances can occur during anaphylaxis. It has long been known that coronary artery spasm and various electrocardiogram (ECG) disturbances are not uncommon. These previously have not been reported during exercise-induced anaphylaxis. Because the differential diagnosis could include myocardial infarction, it is important to be aware that arrhythmias and coronary artery vasospasm with ischemia can occur during exercise-induced anaphylactic events without the presence of intrinsic coronary artery obstruction. In this instance the patient, a man aged 57 years who had a positive family history of atopy and had previously suffered from bronchial asthma, was resuscitated after a cardiac arrest occurred during exercise. An exhaustive cardiovascular work-up, including an ergonovine provocation test, failed to reveal significant arteriosclerotic heart disease, whereas exercise challenge testing consistently provoked flushing, wheezing, sweating, lacrimation, and chest tightness accompanied by a fall in blood pressure. During these anaphylactic events, ECG changes of transmural ischemia followed by ventricular fibrillation occurred in the absence of any coronary artery disease [16].

IDIOPATHIC ANAPHYLAXIS

The original report describing cases of idiopathic anaphylaxis appeared in 1978 [17]. Since that time, idiopathic anaphylaxis has been well chronicled in several large series [18–22]. The number of cases in the United States has been estimated to be approximately 30,000 [21].

The pathogenesis of idiopathic anaphylaxis remains unknown. However, it is clear that mast cell degranulation is involved because both plasma histamine [19] and serum tryptase [23] have been found to be elevated during reactions. The reason for this explosive release of mast cell and perhaps basophil mediators is unknown. Speculation suggests several possibilities [24]. One of these is that there is an intrinsic defect in mast cells and basophils, making them unstable. Such predisposition to degranulation or "hyper-releasability" has been noted in atopic patients with food allergy [25], atopic dermatitis [26], and asthma and bronchopulmonary aspergillosis [27]. This is an interesting concept, because there is an increased incidence of atopy in patients with idiopathic anaphylaxis [28]. If this easy releasability is not due to an intrinsic cellular defect, one could also postulate that the extracellular environment might be the predisposing factor. In this case, there could be circulating histamine-releasing factors or cytokine imbalances. In favor of the extracellular environment theory is that patients with idiopathic anaphylaxis are not more sensitive to skin tests with codeine than are normal individuals [29].

Newer developments regarding idiopathic anaphylaxis include a seemingly increasing frequency in children [30] and the fact that fatalities have now been documented [31]. Although there seems to be an increasing prevalence in children, and although the illness is now known to be potentially fatal, the vast majority of patients can be treated successfully with preventive medical regimens. In addition, the prognosis for idiopathic anaphylaxis appears to be quite good [32]. A total of 61 patients, from an original series of 225 seen between 1971 and 1990, were reported by the Northwestern University Medical School Allergy Division [32]. Of these, 65% percent of patients with infrequent episodes and 91% of patients with frequent episodes went into remission. In addition, there were significant decreases in emergency room visits and hospitalizations with appropriate therapy [32].

A diagnosis of idiopathic anaphylaxis is made after an exhaustive search for etiologic agents has failed to identify a cause. Patients with infrequent and mild episodes occurring three to four times a year probably do not need therapy. With more frequent episodes, such as six to eight times a year, a combination of an H_1 and H_2 antagonist can be instituted on a daily basis. If this regimen fails to produce a response, albuterol or ephedrine can be added to the protocol. In addition, in selected cases, cromolyn sodium may be effective [33]. Ketotifen has proven to be particularly effective in resistant patients deemed to be corticosteroid dependent [34]. Parenteral methotrexate also has been found useful in the management of patients who require large doses of prednisone to prevent life-threatening attacks [35]. In those patients who are corticosteroid dependent, treatment can be initiated with doses of 60 mg per day followed by a gradual tapering of the dose once the episodes are controlled. Most of these patients can be managed on doses of 20 mg or less every other day [33].

Thus, the more recent observations of this illness have confirmed its tendency toward spontaneous remission while simultaneously documenting the fact that it is potentially fatal. In addition, it has been shown to occur in childhood. Finally, the use of ketotifen as an alternative to long-term corticosteroid therapy has been highlighted. Unfortunately, there has been little advance in our understanding of its pathogenesis since its first description.

NITRIC OXIDE

One of the most interesting advances in the understanding of the pathophysiology of immediate hypersensitivity reactions is the identification of nitric oxide (NO) as a central mediator of these events. NO is a diffusable gas that is a messenger of both intra- and intercellular signals.

It has long been known that histamine and other mediators of anaphylaxis act indirectly in an endothelium-dependent fashion to produce vascular permeability and smooth muscle relaxation. In the case of histamine, this effect is mediated through H_1 receptors present on endothelial cells. Originally, the nature of the substance mediating this effect was unknown, but the substance itself, in keeping with its activity, was termed endothelium-derived relaxing factor (EDRF). In 1988, it was first proposed that EDRF was indeed NO [36,37]. NO is synthesized from L-arginine through the activity of nitric oxide synthase (NOS) (Fig. 13-1). There are three isoforms of NOS. Two of these (cNOS) exist constitutively, and the third (iNOS) is inducible. cNOS can be found in endothelium, myocardium, endocardium, skeletal muscle, platelets, and neural tissue. iNOS is

found in macrophages, fibroblasts, neutrophils, and smooth muscle. cNOS is Ca^{2+}\calmodulin-dependent and iNOS is Ca^{2+} independent. iNOS appears to be regulated at the transcriptional level.

Mediators known to induce the synthesis of cNOS can act rapidly, with elevated levels of NO occurring within seconds. These mediators include histamine, platelet activating factor, bradykinin, several of the leukotrienes, and acetylcholine. NO synthesis via iNOS requires gene transcription and can take from minutes to hours. However, once initiated in this fashion, the synthesis can continue for many hours and the amounts of NO produced exceeds that made through the activity of cNOS [38•,39].

The effects of NO are protean. Its effects in anaphylaxis are potentially contradictory (Table 13-2). NO produces smooth muscle relaxation and increases vascular permeability. These two effects can result in profound hypotension. Conversely, smooth muscle relaxation produced by NO exerts a salutary effect on bronchoconstriction and coronary artery vasospasm. In addition, NO can inhibit mediator release from mast cells.

Thus, NO has the potential for both deleterious and beneficial effects during an anaphylactic episode. However, it appears as if the summation effects are hypotension, loss of intravascular volume, and resulting hemoconcentration. At least this is the case in animal models of anaphylaxis, where hypotension can be reversed by the administration of a nitric oxide synthase inhibitor.

THE RENIN-ANGIOTENSIN SYSTEM

During the past decade, it has become evident that the renin-angiotensin system plays an important role in the compensatory response to hypotension during anaphylactic shock (Fig. 13-2). Elevated levels of urinary angiotensin I and angiotensin II have been found in

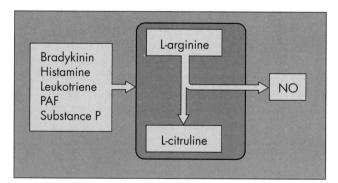

FIGURE 13-1.

Nitric oxide (NO) synthesis. NO synthesis occurs during the conversion of L-arginine to L-citruline, which can be induced by mediators of anaphylaxis. PAF—platelet activating factor. (*Adapted from* Lieberman [37]; with permission.)

patients with anaphylactic reactions to drugs, foods, and food additives [40–42]. In addition, during anaphylactic shock to hymenoptera stings, plasma levels of angiotensin rise in conjunction with those of epinephrine and norepinephrine [43]. It is thus not unexpected that angiotensin-converting enzyme (ACE) inhibitors (and probably angiotensin II-blocking agents as well) might lower the threshold of predisposed individuals to hypotension during anaphylactic reactions. In keeping with this hypothesis, ACE inhibitors have been incriminated as provocateurs in the production of anaphylaxis or anaphylactoid events occurring during plasma exchange with albumin-replacement solutions [44], low-density lipoprotein apheresis using a dextran sulfate cellulose column [45], hemodialysis with synthetic polyacrylonitrile membranes [46] and cuprammonia membranes [47], and during apheresis [48,49]. In addition, ACE inhibitors have been shown to predispose to

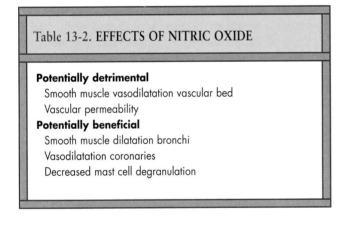

Table 13-2. EFFECTS OF NITRIC OXIDE

Potentially detrimental
Smooth muscle vasodilatation vascular bed
Vascular permeability
Potentially beneficial
Smooth muscle dilatation bronchi
Vasodilatation coronaries
Decreased mast cell degranulation

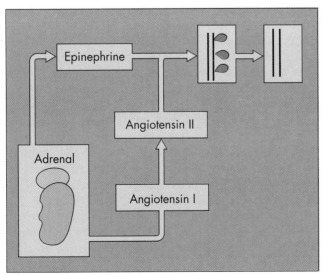

FIGURE 13-2.
The renin-angiotensin system. Angiotensin II synthesis and epinephrine release occur as compensatory responses to hypotension. Each restores vascular integrity, reducing plasma leakage. (*Adapted from* Lieberman [37]; with permission.)

anaphylactic reactions during immunotherapy with hymenoptera venom [50].

Concurrent with these observations are findings suggesting that patients with hymenoptera venom allergy may have an innate defect in their ability to produce angiotensin II in response to hypotension [51–53]. Patients with a history of hymenoptera venom anaphylaxis had significantly lower levels of angiotensin II in their leukocytes than did healthy controls [52] and demonstrated similar decreases in angiotensin I and angiotensin II in plasma [51,53].

Confirming the important role of angiotensin production as a compensatory response to hypotension is the successful treatment of hypotension during anaphylaxis with angiotensinamide, an angiotensin analog [54]. In this instance, the hypotension was refractory to standard vasoconstrictor therapy and fluid but responded to angiotensinamide. This is consistent with the fact that angiotensin is eight to 10 times more potent as a vasoconstricting agent than is norepinephrine, and causes marked vasoconstrictive activity in the blood vessels of the skin, splanchnic area, and renal vasculature. The vasoconstrictive activity of angiotensin occurs through several mechanisms. Angiotensin increases the production and decreases the re-uptake of norepinephrine at sympathetic nerve terminals [55], increases central sympathetic outflow [56], and increases cardiac output via the release of myocardial catecholamines along with an increase in calcium influx that is independent of the β-adrenergic receptor [57].

ACE inhibitors may predispose individuals to anaphylactic reactions through several mechanisms. It is known that inhibitors of ACE inhibit not only the mobilization of angiotensin II, but also the catabolism of bradykinin and substance P [58]. In addition, these drugs activate the cyclooxygenase pathway (presumably through bradykin) with the resultant production of prostanoids [59•]. Thus, prevention of the activity of angiotensin II may not be the sole reason for the role of this class of drugs in the worsening of anaphylactic events.

These collective data have prompted concern regarding the administration of ACE inhibitors and angiotensin II blocking agents to patients at risk for anaphylaxis [60•]. It seems prudent to restrict the administration of these agents to patients with hymenoptera allergy and those with recurrent episodes of idiopathic anaphylaxis. In addition, the *Physicians' Desk Reference* clearly conscripts the use of these agents in patients who are receiving hymenoptera venom immunotherapy. It is not my practice, however, to restrict their use in patients who are receiving pollen immunotherapy. The different approach for patients receiving hymenoptera venom immunotherapy and allergen immunotherapy cannot totally be supported by available data, but there do appear to be qualitative differences between these two groups of patients that lend credence to this practice. As noted, hymenoptera patients have been shown to have defects in the mobilization of the renin-angiotensin system [51–53]. To date, no such abnormality has been found in pollen-allergic subjects. In addition, hymenoptera reactions are anaphylactic in nature and are characterized by hypotension. This of course differs from inhalant reactions to pollen. Finally, to this point, there has been no documentation of ACE inhibitors placing subjects who were receiving pollen immunotherapy at increased risk of anaphylactic events. In a survey of fatalities from skin testing and immunotherapy, there is no mention of ACE inhibitors in this regard. However, it should be noted that the survey did not specifically solicit information regarding the administration of ACE inhibitors [61].

Thus, in summary, ACE inhibitors lower the threshold for anaphylactic events in some settings. The magnitude of this effect has not been determined, and at this time there are no clear-cut recommendations regarding the use of ACE inhibitors and angiotensin blocking agents in patients at risk for anaphylaxis, with the exception of the admonition contained in the *Physicians' Desk Reference* regarding hymenoptera venom immunotherapy. However, it is reasonable to restrict the use of these agents in individuals subject to recurrent episodes of anaphylaxis.

DIAGNOSIS AND TREATMENT

Serum tryptase was proposed as a marker of anaphylaxis in the late 1980s [62]. Since this description, the measurement of tryptase for the diagnosis of anaphylaxis has stood the test of time. Classically, it is thought that tryptase levels peak 1 to 1.5 hours after the onset of anaphylaxis and may be elevated as long as 5 hours after onset [63]. Thus, the best time for measurement is thought to be between 1 to 2 hours but no longer than 6 hours after onset of symptoms [63]. Recently, several investigators have attempted to assess the utility of tryptase in the diagnosis of anaphylaxis both pre- [64–67] and postmortem [68,69].

One of the more salient advances in our understanding of the use of tryptase in establishing a diagnosis of anaphylaxis is the ability to distinguish α-tryptase from β-tryptase. α-tryptase appears to be released constitutively by mast cells, and β-tryptase appears primarily to be released upon degranulation. Original assays of tryptase were based on a radioimmunoassay (RIA) procedure that mainly detected β-tryptase levels. More recently, an enzyme-linked immunosorbent assay (ELISA) has been developed that detects both α- and β-tryptase levels. α-tryptase is released in most cases of biopsy-proven systemic mastocytosis, but in contradistinction, cases of anaphylaxis would be expected to have a relative increase in β-tryptase. Therefore, the use

of the RIA and the ELISA simultaneously may be useful in distinguishing anaphylactic episodes that occur in systemic mastocytosis from those that occur, for example, in idiopathic anaphylaxis [65].

Investigators in Spain have used tryptase levels to assist in the diagnosis of anaphylactic drug reactions. In one instance [67], 18 patients with allergic drug reactions were challenged with the drug in question. Those characterized by anaphylactic symptoms demonstrated elevated serum tryptase levels that correlated with the severity of the reaction. These observations led the authors to conclude that serum tryptase levels would be helpful in making the diagnosis of allergic drug reactions. They later measured serial tryptase levels in six patients with drug-induced anaphylactic events [65]. They found that the time of maximum tryptase levels varied considerably. In three control subjects, the highest tryptase levels were detected within 20 to 30 minutes of the onset of symptoms, whereas in another two, the maximum levels were reached in 2 hours, and in a sixth subject maximum levels were not reached until 3 to 4 hours. In all instances, serum tryptase decreased to basal levels within 24 hours. The time of peak level failed to correlate with the total amount of tryptase detected. Their conclusion was that serial levels may be needed to evaluate mast cell involvement in drug reactions because peak levels are reached at varying time intervals.

Serum tryptase levels have also been used to rule out anaphylactic events. Marshall *et al.* [64] looked at serum tryptase levels in intensive care patients who had experienced unexplained episodes of hypotension. Serum was obtained from 22 consecutive patients at 0, 12, and 24 hours after unexplained hypotension. Samples were analyzed by RIA. Only three of 22 patients had detectable levels of tryptase at 0 and 12 hours. A retrospective chart review found that all three patients had previous drug allergy histories and were receiving suspect antimicrobials. The highest serum tryptase level (12.9 ng/mL) occurred in a patient with a history of penicillin allergy who had been administered cephaclor immediately prior to the onset of hypotension. The authors concluded that anaphylaxis is a relatively uncommon cause of hypotension in the intensive care setting, and their data supported the specificity of serum tryptase as an indicator of anaphylaxis in patients experiencing unexplained hypotension in the intensive care unit.

Serum tryptase may also be used to make a postmortem diagnosis of anaphylaxis. Becker *et al.* [68] assayed tryptase in samples of ante- and postmortem sera from 50 patients. No patient had died of anaphylaxis or asthma. Serum tryptase was not detectable in any pre-mortem sample, but tryptase was detectable in 17 postmortem samples. An analysis of trend indicated a highly significant increase in postmortem serum tryptase from samples obtained more than 15 hours after death. The authors concluded that serum tryptase could be a valuable laboratory aid for the diagnosis of anaphylaxis, but only when postmortem samples were obtained within 15 hours of death. In another example of the use of serum tryptase postmortem, serum was obtained from a subject who died during an anaphylactoid reaction to radiocontrast media [69]. Both tryptase and eosinophilic cationic protein were markedly elevated. The authors, therefore, concluded that serum tryptase is a useful tool, when obtained postmortem, to establish a diagnosis of anaphylaxis.

One area of great debate is the equipment necessary to treat an episode of anaphylaxis in the office. Several attempts at forming consensus lists have been made [70–72]. More recently, a different approach has been taken by the Anaphylaxis Committee of the American Academy of Allergy, Asthma and Immunology [73]. The committee used a survey to assess the medication and devices available to treat anaphylaxis in allergists' offices. There were 477 responding office practices; 83% to 92% of these did contain items recommended by the most recent position statement of the American Academy of Allergy, Asthma and Immunology [72]. These items included stethoscope, blood pressure cuff, tourniquet, syringes, oxygen, epinephrine, diphenhydramine, ambu bag/oral airway, intravenous set-up, and corticosteroid for intravenous injection. However, intravenous fluids were only available in 68% of offices, intravenous pressors only in 23% to 55%, aminophylline in 65%, and a laryngoscope/endotracheal tube in 61%. Atropine was present in 60%, lidocaine in 55%, sodium bicarbonate in 51%, calcium gluconate in 42%, glucagon in 36%, dopamine in 35%, neuroleptics in 33%, and an H2 antagonist in 31%. An ECG was present in 36% of the offices, suction in 35%, equipment for intracardiac injection in 22%, and a defibrillator in 18%; 79% of the offices had all equipment organized in a single place, and the staff were trained in cardiopulmonary resuscitation (CPR) in 76%. The authors concluded that most offices were "almost but not fully compliant with current guidelines." The most conspicuous absences were intravenous fluids and certain medications. Table 13-3 lists agents that have been suggested as tools for the management of anaphylaxis in the office, along with the percent of allergists who had them available.

Very little new information has been presented regarding therapy of the acute episode. The debate regarding the dose and route of administration of epinephrine continues. Simons *et al.* [74] have shed some scientific light on this debate in a prospective study of epinephrine absorption in children with a history of anaphylaxis. They evaluated the rate of absorption of epinephrine after injection in 17 children with a history of anaphylaxis. Epinephrine was injected intramuscularly from an EpiPen (Dey

Laboratories, Napa, CA) auto-injector or subcutaneously using an epinephrine syringe. Intramuscular injection was judged superior to subcutaneous injection with regard to attaining peak plasma levels rapidly. The authors concluded that these findings might have important clinical implications regarding the route of administration of epinephrine during anaphylaxis.

DIFFERENTIAL DIAGNOSIS

The classical differential diagnosis of anaphylaxis and anaphylactoid events is seen in Table 13-4. Recent

Table 13-3. EQUIPMENT AND MEDICATION FOR THERAPY OF ANAPHYLAXIS IN OFFICE	
Equipment	Percent, %*
Primary	
Tourniquet	83 to 92
1- and 5-mL disposable syringes	83 to 92
Oxygen tank and mask/nasal prongs	83 to 92
Epinephrine solution (aqueous) 1:1000	83 to 92
Diphenhydramine, injectable	83 to 92
Ranitidine or cimetidine, injectable	31
Injectable corticosteroids	83 to 92
Ambu bag, oral airway	83 to 92
Intravenous setup with large-bore catheter	83 to 92
Intravenous fluids; 2000 mL crystalloid, 1000 mL hydroxyethyl starch	68
Aerosol b_2 bronchodilator and compressor nebulizer	
Glucagon	36
Electrocardiogram	36
Normal saline, 10 mL vial for epinephrine dilution	
Stethoscope	83 to 92
Blood pressure cuff	83 to 92
Laryngoscope/endotracheal tube	61
Supporting	
Suction apparatus	35
Dopamine or other pressor	23 to 55
Sodium bicarbonate	51
Aminophylline	65
Atropine	60
Optional	
Defibrillator	15
Calcium gluconate	42
Neuroleptics for seizures	33
Lidocaine	55

Percent of allergists that had this equipment and medication available in office

Data from *The American Academy of Pediatrics Committee on Drugs* [70], *The Journal of Allergy and Clinical Immunology* [71,72], *and Golden and Schwartz* [73].

Table 13-4. DIFFERENTIAL DIAGNOSIS

Anaphylaxis and anaphylactoid reactions
Anaphylaxis and anaphylactoid reactions to
  exogenously administered agents
Physical factors
  Exercise
  Cold, heat, sunlight
Idiopathic

Vasodepressor reactions

Flush syndromes
Carcinoid
Postmenopausal
Chlorpropamide—alcohol
Medullary carcinoma thyroid, oat cell carcinoma,
  pancreatic tumors
Autonomic epilepsy
Pheochromocytoma

"Restaurant syndromes"
Monosodium glutamate
Sulfites
Scombroidosis

Other forms of shock
Hemorrhagic
Cardiogenic
Endotoxic

Excess endogenous production of histamine syndromes
Systemic mastocytosis
Urticaria pigmentosa
Basophilic leukemia
Acute promyelocytic leukemia (tretinoin treatment)
Hydatid cyst

Nonorganic disease
Panic attacks
Munchausen's stridor
Vocal chord dysfunction syndrome
Globus hystericus

Miscellaneous
Hereditary angioedema
"Progesterone" anaphylaxis
Urticarial vasculitis
Capillary leak syndrome
Hyperimmunoglobulin E, urticaria syndrome
Neurologic (seizure, stroke)
Pseudoanaphylaxis
Red man syndrome (vancomycin)

decaying flesh of scombroid fish, especially tuna. Enzymatic decarboxylation of histidine is produced by bacterial degradation of blue fish flesh. This degradation occurs optimally between 20° and 30°C and can be inhibited by preservatives or refrigeration. It is thought that a level of histamine exceeding 50 mg per 100 gm of fish flesh can produce symptoms [78].

Symptoms of scombroid poisoning are identical to those due to histamine release from mast cells and basophils and include abdominal cramping with nausea, vomiting and diarrhea, flush, headache, and dizziness. The symptoms usually begin within a few minutes to a few hours after ingestion of the fish. A telltale finding suggesting the diagnosis is the occurrence of anaphylactic-like symptoms in more than one person at the meal.

In a recent study, the authors were able to determine serum and urinary histamine, 24-hour urinary methylhistamine, and serum tryptase levels. As expected, serum histamine, urine histamine, and 24-hour urinary methylhistamine levels were increased, whereas serum tryptase levels were normal. None of the patients studied exhibited specific IgE to fish either by in vivo or ex vivo tests.

The capillary leak syndrome is a rare and potentially fatal disorder with systemic symptoms suggestive of anaphylaxis (hypotension, swelling suggesting angioedema, and gastrointestinal symptoms). It usually is associated with a monoclonal gammopathy. A recent report described a woman, 47 years of age, with this disorder who had experienced six life-threatening bouts of diarrhea, vomiting, angioedema, and shock [76].

A recent review and case report highlighted the importance of flushing episodes in the differential diagnosis [77•]. Of importance is the recognition that carcinoid-like symptoms can be produced not only by carcinoid tumors, but also by malignancies such as medullary carcinoma, oat cell carcinoma of the lung, and a number of different pancreatic tumors including insulinoma, glucagonoma, vasoactive intestinal polypeptide secreting tumor, and gastrinoma. Perhaps the most common of these is medullary carcinoma of the thyroid, which is a tumor of parafollicular cells. With medullary carcinoma of the thyroid, there is often a secretory diarrhea and spontaneous flushing attacks. Several vasoactive mediators can be produced by medullary carcinomas.

Although pheochromocytoma classically produces hypertension, paradoxical hypotension can occur. Because pheochromocytoma can be associated with flushing (along with diaphoresis and palpitations), this entity should be included in the diagnosis of puzzling cases of anaphylaxis.

Of note is the fact that in addition to the measurement of serotonin and catecholamines to evaluate the possibility of carcinoid syndrome and pheochromocytoma, nuclear scanning with octreotide (for carcinoid syndrome) and 131I-metaiodobenzylguanidine (for

reports have highlighted three entities in the differential diagnosis and have presented interesting cases in this regard [75,76,77•].

A detailed report of four cases of scombroid fish poisoning is of note [78]. Scombroid poisoning is due to the ingestion of high levels of histamine found in the pheochromocytomas) can be performed. In addition, there are commercially available assays for other vasoactive mediators such as vasoactive intestinal polypeptide, substance P, and so forth.

REACTIONS TO HIDDEN AGENTS

One of the most intriguing areas regarding anaphylaxis is the description of cryptic agents disguised in foods and drugs that are responsible for anaphylactic reactions. Reading case reports of these reactions engenders appreciation of the "murder mystery" type of detective work of the authors and alerts the readers to the possibility that similar such cases might be seen in their practice. Recent reports include the description of anaphylaxis to mites contained in wheat flour [79], to carmine dye contained in a popsicle [80], to mustard in "chicken dips" [81], to coriander in teriyaki sauce [82], to *Anisakis simplex* in fish [83], and to carboxymethyl-cellulose as a component of barium sulfate administered for a gastrointestinal contrast study [84]. A detailed review of such reactions to "hidden" allergens is offered by Steinman [85••].

In keeping with the discovery of unexpected agents that cause anaphylaxis is the discovery of the importance of gelatin in the production of anaphylactic reactions to vaccines [86], with the simultaneous documentation of the lack of importance of egg allergy [87,88].

Finally, of note is the recent report of the possibility that deaths in heroin addicts could be due to anaphylactoid reactions to heroin, presumably acting through opiate mast cell receptors. The hypothesis that these deaths were anaphylactoid in nature rested on the finding that postmortem tryptase levels were elevated [89].

REFERENCES AND RECOMMENDED READING

Recently published papers of particular interest have been highlighted as:
• Of interest
•• Of outstanding interest

1.•• Lieberman P: Specific and idiopathic anaphylaxis: pathophysiology and treatment. In *Allergy, Asthma and Immunology from Infancy to Adulthood* edn 3. Edited by Bierman W, Pearlman D, Shapiro G, Busse W. Philadelphia: WB Saunders; 1996:297–320.
This is a comprehensive review of anaphylaxis and anaphylactoid reactions, a detailed sources of references, and a complete description of therapy of the acute episode and differential diagnosis.

2. Lieberman P: Distinguishing anaphylaxis from other serious disorders. *J Respir Dis* 1995, 16:411–420.

3. Lieberman P: Anaphylaxis. *MedScape Respiratory Care.* Edited by Bierman CW, 1997. Available at: http://medscape.com.

4. Lieberman P: Anaphylaxis and anaphylactoid reactions. In *Allergy: Principles and Practice* vol 2, edn 5. Edited by Middleton E, Ellis EF, Yuninger JW, *et al.* St. Louis: Mosby Yearbook; 1998:1079–1092.

5. Yocum MW, Khan DA: Assessment of patients who have experienced anaphylaxis: a 3-year survey. *Mayo Clin Proc* 1994, 69:16–23.

6. Perez C, Tejedor MA, Hoz A, Puras B: Anaphylaxis: a descriptive study of 182 patients [abstract]. *J Allergy Clin Immunol* 1995, 95:368.

7. Kemp SF, Lockey RF, Wolf BL, Lieberman P: Anaphylaxis: a review of 266 cases. *Arch Int Med* 1995, 155:1749–1754.

8. Kagy L, Blaiss M, Lieberman P: Clinical profile of 380 cases of anaphylaxis. *Ann Allergy Asthma Clin Immunol* 1988: in press.

9. Yocum MW, Silverstein M, Klein J: Anaphylaxis in Olmstead County. *J Allergy Clin Immunol* 1996, 97:149–213.

10. Lenler-Petersen P, Hansen D, Andersen M, *et al.*: Drug-related fatal anaphylactic shock in Denmark 1968–1990: a study based on notifications to the Committee on Adverse Drug Reactions. *J Clin Epidemiol* 1995, 48:1185–1188.

11. Van der Klauw MM, Wilson JHP, Stricker BHCh: Drug-associated anaphylaxis: 20 years of reporting in the Netherlands (1974–1994) and review of literature. *Clin Exp Allergy* 1996, 26:1355–1363.

12. Van der Klauw MM, Stricker BHCh, Herings RMC, *et al.*: A population-based case-cohort study of drug-induced anaphylaxis. *Br J Clin Pharmacol* 1993, 35:400–408.

13. Stricker BHCh, De Groot RRM, Wilson JHP: Glafenine-associated anaphylaxis as a cause of hospital admission in the Netherlands. *Eur J Clin Pharmacol* 1991, 40:367–371.

14. Lefevre N, Delaunay L, Hingot JL, Bonnet F: Bilateral massive adrenal haemorrhage complicating anaphylactic shock: a case report. *Intensive Care Med* 1996, 2:447–449.

15. Woltsche-Kahr I, Dranke B: Recurrent losses of consciousness in anaphylactic reactions. *DTW Dtsch Med Wochenschr* 1997, 122:747–750.

16. Attenhofer C, Rudolf S, Salomon F, *et al.*: Ventricular fibrillation in a patient with exercise-induced anaphylaxis, normal coronary arteries and a positive ergonovine test. *Chest* 1994, 105:620–622.

17. Bacal E, Patterson R, Zeiss CR: Evaluation of severe (anaphylactic) reactions. *Clin Allergy* 1978, 8:295–304.

18. Ditto AM, Harris KE, Krasnick J, Miller MA, Patterson R: Idiopathic anaphylaxis: a series of 335 cases. *Ann Allergy Asthma Immunol* 1996, 77:285–291.

19. Lieberman P, Taylor WW: Recurrent idiopathic anaphylaxis. *Arch Intern Med* 1979, 139:1032–1034.

20. Wiggins CA, Dykewicz MS, Patterson R: Idiopathic anaphylaxis: classification, evaluation, and treatment of 123 patients. *J Allergy Clin Immunol* 1988, 82:849–855.

21. Patterson R, Hogan MB, Yarnold PR, Harris KE: Idiopathic anaphylaxis: an attempt to estimate the incidence in the United States. *Arch Intern Med* 1995, 155:869–871.

22. Patterson R, Stoloff RS, Greenberger PA, *et al.*: Algorithms for the diagnosis and management of idiopathic anaphylaxis. *Ann Allergy* 1993, 71:40–44.

23. Tanus T, Atkins PC, Levinson AI: Serum tryptase in idiopathic anaphylaxis: a case report and review of the literature. *Ann Emerg Med* 1994, 24:104–107.

24. Patterson R, Greenberger PA, Grammar LC, *et al.*: Idiopathic anaphylaxis (IA): suggested theories relative to the pathogenesis and response to therapy. *Allergy Proc* 1993, 14:365–367.

25. Frieri M, Madden J, Nolte H: Spontaneous basophil histamine release (BHR) in atopic patients with food hypersensitivity [abstract]. *J Allergy Clin Immunol* 1992, 89:195.

26. Sampson HA, Broadbent K: "Spontaneous" histamine release and histamine releasing factor in patients with atopic dermatitis and food hypersensitivity [abstract]. *J Allergy Clin Immunol* 1987, 79:294.

27. Patterson R, Pruzansky JJ, Dykewicz MS, Lawrence ID: Basophil-mast cell response syndromes: a unified clinical approach. *Allergy Proc* 1988, 9:611–620.

28. Kemp SF, Lockey RF, Wolf BL, Lieberman P: Anaphylaxis: a review of 266 cases. *Arch Intern Med* 1995, 155:1749–1754.

29. Friedman BS, Steinberg SC, Meggs WJ, *et al.*: Analysis of plasma histamine levels in patients with mast cell disorders. *Am J Med* 1989, 87:649–654.

30. Ditto, AM, Krasnick J, Greenberger PA, *et al.*: Pediatric idiopathic anaphylaxis: experience with 22 patients. *J Allergy Clin Immunol* 1997, 100:320–326.

31. Krasnick J, Patterson R, Meyers GL: A fatality from idiopathic anaphylaxis. *Ann Allergy Asthma Immunol* 1996, 76:376–378.

32. Krasnick J, Patterson R, Harris KE: Idiopathic anaphylaxis: long-term follow-up cost and outlook [abstract]. *J Allergy Clin Immunol* 1996, 97:349.

33. Greenberger PA: Idiopathic anaphylaxis. *Immunol Allergy Clin North Am* 1992, 12:571–583.

34. Wong S, Patterson R, Harris KE, Dykewicz MS: Efficacy of ketotifen in corticosteroid-dependent idiopathic anaphylaxis. *Ann Allergy* 1991, 67:359–369.

35. Lee TM, Britton L: Use of methotrexate (MTX) in corticosteroid (CS)-dependent idiopathic anaphylaxis (IA) [abstract]. *J Allergy Clin Immunol* 1993, 91(suppl):155.

36. Furchgott RF: The discovery of endothelium-derived relaxing factor and its importance in the identification of nitric oxide. *JAMA* 1996, 276:1186–1188.

37. Liebermann P: Anaphylaxis and anaphylactoid reactions: slide presentation. Current Views, November 1996.

38.• Lyons CR: Emerging roles of nitric oxide in inflammation. *Hosp Pract* 1996, 31:69–86.
This is a very readable review of the role of NO in the production of inflammation and a detailed explanation of its role in anaphylactic events.

39. Liggett SB, Levi R, Metzger H: G-protein coupled receptors, nitric oxide, and the IgE receptor in asthma. *Am J Respir Crit Care Med* 1995, 152:394–402.

40. Rittweger R, Hermann K, Ring J: Increased urinary excretion of angiotensin during anaphylactoid reactions. *Int Arch Allergy Immunol* 1994, 104:255–261.

41. Hermann K, Ring J: Changes in angiotensin peptides in plasma and urine in patients with anaphylaxis. *Int Arch Allergy Immunol* 1992, 99:446–448.

42. Hermann K, Rittweger R, Phillips MI, Ring J: Presence of angiotensin peptides in human urine. *Clin Chem* 1992, 38:1768–1772.

43. Van der Linden P, Struyvenberg A, Kraaijenhagen R, *et al.*: Anaphylactic shock after insect-sting challenge in 138 persons with a previous insect-sting reaction. *Ann Intern Med* 1993, 118:161–168.

44. Owen HG, Brecher ME: Atypical reactions associated with use of angiotensin-converting enzyme inhibitors and apheresis. *Transfusion* 1994, 34:891–894.

45. Koga N, Nagano T, Sato T, Kagasawa K: Anaphylactoid reactions and bradykinin generation in patients treated with LDL-apheresis and an ACE inhibitor. *ASAIO J* 1993, 39:M288–M291.

46. Verresen L, Fink E, Lemke H, Vanrenterghem Y: Bradykinin is a mediator of anaphylactoid reactions during hemodialysis with AN69 membranes. *Kidney Int* 1994, 45:1497–1503.

47. Korashe GK, Shinenberger JH, Klaustenmeyer WB: Severe hypersensitivity reaction during hemodialysis. *Ann Allergy Asthma Immunol* 1997, 78:217–220.

48. Olbricht CJ, Schaumann D, Fischer D: Anaphylactoid reactions, LDL apheresis with dextran sulphate, and ACE inhibitors [letter]. *Lancet* 1992, 340:908–909.

49. Kroon AA, Mol MJ, Stalenhoff AF: ACE inhibitors and LDL-apheresis with dextran sulphate absorption [letter]. *Lancet* 1992, 340:1476.

50. Tunon-de-Lara JM, Villanueva P, Marcus M, Taytard A: ACE inhibitors and anaphylactoid reactions during venom immunotherapy [letter]. *Lancet* 1992, 340:908.

51. Hermann K, Ring J: Hymenoptera venom anaphylaxis: may decreased levels of angiotensin peptides play a role? *Clin Exp Allergy* 1990, 20:569–570.

52. Hermann K, Donhauser S, Ring J: Angiotensin in human leukocytes of patients with insect venom anaphylaxis and healthy volunteers. *Int Arch Allergy Immunol* 1995, 107:385–386.

53. Hermann K, von Tschirschnitz M, von Eschenbach C, Ring J: Histamine, tryptase, norepinephrine, angiotensinogen, angiotensin-converting enzyme, angiotensin I and II in plasma of patients with hymenoptera venom anaphylaxis. *Int Arch Allergy Immunol* 1994, 104:379–384.

54. McKinnon RP, Sinclair CJ: Angiotensinamide in the treatment of probable anaphylaxis to succinylated gelatin (gelofusine). *Anaesthesia* 1994, 49:309–311.

55. Zimmerman BG: Actions of angiotensin on adrenergic nerve endings. *Fed Proc* 1978, 37:199–202.

56. Reid IA: Actions of angiotensin II on the brain: mechanisms and physiologic role. *Am J Physiol* 1984, 246:F533–F543.

57. Peach MJ: Molecular actions of angiotensin. *Biochem Pharmacol* 1981, 30:2745–2751.

58. Israili ZH, Hall WD: Cough and angioneurotic edema associated with angiotensin-converting enzyme inhibitor therapy: a review of the literature and pathophysiology. *Ann Intern Med* 1992, 117:234–242.

59.• Malini P, Zanardi M, Milani M, Amlosioni E: Thromboxane antagonism and cough induced by angiotensin-converting enzyme inhibitor. *Lancet* 1997, 350:15–18.
This is an interesting discussion of the mechanism of action of ACE inhibitors and their potential role in worsening hypotensive anaphylactic episodes.

60.• Kemp SF, Lieberman P: Inhibitors of angiotensin II: potential hazards for patients at risk for anaphylaxis? *Ann Allergy Asthma Immunol* 1997, 78:527–529.
This is a readable and detailed review of the role of ACE inhibitors in worsening anaphylactic episodes.

61. Reid MJ, Lockey RF, Turkeltaub PC, Platts-Mills TAE: Survey of fatalities from skin testing and immunotherapy 1985–1989. *J Allergy Clin Immunol* 1993, 92:6–15.

62. Schwartz LB, Metcalfe DD, Miller JS, *et al.*: Tryptase levels as an indicator of mast cell activation in systemic anaphylaxis and mastocytosis. *N Engl J Med* 1987, 316:1622–1626.

63. LaRoche D, Vergnaud M, Sillard B, *et al.*: Biochemical markers of anaphylactoid reactions to drugs: comparison of plasma histamine and tryptase. *Anesthesiology* 1991, 75:945–949.

64. Marshall GD, Calabrese DM, Schwartz LB: Serum tryptase levels in ICU patients with unexplained acute hypotension [abstract]. *J Allergy Clin Immunol* 1996, 97:329.

65. Ordoqui E, Aranzabal A, Zubeldia JM, *et al.*: Latent period of tryptase serum peak levels in allergic drug reactions [abstract]. *J Allergy Clin Immunol* 1996, 97:351.

66. Carias K, Abernathy C, Schwartz LB: Serum α-tryptase, an update on its use to screen for systemic mastocytosis [abstract]. *J Allergy Clin Immunol* 1996, 97:269.

67. Ordoqui E, Rodriguez V, Zubeldia JM, *et al.*: Serum tryptase levels in allergic drug reactions [abstract]. *J Allergy Clin Immunol* 1995, 95:172.

68. Becker AB, Mactavish G, Frith E, *et al.*: Postmortem stability of serum tryptase and immunoglobulin E [abstract]. *J Allergy Clin Immunol* 1995, 95:369.

69. Brockow K, Vieluf D, Ring J: Postmortem diagnosis of an anaphylactoid reaction due to nonionic radiocontrast media by serum tryptase analysis: a case report [abstract]. *J Allergy Clin Immunol* 1996, 97:363.

70. The American Academy of Pediatrics Committee on Drugs: Anaphylaxis. *Pediatrics* 1973, 51:136–140.

71. The Journal of Allergy and Clinical Immunology: Position statement. *J Allergy Clin Immunol* 1986, 77:271–273.

72. The Journal of Allergy and Clinical Immunology: Position statement: guidelines to minimize the risk from systemic reactions caused by immunotherapy with allergenic extracts. *J Allergy Clin Immunol* 1994, 93:811–812.

73. Golden DB, Schwartz HJ: Anaphylaxis in the allergy office [abstract]. *J Allergy Clin Immunol* 1996, 97:351.

74. Simons KJ, Roberts JR, Gu X, *et al.*: Prospective study of epinephrine (EPI) absorption in children with a history of anaphylaxis [abstract]. *J Allergy Clin Immunol* 1997, 99:S494.

75. Sanchez-Guerrero IM, Vidal JB, Escudero AI: Scombroid fish poisoning: a potentially life-threatening allergic-like reaction. *J Allergy Clin Immunol* 1997, 100:433–434.

76. Cogen F, Greipp P: Capillary leak syndrome (CLS) presenting as idiopathic anaphylaxis (A) [abstract]. *J Allergy Clin Immunol* 1995, 95:367.

77.• Suchard JR: Recurrent near-syncope with flushing. *Acad Emerg Med* 1997, 4:718–724.
This is a good review of causes of flushing.

78. Taylor SL, Stratton JE, Nordlec JA: Histamine poisoning (scombroid fish poisoning): an allergic-like intoxication. *J Toxicol Clin Toxicol* 1989, 27:225–240.

79. Blanco C, Quiralte J, Castillo R, Delgado J, *et al.*: Anaphylaxis after ingestion of wheat flour contaminated with mites. *J Allergy Clin Immunol* 1997, 99:308–313.

80. Baldwin JL, Chou AH, Solomon WR: Popsicle-induced anaphylaxis due to carmine allergy. *Ann Allergy Asthma Immunol* 1997, 79:415–419.

81. Kanny G, Fremont S, Talhouarne G, *et al.*: Anaphylaxis to mustard as a masked allergen in "chicken dips." *Ann Allergy Asthma Immunol* 1995, 75:340–342.

82. Bock SA: Anaphylaxis to coriander: a sleuthing story. *J Allergy Clin Immunol* 1993, 91:1232–1233.

83. Audicana MT, Fernandez de Corres L, Munoz D, *et al.*: Recurrent anaphylaxis caused by Anisakis simplex parasitizing fish. *J Allergy Clin Immunol* 1995, 96:558–560.

84. Muroi N, Nishibori M, Fujii T, *et al.*: Anaphylaxis from the carboxymethylcellulose component of barium sulfate suspension. *N Engl J Med* 1997, 337:1275–277.

85.•• Steinman H: "Hidden" allergens in food. *J Allergy Clin Immunol* 1997, 98:241–250.
This paper provides interesting insights into the role of hidden allergens in foods and a comprehensive list of such allergens.

86. Sakaguchi M, Nakayama T, Inouye S: Food allergy to gelatin in children with systemic immediate-type reactions, including anaphylaxis, to vaccines. *J Allergy Clin Immunol* 1996, 98:1058–1061.

87. James JM, Burks AW, Roberson PK, *et al.*: Safe administration of the measles vaccine to children allergic to eggs. *N Engl J Med* 1995, 332:1262–1266.

88. James JM, Zeiger RS, Lester MR, *et al.*: Safe administration of influenza vaccine to egg allergic patients [abstract]. *J Allergy Clin Immunol* 1996, 97:239.

89. Edston E, van Hage-Hamsten M: Anaphylactoid shock a common cause of death in heroin addicts? *Allergy* 1997, 52:950–954.

Table 14-1. CLASSIFICATION OF PHYSICALLY INDUCED OR PHYSIOLOGICALLY RELATED URTICARIAL DISEASE AND ANGIOEDEMA

Thermomechanical stimuli
  Vibratory angioedema
  Dermographism
  Pressure-induced urticaria and angioedema (delayed)
  Cold-induced urticaria
    Idiopathic cold urticaria
    Urticaria associated with cryopathies, such as cryoglobulinemia, cold agglutinins, and cryofibrinoginemia
  Heat-induced urticaria
    Cholinergic urticaria
    Local heat urticaria
  Solar urticaria
Physiologic stimuli
  Exercise-induced urticaria and anaphylaxis

developing during exposure to warm environments capable of elevating core body temperatures are deemed cholinergic urticaria in the absence of exercise.

Differential diagnosis and etiologic considerations

Acute urticaria and angioedema

These are common occurrences in children and are less frequent in adults. Acute urticaria is a self-limited eruption caused by mast cell degranulation, which is usually an isolated event or is not protracted beyond several weeks. Patients have mild-to-severe pruritus with urticaria that is localized or generalized. Angioedema can be present as well as dermographism. Etiologic considerations for acute urticaria focus on identifiable inciting events [4]. In children, acute viral illnesses are known to be associated with urticarial eruptions. These episodes are transient and tend to improve with the resolution of the viral infection.

Other acute events that may result in urticaria and angioedema include IgE–mediated reactions to foods or drugs. Classically, penicillin has been associated with IgE-mediated hypersensitivity and can result in an urticarial eruption, which can progress to anaphylaxis [5]. However, virtually any food or drug can result in an IgE-mediated reaction, and the patients are often aware of the connection between the food or medication and the episode. Occasionally, ingredients, such as eggs, milk, or soy, that are found in multiple types of food can cause confusion. In some cases, the surreptitious ingestion of foods or drugs can result in a patient developing recurrent episodes of acute urticaria, which can lead erroneously to a diagnosis of chronic urticaria.

Such instances are those in which people continue to ingest the foods or medications that result in urticarial lesions. This is the case, for instance, in inadvertent exposure to penicillin, a drug commonly used in the swine and dairy industries. Exposure to penicillin may be a consideration for individuals who are highly allergic to this drug and develop mild acute outbreaks on a sporadic basis despite the absence of apparent exposure to β-lactam antibiotics.

In the patient who experiences an episode of acute urticaria or angioedema, attention to specific historical events is necessary. The ingestion of specific foods or medications may be the etiologic factor resulting in mast cell degranulation. Recurrent acute episodes could reflect the inadvertent ingestion of the same material on multiple occasions. In the child with an upper respiratory tract infection, the possibility that the acute urticaria is related to the viral illness must be entertained. However, in children in whom a viral infection has resulted in symptoms for which an antibiotic has been prescribed, a β-lactam antibiotic could be the cause of the urticarial process. This can be a frustrating situation, and can be avoided or at least simplified if judicious use of antibiotics is observed.

Non-IgE–mediated reactions can also result in acute urticaria or angioedema [6]. Included in this etiologic consideration is the development of an anaphylactoid or non-IgE–mediated reaction to intravenous radiocontrast media (RCM). The first-generation agents used previously resulted in a significant osmolar change, and this, in turn, caused nonspecific degranulation of mast cells. Patients develop urticarial lesions and angioedema temporally related to the infusion of the RCM. Similarly, the use of codeine or related opiod drugs also can also cause nonspecific degranulation of mast cells without IgE involvement, resulting in an acute urticarial event [7]. Finally, aspirin and nonsteroidal anti-inflammatory drugs (NSAIDs), which are capable of altering arachidonic acid metabolism, can result in urticaria or angioedema in the absence of a specific interaction between IgE and the pharmacologic agent.

Chronic urticaria and angioedema

This is a designation restricted to patients with lesions recurring for greater than 6 weeks. These patients rarely have immediate hypersensitivity (IgE-mediated) reactions to food or drugs as causative factors unless the causative agent has not been identified or discontinued. Etiologic considerations for chronic urticaria and angioedema are diverse, including underlying systemic illness, complement-mediated diseases, the perturbation of bradykinin metabolism by therapeutic agents, and, by exclusion, "idiopathic" mechanisms. The group of chronic urticaria that has been previously deemed idiopathic (Fig. 14-1) has been quite large, accounting for over 90% of chronic urticaria patients if all physically-induced urticarias are excluded [8]. However, this percentage continues to shrink as research elucidates etiologic mechanisms.

The aforementioned IgE-mediated reactions to foods, drugs, or food additives rarely cause chronic urticaria [9]. Generally, the patients are able to correlate the ingestion of a food or the use of a medication with the onset of their cutaneous eruptions. Rarely does an ingredient in a food or a pharmacologic agent used in veterinary medicine result in such lesions. Often, these possibilities can be further assessed by the use of a careful diet diary or by food-elimination diet.

Recurrent acute episodes of urticaria can be the result of non-IgE–mediated reactions to drugs, which generally include the widely available category of drugs that alter arachidonic acid metabolism. Aspirin and aspirin-containing over-the-counter products as well as NSAIDs can result in urticarial eruptions or angioedema, which are believed to be related to their alteration of prostaglandin

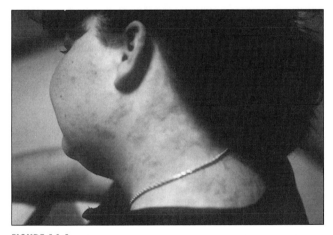

FIGURE 14-1.
Typical lesions seen in chronic idiopathic urticaria.

synthesis (Fig. 14-2). However, patients generally identify the relationship between their use of the medication and the development of hives or swelling.

A group of physically-induced urticarias can result in chronic disease, but the appearance and duration of the individual lesions are quite different from what one observes with chronic urticaria [10]. Dermographism, which designates the occurrence of hives or linear urticarial lesions with tensile movement of the skin, can recur for months to years (Fig. 14-3). The etiologic event resulting in this altered skin response is generally unidentified. Another physical urticaria that can be chronic in occurrence is cold urticaria, which will result in lesions when the individual is exposed to either cold weather or cold items [11]. Patients suffering from cold urticaria develop urticarial lesions on the face and hands if they are in a cold climate and if they are not using appropriate clothing to protect themselves from the cold. In addition, if they handle cold items, such as meats during food preparation or cold beverages, they develop swelling of the hands. Histamine and tumor necrosis factor-α are found elevated in the blood of these patients following cold exposure [12•]. The chronic nature of the urticaria is dependent on the necessary direct exposure to a cold stimulus. Solar urticaria results from the exposure of the skin to ambient light [13]. Thus, an individual exposed on a regular basis would have chronic urticarial lesions. The multiple types of solar urticaria are outlined in Table 14-2.

Cholinergic urticaria

Another form of physically-induced, physiologically-related urticaria that can result in chronic disease in children and adults is cholinergic urticaria [14]. Cholinergic urticaria manifests as small, punctate urticarial lesions that are intensely pruritic. They develop when the individual is exposed to a warm environment or performs an

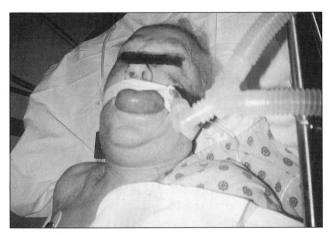

FIGURE 14-2.
Glossal angioedema caused by nonsteroidal anti-inflammatory drug.

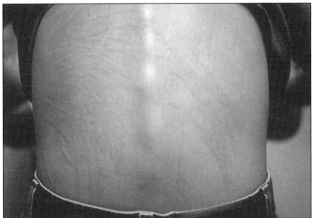

FIGURE 14-3.
Linear urticaria caused by scratching on back of patient with dermographism.

Table 14-2. DESIGNATIONS OF SOLAR URTICARIA BASED ON WAVELENGTH OF LIGHT INCITING CUTANEOUS ERUPTION	
Type of solar urticaria	Wavelength of light
1	280 to 320 nm (ultraviolet B)—may be passively transferred
2	320 to 400 nm (ultraviolet A)
3	400 to 500 nm (visible)
4	400 to 500 nm (visible)—may be passively transferred
5	280 to 500 nm (ultraviolet A, B, and visible)
6	400 to 500 nm*

* Erythropoietic protoporphria will cause urticarial skin lesions with frank necrosis of skin if exposed to light in the 400- to 500-nm spectrum.

activity sufficient to raise core body temperature. These lesions occur when an individual takes a hot shower or performs exercise. Sweating often occurs concomitantly with hive formation. In contrast, exercise-induced urticaria will result in chronic disease in the individual whose threshold for hives with aerobic activity is low, resulting in development of urticarial lesions with minimal activity, such as walking briskly. This individual, however, will not develop urticaria when taking a hot shower, and must be involved in some degree of physical activity to elicit exercise-induced lesions.

Chronic urticaria and infectious diseases

Chronic urticaria may be occasionally associated with a coincident infectious process. Enteric parasitic disease found in immigrants from underdeveloped countries or individuals with travel histories can result in urticarial eruptions. These patients often complain of diarrhea and loose stools and are found to have ova and parasites in their fecal material. Generally, they are found to have elevated eosinophil counts. Other parasites, such as larvae migrans, can result in urticaria. Patients who are immunosuppressed or on systemic corticosteroids are also at risk for parasitic infections, such as pulmonary *Strongyloides*. These patients can also develop urticarial lesions [3].

Chronic urticaria versus vasculitis

Chronic lesions that appear urticarial and leave residual scarring or that have a petechial nature can actually be caused by a vasculitic process. Autoimmune processes, such as systemic lupus erythematosus, Sjögrens syndrome, rheumatoid arthritis, and cryoglobulinemia as well as other primarily vasculitic processes, can cause

lesions that can be mistakenly identified as urticarial; a skin biopsy is needed to demonstrate the underlying vasculitis. Occasionally, these autoimmune diseases can result in immune-complex deposition with complement consumption and the degranulation of mast cells by products of complement activation (C3a, C5a) [2••].

Chronic urticaria, thyroid disease, and autoimmunity

For the past decade, an increasing body of evidence suggests an association of thyroid disease with chronic urticaria. Studies from the late 1980s revealed an association of elevated autoimmune thyroid serologies and chronic hives [15,16]. Elevated antimicrosomal (antiperoxidase) antibodies and antithyroglobulin antibodies were demonstrated in approximately 12% of patients even if they were euthyroid; many, however, have Hashimoto's thyroiditis. This finding has been investigated further and more recent data in those individuals with severe chronic urticaria suggest an incidence of antithyroid antibodies in approximately 20% to 25% of patients, most of whom are women [17]. Furthermore, an association has been demonstrated recently between the presence of antibodies against the α subunit of the high-affinity IgE receptor (FcεRI) on mast cells and the presence of urticaria [18••–20••]. This high-affinity receptor and its tetrameric chains are shown in Figure 14-4. The autoimmune antibody apparently has the capability to cause degranulation of mast cells and basophils through the cross-linking of two α subunits from two separate receptors, as depicted in Figure 14-5. Its specific relationship to the clinical disease seen in chronic idiopathic urticaria is under careful investigation, but an incidence of IgG anti-FcεRI-α subunit of 45% has been reported. The measurement of antibodies against the IgE receptor subunit is still an investigative tool; however, extension into the clinical arena is expected. Large-scale epidemiologic studies establishing titers in both normal and disease populations have yet to be performed.

Etiology of chronic urticaria and chronic angiodema

When considering the etiology of chronic urticaria, a careful history and physical examination are paramount. One must search for the specific physical stimuli that can be etiologic in recurrent lesions, such as exposure to the cold, sun, or various physiologic stresses, such as exercise or passive heating. The history of the patient should disclose the possibility of enteric parasitic pathogens. The frequent use of NSAIDs for musculoskeletal problems could relate to recurrent acute angioedema. The presence of systemic symptoms or other findings suggestive of the systemic autoimmune disease can reflect the possibility of a vasculitic process. Therefore, laboratory data that include a complete blood count, erythrocyte sedimentation rate, antinuclear antibodies, rheumatoid factor, and

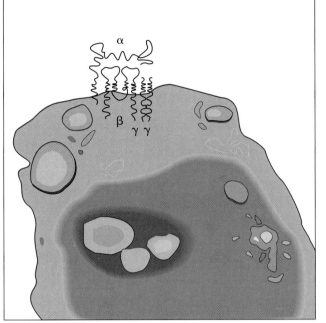

FIGURE 14-4.
The subunit chains of the FcϵRI on basophils and mast cells.

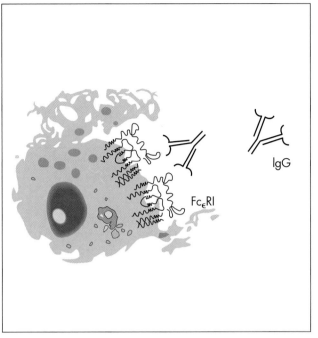

FIGURE 14-5.
IgG autoantibody specific for the FcϵRI receptor causing mast cell degranulation.

serum chemistries would be advantageous. A urinalysis, as well as complement studies (C3, C4, CH_{50}), may be indicated for appropriate patients. Finally, the recent finding of an association between autoimmune thyroiditis and chronic urticaria warrants the investigation of antithyroid antibodies (antiperoxidase, antithyroglobulin) and investigation of thyroid function (thyroxin, thyroid-stimulating hormone). Further, serologic analysis of antibodies against the IgE receptor (α subunit) also would serve as an appropriate investigative tool.

Chronic angioedema can occur in the absence of urticarial lesions, and it is rarely associated with the presence of an inheritable deficiency of the C1-inhibitor (C1-INH) [3,21,22]. Since hereditary angioedema has no association with urticaria, patients with both hives and swelling do not require evaluation of C1-INH deficiency. Hereditary angioedema can be the result of either a lack of production of the C1-INH protein, or the production of a dysfunctional protein. Type I hereditary angioedema has been arbitrarily assigned to the congenital absence of the protein, and the designation of type II hereditary angioedema denotes the presence of a dysfunctional protein [3,21]. In their younger years or teens, these patients generally present with visceral complaints (abdominal pain simulating an acute abdomen) and laryngeal edema. Often, the family history can reveal other family members with a similar disease.

Chronic angioedema can also occur in another population of patients who have an acquired C1-INH deficiency [23]. These patients generally are older individu-

als who have lymphoproliferative malignancies. In one group, the patients with lymphoproliferative disease have anti-idiotypic antibodies to a monoclonal paraprotein. Their combination results in high levels of complement-activating complexes that bind C1q, thereby activating C1 (C1r and C1s) and consuming the C1-INH. Another uncommon form of acquired C1-INH deficiency is due to an IgG autoantibody which binds C1-INH. It is digested by enzymes but can no longer inactivate C1 esterase. Thus, a low molecular weight C1-INH is found in the circulation, which distinguishes it from the other types of hereditary or acquired C1-INH deficiency. In assessing whether a patient with chronic angioedema has either a primary or secondary deficiency of the C1-INH, obtaining functional assays is useful. A CH_{50}, C4, and C1q often can delineate which etiology is responsible, as seen in Table 14-3. Note that a depressed C1q complement component with a depressed C1 esterase inhibitor, or CH_{50} in an older patient, is a lymphoproliferative process until proven otherwise. Some connective tissue diseases with circulating immune complexes (systemic lupus erythematosus) can cause angioedema by the same mechanism.

A common problem in the development of angiodema is the widespread use of angiotensin-converting enzyme inhibitors (ACEI) [24]. ACEI are widely used in the treatment of hypertension and in congestive heart failure. They have the capability of inhibiting the kininase enzyme, which is responsible for the degradation of bradykinin and substance P. Elevated levels of

Table 14-3. LABORATORY EVALUATION OF COMPLEMENT-MEDIATED ANGIOEDEMA

C_1 esterase inhibitor (antigenic assay)

Decreased	Type I hereditary angioedema
Normal*	Type II hereditary angioedema
Decreased	Acquired C_1 esterase deficiency

C_1-esterase inhibitor (functional assay)

Decreased	Types I and II hereditary angioedema
Decreased	Acquired C_1 esterase deficiency

CH_{50}

Decreased	Types I and II hereditary angioedema
Decreased	Acquired C_1 esterase deficiency

C4

Decreased	Types I and II hereditary angioedema
Decreased	Acquired C_1 esterase deficiency

C_{1q}

Normal	Types I and II hereditary angioedema
Decreased*	Acquired C_1 esterase deficiency

Denotes differentiating lab finding.

bradykinin and substance P are capable of degranulating mast cells. The ability of ACEI to magnify bradykinin-induced wheals indirectly supports this scenario. Therefore, in an individual with chronic angioedema, a careful history of medications used for hypertension or heart disease must be obtained to rule out this possible cause of swelling. The development of angioedema can occur at any time during the treatment with an ACEI and a latency period of years can be observed. In addition, angioedema episodes can be separated by significant intervals of time. Other coincidental or ancillary factors that can contribute to angioedema have yet to be identified, and could include such factors as the effect of α- and β-adrenergic receptor blockers and coincident viral infections.

Melkersson-Rosenthal syndrome

This syndrome represents a disorder that may be incorrectly interpreted as chronic angioedema [25,26]. It is a persistent, nonremitting, angioedema-like swelling of the lips and perioral tissue. Biopsy of this tissue reveals a granulomatous process. The specific inciting event or pathogen resulting in the granulomatous infiltration has yet to be identified. The swelling persists despite treatment with high dose antihistamines; it may respond partially to oral or injected corticosteroids, but this is usually transient and incomplete. Clofazamine has been used with some success [27].

NEW CONCEPTS IN THE PATHOBIOLOGY OF CHRONIC URTICARIA

The specific interaction of an antigen with the IgE affixed to mast cells and basophils leads to cell activation with degranulation. There is agreement that such a mechanism is involved when an antigen, such as penicillin, or a food allergen, such as peanut, results in the degranulation of mast cells or basophils and causes urticaria. However, there has not been a satisfactory explanation of the protracted urticarial state seen in chronic idiopathic urticaria. An exhaustive research effort has been undertaken to look for a factor or factors that could result in the degranulation of basophils or mast cells and could be responsible for the mast cell degranulation seen in this disorder. Such a factor has been loosely termed histamine-releasing factor (HRF) [28,29]. HRF-type substances were sought in various cell types that might be involved in the pathogenesis of chronic urticaria. The presence of a perivascular non-necrotizing mononuclear infiltrate seen in chronic urticaria spurred interest in assessing whether mononuclear cells could be the source of HRF [30].

The first cytokine found to have HRF-like ability was interleukin (IL)-1 [31]. IL-1 was demonstrated to have weak histamine-releasing activity from in vitro preparations of basophils. Further efforts using supernatants obtained from mononuclear cell preparations revealed that IL-3 and granulocyte-macrophage colony-stimulating factor (GM-CSF) also have the capability of releasing histamine from basophils [32]. This work was extended, and subsequently determined that these agents also could act as priming agents (eg, augment basophil secretion dose to other agonists including IgE plus antigen). IL-8 obtained from lymphocytes was found to have the opposite effect on basophils and resulted in inhibition of basophil histamine release [33]. Over a period of approximately 10 years, a myriad of cytokines and mediators of inflammation have demonstrated some effect on the secretion of histamine from basophil and mast cell preparations (Table 14-4) [34••–36••]. The degree to which these secretagogues contribute to the clinical disease seen in chronic urticaria and angioedema has not been fully established. Studies have shown that fluid obtained from iatrogenically-induced blisters in patients with chronic idiopathic urticaria can demonstrate the presence of various cytokines and their HRF-activity [37,38,39••,40••]. However, the specific factors that can stimulate basophil and mast cell degranulation have not been identified.

In the late 1980s, Leznoff et al. [15,16] demonstrated an increased incidence of antithyroid (antimicrosomal, antithyroglobulin) antibodies in individuals with chronic idiopathic urticaria. They assessed the presence of these antibodies in patients who exhibited chronic urticaria and found that approximately 12% of these patients did demonstrate the presence of elevated titers. More recently, we have assessed the presence of antithyroid antibodies

Table 14-4. CYTOKINES REPORTED TO ACTIVATE OR PRIME BASOPHILS FOR HISTAMINE RELEASE

Interleukin-1

Interleukin-3

Granulocyte-macrophage colony-stimulating factor

Connective tissue activating peptide III

Macrophage inflammatory protein 1-α and 1-β

Neutrophil activating peptide-2

Monocyte chemotactic and activating factor/monocyte chemoattractant protein-1

Regulated upon activation, normal T-cell expressed and secreted (RANTES)

(antiperoxidase, antithyroglobulin) in severe chronic urticaria patients referred to our clinical facility (The National Urticaria Research and Treatment Center Inc, Charleston, SC) and have revealed an incidence of approximately 20% to 25% [17]. Whether this higher incidence of autoimmune thyroid serologies in our population reflects a different patient cohort, differences in methodology, or a different reference interval is not clear [41••]. Presently, no evidence suggests that a direct causative relationship exists between the elevated antithyroid autoantibodies and the presence of mast cell degranulation or urticaria (ie, it is an associated rather than "cause and effect" phenomenon) [42].

Studies attempting to attenuate the urticarial disease with the administration of thyroid hormone in euthyroid patients with chronic idiopathic urticaria and antithyroid antibodies have not shown any major change in the natural course of the disease with the use of thyroid replacement. Limited studies and anecdotal reports have shown that the use of thyroid replacement had variable benefit to the severity or duration of the urticarial lesions [43•,44]. During the same period, studies began to assess the possibility that an autoantibody against the IgE molecule could result in cross-linking of IgE on mast cells and basophils and cause subsequent degranulation. Initial studies demonstrated the presence of autoantibodies against the IgE molecule in patients with chronic idiopathic urticaria [45,46]; however, the incidence was only 5% to 10%. Moreover, autoantibodies directed against the IgE molecule were also found in other disease states not associated with urticarial lesions, such as atopic dermatitis. With the identification and purification of FcεRI, studies next addressed the possibility that such an autoantibody could result in activation of the basophils or mast cells by cross-linking this high-affinity receptor. Soon thereafter, the IgG fraction of sera from chronic idiopathic urticaria patients was shown to initiate basophil or mast cell degranulation in about one third of patients [47,48].

In several laboratories, various methodologies have demonstrated that autoantibodies against the IgE receptor do indeed exist. These include degranulation of rat basophil leukemic cells transfected with the α-subunit of the IgE receptor; degranulation of human basophils; degranulation of cutaneous mast cells; and binding to cloned α-subunit by immunoblot [18••–20••]. Recent studies suggest that this anti-IgE receptor autoantibody is present in 45% to 50% of chronic idiopathic urticaria patients [20••]. Thus, the characteristic histopathology one associates with chronic urticaria must be secondary to autoantibody activation of cutaneous mast cells. Studies are investigating its incidence in the normal population as well as other disease states, including autoimmune entities, such as systemic lupus erythematosus. Efforts are also under way to determine appropriate reference intervals and mechanisms through which the autoantibody may be selectively directed against dermal mast cells rather than mast cells in other tissues.

EVALUATION
History and physical examination

As with the assessment of any patient for the presence of a clinical disease, the history and physical examination are critically important. The history usually reveals information regarding the duration of the disease and its relationship to specific physical stimuli or activities. Whether the lesions are of a chronic nature or whether they represent recurrent acute episodes must be appreciated. A careful dietary and medication history must be obtained to ascertain the possibility that foods or therapeutic agents are resulting in either IgE-mediated or non-IgE–mediated degranulation of mast cells. The inquiry must also include the assessment of travel to areas endemic for parasitic disease. The review of systems must include the possibility of other systemic symptoms, which could reflect an occult systemic disease. The presence of constitutional symptoms, frank arthritis, gastrointestinal complaints, or others may be evidence of a coincident disease process. The physical examination must be in depth and complete. Findings of mucosal lesions, adenopathy, abnormal lung or heart sounds on auscultation, hepatosplenomegaly, or joint findings, such as synovitis, expand the diagnostic considerations.

In the patient with acute urticaria or angioedema, the history and physical examination will be the most revealing. Ruling out the use of antibiotics or analgesics as the cause is imperative for proper diagnosis and treatment. Occasionally, food skin tests will confirm the suspicion that a dietary constituent resulted in the urticarial eruption. Penicillin skin testing can be used to confirm the presence of an IgE-mediated hypersensitivity to β-lactam antibiotics.

The evaluation for chronic urticaria and angioedema is different from that for acute urticaria and angioedema.

Certainly, the history and physical examination are once again paramount to developing the differential diagnostic list. Attention must be directed to signs and symptoms that suggest underlying systemic disease. One must be vigilant to eliminate the possibility of recurrent acute episodes of mast cell degranulation due to therapeutic agents, such as ACEI. Generally, IgE-mediated reactions to foods or drugs are not causative in chronic urticaria and angioedema, because this relationship is generally identified by the patient. However, food skin tests and avoidance diets are often indispensable to convince both the patient and referring physicians that these agents are not responsible for the patient's cutaneous disease.

Laboratory studies

Various laboratory studies can be helpful in a patient with a protracted disease, such as chronic idiopathic urticaria. A complete blood count, urinalysis, and erythrocyte sedimentation rate can display findings consistent with systemic disease processes. Serum chemistries can disclose the presence of hepatic or renal disease. Thyroid function tests are recommended, because studies have shown that 15% of individuals with chronic idiopathic urticaria will have an abnormal serum thyroxine (T4) or thyroid-stimulating hormone [17]. Autoimmune thyroid serologies, including antiperoxidase and antithyroglobulin antibodies, should be assessed. In individuals with evidence of elevated autoimmune thyroid antibodies, the development of clinical hypothyroidism should be followed in light of its annual incidence of approximately 2.5% to 4.5% [49,50]. If a suspicion exists of coincident autoimmune disease, an antinuclear antibody and rheumatoid factor might be obtained.

Skin biopsy

The histopathology of an acute urticarial lesion is merely one of dermal edema, which is a nonspecific finding. However, if the diagnosis of chronic urticaria is in question, a biopsy may be useful. The biopsy should reveal the presence of a perivascular mononuclear infiltrate with an increased number of mast cells. If any unusual characteristics of the urticarial lesion appear, such as residual scarring or associated petechial rash, a biopsy should be obtained. Infiltration of the dermal vessels with neutrophils, in combination with leukocytoclasis, nuclear debris, and immunoprotein deposition, would be consistent with the diagnosis of vasculitis. It is then necessary to distinguish the various types of cutaneous vasculitis from a systemic disorder of which cutaneous vasculitis is one manifestation.

TREATMENT OF CHRONIC URTICARIA AND ANGIOEDEMA
Nonpharmacologic approaches

Acute urticaria caused by a specific food or medicinal agent is merely treated by avoidance of that agent.

Symptomatic improvement will occur within 12 to 24 hours if no further allergen exposure is encountered. Often, the intense pruritus can be symptomatically improved with the use of oatmeal baths. Ingestion of alcohol-containing beverages should be discouraged, because the vasodilation that is produced by ethanol will often exacerbate the discomfort.

The physical stimulus or physiologic activity resulting in the urticarial lesions should be avoided. Patients who have cold-induced urticaria should take precautions to limit their exposure to cold environments. In colder climates, gloves, hats, and scarves should be used. Often, a ski mask will help to exclude the development of urticaria on an exposed face. Patients with cold-induced urticarial disease should refrain from holding cold objects, such as soft-drink cans. They can use vinyl gloves with cotton inserts during preparation of cold foods. They must take specific action to avoid either bathing or swimming in cold water because systemic hypotension can occur, with fatalities due to syncope and drowning. Finally, individuals who have a predisposition for urticaria and angioedema as a result of IgE-mediated processes to foods or drugs or have severe physical urticaria should avoid the use of β-adrenergic blockers. These agents often exacerbate the systemic hypotension and vascular vasodilation that can occur with mast cell or basophil degranulation.

Pharmacologic therapy

Acute urticaria and chronic urticaria are symptomatically improved with the use of antihistamines. An extensive armamentarium of H_1 histamine blockers can be employed in the symptomatic improvement of urticaria and angioedema [51••,52]. First-generation antihistamines do result in improvement in the urticarial lesions; however, they have the unwanted side effects of sedation and mucosal drying [53]. Newer second-generation antihistamines (eg, cetirizine, fexofenadine and loratadine) have less soporific effects and have been shown to be safe and effective in the treatment of chronic urticaria [54–58]. Doxepin, which traditionally is used as an antidepressive agent, has been found to have significant antimuscarinic, antiserotoninergic, and antihistaminic activity (H_1 and H_2). Its use in chronic urticaria is limited by its excessive soporific effects. Cyproheptadine, an antiserotoninergic agent, is often helpful in the treatment of cold-induced urticaria. However, cyproheptadine can stimulate the appetite and result in significant weight gain.

H_2 antihistamines have been employed in the treatment of chronic urticaria and angioedema. It is believed that approximately 15% of histamine receptors found on endothelial cells are of the H_2 subtype. Studies investigating the use of H_2 antihistamines have revealed limited beneficial effects in chronic urticaria [59–62]. Thus,

H_2 antihistamines can be added to H_1 antihistamines in cases of refractory urticarial disease.

Systemic corticosteroids will attenuate the symptoms and signs of chronic urticaria. The perivascular infiltrates seen in chronic urticarial skin biopsies reflect the inflammatory nature of the disorder. The presence of antithyroid antibodies as well as anti-IgE receptor antibodies emphasizes the immune deregulation present. Although systemic corticosteroids do not directly affect the titers of pathogenic autoantibodies nor inhibit mast cell degranulation, they do modulate the secretion of cytokines or HRF-type substances that contribute to local inflammatory response, including the recruitment of T lymphocytes, monocytes, eosinophils, and basophils [63••]. No studies have established steroid regimens as helpful in the attenuation of chronic urticaria and it is felt that the prolonged use of systemic corticosteroids is not appropriate. Thus, consideration of alternative therapies should be pursued aggressively. However, a regimen of alternate-day steroids with a gradual decreasing dose over 3 to 4 months has been advocated for severe cases where there is clear disruption of work and activities of daily living [64••]. Daily steroids are avoided except for an initial 1 to 2 weeks steroid burst, after which an alternate-day regimen would be established.

With the understanding that a proportion of patients' chronic idiopathic urticaria is related to autoimmune disease (anti-IgE receptor antibodies) or immune deregulatory processes reflected by the presence of other autoimmune antibodies (antithyroid antibodies), one must consider the possibility of immunomodulators [65•]. These are generally employed in the attempt to minimize the use of systemic corticosteroids. If the use of both H_1 and H_2 antihistamines is ineffective in controlling the disease and prolonged use of systemic corticosteroids is anticipated, alternative agents may be considered. Unfortunately, there are no trials that indicate the safety or efficacy of any immunomodulators in the treatment of chronic idiopathic urticaria other than anecdotal reports on small numbers of patients. Immunomodulators are employed based on their efficacy in other autoimmune and immune deregulatory diseases. Agents that have been considered for use as immunomodulators in other autoimmune diseases include methotrexate, hydroxychloroquine, dapsone, and cyclosporine. Cyclosporine has been advocated for refractory urticaria [66•]; however, at this stage, it is not recommended other than as part of an investigational study. Significantly, no controlled studies are presently available to guide the clinician caring for an individual with severe refractory chronic idiopathic urticaria of a suspected autoimmune etiology.

Theoretically, the consideration of plasmapheresis to remove an autoantibody responsible for mast cell degranulation is possible. Plasmapheresis has been employed in disease states associated with autoimmune processes with varying success. If, indeed, one were able to remove substantial amounts of an autoantibody active in mast cell degranulation, the effect would be short-lived. The volume of distribution extends beyond the intravascular compartment, and there would be movement of IgG from other areas to the intravascular compartment. Additionally, the B cells responsible for the elaboration of the autoantibody would remain viable. As such, they would be capable of reconstituting the ambient level of IgG. Controlled studies will be necessary to determine if there is any short-term benefit or applicability of plasmaphersis in chronic idiopathic urticaria associated with a pathogenic autoimmune antibody resulting in mast cell degranulation.

Treatment of hereditary angioedema

Hereditary angioedema is a potentially life-threatening disease with severe swelling. Symptoms often include prominent swelling of the extremities, facial structures, and vocal cords, and edema of the bowel wall. The use of attenuated androgens (danazol, stanozolol) has had some considerable effects [67,68]. These agents are believed to up-regulate the synthetic capability of hepatic cells responsible for elaborating the C1-INH. With the congenital absence of one allele, these attenuated androgens can stimulate increased production of the C1-INH by the remaining gene. Significant side effects are associated with attenuated androgens, including hirsutism, weight gain, abnormal liver function, and a procoagulant effect. Their use is limited in female patients due to the hirsutism or concerns regarding menarche. Generally, these agents can be used regularly to control active disease or prophylactically before stress events, such as elective surgery. Attenuated androgens should be used at increased dosages 4 to 5 days before elective surgery and dental procedures to ensure adequate levels of the C1-INH. Esterase-inhibiting drugs, such as epsilon aminocaproic acid and tranexamic acid, have been used to slow complement activation [2]. Their use is limited by their effects on musculoskeletal system.

Previously, plasma has been used to provide a source of C1-INH. Its use is limited by infectious disease issues when blood products are employed. With this concern in mind, a C1-INH bioengineered protein is being developed. In lieu of its availability, a C1-INH concentrate harvested from plasma can be administered [69•]. It can be used in cases of life-threatening angioedema or as an immediate preoperative administration for emergent surgery. Elective surgery should be scheduled in order to allow for the administration of attenuated androgens for 4 to 5 days prior to the surgical procedure.

CONCLUSIONS

Urticaria and angioedema can result from a myriad of pathobiologic mechanisms. They include classic IgE-mediated hypersensitivity with an acute, immediate hypersensitivity-type response. They can also result from nonspecific mast cell degranulation that can occur following the use of RCM or substances that alter arachidonic metabolism. Complement activation can elaborate C3a and C5a and degranulate mast cells in a fashion similar to the many HRFs presently identified. Finally, perturbation of bradykinin metabolism by therapeutic agents, such as ACEIs, can also result in angioedema. Most recently, a large subgroup of chronic urticaria, previously deemed idiopathic, has been found to be related to autoimmune processes. The relationship to the autoimmune mechanisms has not been fully clarified and, as such, could represent either an epiphenomenon or causal relationship.

In the treatment of patients with urticaria and angioedema, the traditional approach of obtaining a careful history and physical examination is most important. Laboratory studies can be helpful for further evaluation of either occult or coincident disease. Ultimately, laboratories that investigate the autoimmune nature of this disease could be important in determining etiology, prognosis, and treatment.

Treatment modalities will continue to depend heavily on the use of antihistamines for symptomatic relief. Protocols investigating immunosuppressives, such as systemic corticosteroids, would be helpful in the establishment of guidelines for their use. An initial trial of systemic corticosteroids may be appropriate to induce remission and suppress disease manifestations of a self-perpetuating cascade involving the initial mast cell degranulation by an autoantibody with a subsequent perpetuation of the process by cell recruitment and HRFs (Figure 14-6). As this explanation is entirely speculative, it requires further research.

Finally, studies will need to be performed that focus on the use of immunomodulators as steroid-sparing agents in severe refractory disease. With the elucidation of the mechanisms or relevance of the immune deregulation documented in chronic idiopathic urticaria, novel therapies can be developed to address this most challenging disease.

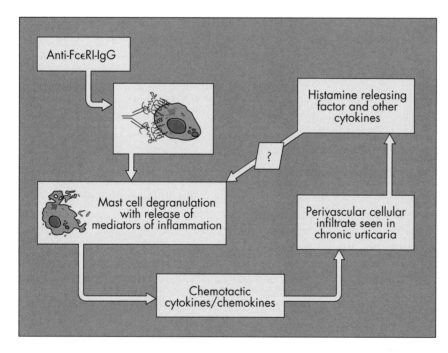

FIGURE 14-6.
Theoretical considerations for the pathophysiology of chronic autoimmune urticaria.

REFERENCES AND RECOMMENDED READING

Recently published papers of particular interest have been highlighted as:

• Of interest

•• Of outstanding interest

1. Soter NA: Acute and chronic urticaria and angioedema. *J Am Acad Dermatol* 1991, 25:146–154.

2.•• Kaplan AP: Urticaria and angioedema. In *Allergy*. Philadelphia: WB Saunders; 1997:573–592.
This is a comprehensive review of urticaria and angioedema.

3. Cooper KD: Urticaria and angioedema: diagnosis and evaluation. *J Am Acad Dermatol* 1991, 25:166–176.

4. Ghosh S, Kanwar AJ, Kaur S: Urticaria in children. *Pediatr Dermatol* 1993, 10:107–110.

5. Margolius CF, Nisi R: Urticaria in a family practice. *J Fam Pract* 1985, 20:57–64.

6. Huston DP, Bressler RB: Urticaria and angioedema. *Med Clin North Am* 1992, 76:805–840.

7. Barke KE, Hough LB: Opiates, mast cells and histamine release. *Life Sci* 1993, 53:1391–1399.

8. Kaplan AP: Urticaria and angioedema. In *Allergy: Principles and Practice*. Edited by Middleton E, Reed CE, Ellis EF, *et al.* St. Louis: Mosby; 1993:1553.

9. Ormerod AD: Urticaria: recognition, causes, and treatment. *Drugs* 1994, 48:717–730.

10. Orfan NA, Kolski GB: Physical urticarias. *Ann Allergy* 1993, 71:205–211.

11. Wanderer AA: Cold urticaria syndromes: historical background, diagnostic classification, clinical and laboratory characteristics, pathogenesis, and management. *J Allergy Clin Immunol* 1990, 85:965–981.

12.• Tillie-Leblond I, Gosset P, Janin A, *et al.*: Tumor necrosis factor-α release during systemic reaction in cold urticaria. *J Allergy Clin Immunol* 1994, 93:501–509.
The authors investigate the release of a cytokine, tumor necrosis factor-α, by mast cells in patients with cold-induced urticaria. The release was significant in patients with systemic symptoms, implicating this cytokine in the shock-like reactions of cold urticaria.

13. Leenutaphong V, Holze E, Plewig G: Pathogenesis and classifications of solar urticaria: a new concept. *J Am Acad Dermatol* 1989, 21:237–240.

14. Zuberbier T, Althaus C, Chantraine-Hess S, Czarnetski B: Prevalence of cholinergic urticaria in young adults. *J Am Acad Dermatol* 1994, 31:978–981.

15. Leznoff A, Josse RG, Denburg J, Dolovich J: Association of chronic urticaria and angioedema with thyroid autoimmunity. *Arch Dermatol* 1983, 119:636–640.

16. Leznoff A, Sussman GL: Syndrome of idiopathic chronic urticaria and angioedema with thyroid autoimmunity: a study of 90 patients. *J Allergy Clin Immunol* 1989, 84:66–71.

17. Finn AF, Levy A, Banov CH: Autoimmune thyroid antibodies and thyroid function test in chronic urticaria and angioedema. *J Allergy Clin Immunol* 1997, 99:334.

18.•• Fiebiger E, Maurer D, Holub H, *et al.*: Serum IgG autoantibodies directed against the α chain of FcεRI: a selective marker and pathogenic factor in a distinct subset of chronic urticaria patients. *J Clinical Invest* 1995, 96:2606–2612.
This study demonstrated the specificity of the IgG autoantibody in chronic idiopathic urticaria patients for the α subunit of the tetrameric high-affinity IgE receptor, FcεRI.

19.•• Nimi N, Francis DM, Kerman F, *et al.*: Dermal mast cell activation by autoantibodies against the high-affinity IgE receptor in chronic urticaria. *J Invest Dermatol* 1996, 106:1001–1006.
The investigators demonstrate activity of the anti-IgE receptor autoantibody from chronic idiopathic urticaria patients on skin mast cells.

20.•• Tong LF, Balakrishnan G, Kochan JP, *et al.*: Assessment of autoimmunity in chronic urticaria. *J Allergy Clin Immunol* 1997, 99:461–465.
The authors present data revealing the prevalence of functional autoantibodies (anti-IgE, anti-FcεRI-α) in chronic urticaria patients.

21. Greaves M, Lawlor F: Angioedema: manifestations and management. *J Am Acad Dermatol* 1991, 25:155–165.

22. Stoppa-Lyonnet D, Tosi M, Laurent J, *et al.*: Altered C1-inhibitor genes in type I hereditary angioedema. *N Engl J Med* 1987, 317:1–6.

23. Alsenz J, Bork K, Loos M: Autoantibody-mediated acquired deficiency of C1-inhibitor. *N Engl J Med* 1987, 316:1360–1366.

24. Kobza-Black AK, Greaves MW, Champion RH, Pye RJ: The urticarias 1990. *Br J Dermatol* 1991, 124:100–108.

25. Minor MW, Fox RW, Bukantz SC, Lockey RF: Melkersson-Rosenthal syndrome. *J Allergy Clin Immunol* 1987, 80:64–67.

26. Greene RM, Rogers RS III: Melkersson-Rosenthal syndrome: a review of 36 patients. *J Am Acad Dermatol* 1989, 21:1263–1270.

27. Podmore P, Burrows D: Clofazamine: an effective treatment for Melkersson-Rosenthal syndrome. *J Am Acad Dermatol* 1986, 11:173–178.

28. Thueson DO, Speck LS, Lett-Brown MA, Grant JA: Histamine-releasing activity (HRA) I: production by mitogen or antigen stimulated human mononuclear cells. *J Immunol* 1979, 122:623–632.

29. Thueson DO, Speck LS, Lett-Brown MA, Grant JA: Histamine-releasing activity (HRA) II: interaction with basophils and physiochemical characterization. *J Immunol* 1979, 122:633–639.

30. Elias J, Boss E, Kaplan AP: Studies of the cellular infiltrate of chronic idiopathic urticaria: prominence of T-lymphocytes, monocytes, and mast cells. *J Allergy Clin Immunol* 1986, 78:914–918.

31. Haak-Frendscho M, Dinarello C, Kaplan AP: Recombinant interleukin-1 β causes histamine release from human basophils. *J Allergy Clin Immunol* 1988, 82:218–233.

32. Haak-Frendscho M, Arai N, Arai K-I, *et al.*: Human recombinant granulocyte-macrophage colony-stimulating factor and interleukin-3 cause basophil histamine release. *J Clin Invest* 1988, 82:17–20.

33. Kuna P, Reddigari SR, Kornfeld D, Kaplan AP: IL-8 inhibits histamine release from human basophils induced by histamine releasing factors, connective tissue activating peptide III, and IL-3. *J Immunol* 1991, 147:1920–1924.

34.•• Kuna P, Kaplan AP: Relationship of histamine-releasing factors and histamine-releasing inhibitory factors of chemokine group of cytokines. *All Asthma Proceedings* 1996, 17:5–11.
This is a comprehensive discussion focused on cytokines that modulate histamine release by basophils and mast cells. Their structural relationships, relative potency, and potential contribution to clinical disease are reviewed.

35.•• Alam R: Chemokines in allergic inflammation. *J Allergy Clin Immunol* 1997, 99:273–277.
This is a concise review of chemotactic cytokines in allergic disease.

36.•• Luster AD: Chemokines: chemotactic cytokines that mediate inflammation. *N Engl J Med* 1998, 338:436–445.
This is an updated review of chemokines and their involvement in the pathophysiology of inflammation.

37. Jacques P, Lavoid A, Bedard PM, *et al.*: Chronic idiopathic urticaria: profiles of skin mast cell histamine release during active disease and remission. *J Allergy Clin Immunol* 1992, 89:1139–1143.

38. Claveau J, Lavoie A, Brunet C, *et al.*: Chronic idiopathic urticaria: possible contribution of histamine-releasing factor to pathogenesis. *J Allergy Clin Immunol* 1993, 92:132–137.

39.•• Claveau J, Lavoie A, Brunet C, *et al.*: Comparison of histamine-releasing factor recovered from skin and peripheral blood mononuclear cells of patients with chronic idiopathic urticaria. *Ann Allergy Asthma Immunol* 1996, 77:475–479.
This report documents the presence of increased levels of HRFs in the normal skin of patients with chronic urticaria but lesser levels in the peripheral blood. An explanation offered for this interesting observation is the migration of activated T cells to the skin, where they elaborate HRFs.

40.•• Zweiman B, Valenzano M, Atkins PC, *et al.*: Characteristics of histamine-releasing activity in the sera of patients with chronic idiopathic urticaria. *J Allergy Clin Immunol* 1996, 89:89–98.
The investigators characterized histamine-releasing activity in a large group of chronic idiopathic urticaria patients. They found the activity in the IgG fraction of serum and found it directed against the IgE receptor.

41.•• Turktas I, Gokcora N, Demirsoy S, *et al.*: The association of chronic urticaria and angioedema with autoimmune thyroiditis. *Int J Dermatol* 1997, 36:187–190.
This paper reports the results of a study conducted in Turkey, assessing the prevalence of autoimmune thyroid disease in a cohort of chronic urticaria patients.

42. Finn A, Balakrishan G, Reddigari S, Kaplan A: Investigation of chronic urticaria with autoimmune thyroid disease and rat basophil leukemic cell degranulation. *J Allergy Clin Immunol* 1996, 97:366.

43.• Rumbyrt JS, Katz JL, Schocket AL: Resolution of chronic urticaria in patients with thyroid autoimmunity. *J Allergy Clin Immunol* 1995, 96:901–905.
This study assesses the benefit of using thyroid replacement in a small group of euthyroid patients with chronic urticaria.

44. Bommanna V, Cumella J, Ballow MD, Ramesh S: Chronic urticaria associated with antithyroid antibodies. *Ann Allergy Asthma Immunol* 1998, 80:134.

45. Gruber BL, Baeza M, Marchese M, *et al.*: Prevalence and functional role of anti-IgE autoantibodies in urticarial syndromes. *J Invest Dermatol* 1988, 90:213–217.

46. Grattan CEH, Francis DM, Hide M, Greaves MW: Detection of circulating histamine-releasing autoantibodies with functional properties of anti-IgE in chronic urticaria. *Clin Exp Allergy* 1991, 21:695–704.

47. Hide M, Francis DM, Grattan CEH, *et al.*: Autoantibodies against the high-affinity IgE receptor as a cause of histamine release in chronic urticaria. *N Engl J Med* 1993, 328:1599–1604.

48. Hide M, Francis DM, Grattan CEH, *et al.*: The pathogenesis of chronic idiopathic urticaria: new evidence suggests an autoimmune basis and implications for treatment. *Clin Exp Allergy* 1994, 24:624–627.

49. Woeber KA: Subclinical thyroid dysfunction. *Arch Intern Med* 1997, 157:1065–1068.

50. Dayan CM, Daniels GH: Chronic autoimmune thyroiditis. *N Engl J Med* 1996, 335:99–107.

51.•• Greaves MW: Chronic urticaria. *N Engl J Med* 1995, 332:1767–1772.
This author provides a broad review of the topic of chronic urticaria.

52. Soter NA: Urticaria: current therapy. *J Allergy Clin Immunol* 1990, 86:1009–1014.

53. Monroe EW: The role of antihistamines in the treatment of chronic urticaria. *J Allergy Clin Immunol* 1990, 86:662–665.

54. Monroe EW: Nonsedating H$_1$ antihistamines in chronic urticaria. *Annals of Allergy* 1993, 71:585–591.

55. Townley RG: Cetirizine: a new H$_1$ antagonist with anti-eosinophilic activity in chronic urticaria. *J Am Acad Dermatol* 1991, 25:668–674.

56. Pierson WE: Cetirizine: a unique second-generation antihistamine for treatment of rhinitis and chronic urticaria. *Clin Ther* 1991, 13:92–99.

57. Monroe EW, Fox RW, Green AW: Efficacy and safety of loratadine in the management of idiopathic chronic urticaria. *J Am Acad Derm* 1988, 19:138–139.

58. Monroe EW: Relative efficacy and safety of loratadine, hydroxyzine, and placebo in chronic idiopathic urticaria and atopic dermatitis. *Clin Ther* 1992, 14:17–21.

59. Phanuphak P, Schocket A, Kohler PF: Treatment of chronic idiopathic urticaria with combined H$_1$ and H$_2$ blockers. *Clin Allergy* 1978, 8:429–433.

60. Monroe EW, Cohen SH, Kalbfleisch J, Schulz CI: Combined H$_1$ and H$_2$ antihistamine therapy in chronic urticaria. *Arch Dermatol* 1981, 117:404–407.

61. Paul E, Bodeker RH: Treatment of chronic urticaria with terfenadine and ranitidine: a randomized double-blind study in 45 patients. *Eur J Clin Pharmacol* 1986, 31:277–280.

62. Bleehen SS, Thomas SE, Breaves MW, *et al.*: Cimetidine and chlorpheniramine in the treatment of chronic idiopathic urticaria: a multicentre randomized double-blind study. *Br J Dermatol* 1987, 117:81–88.

63.•• Paradis L, Lavoie A, Brunet C, *et al.*: Effects of systemic corticosteroids on cutaneous histamine secretion and histamine-releasing factor in patients with chronic idiopathic urticaria. *Clin Exp Allergy* 1996, 25:815–820.
The authors present findings that reveal the ability of systemic corticosteroids to decrease production of HRFs in the skin of patients with chronic idiopathic urticaria. This decreased production of HRF was in association with improved symptoms.

64.•• O'Donnell BF, Lawlor F, Simpson J, *et al.*: The impact of chronic urticaria on the quality of life. *Br J Dermatol* 1997, 136:197–201.
This study investigated the issue of quality of life in chronic urticaria patients. This investigation is the first to document significant disability, handicap, and impact on quality of life in patients with chronic urticaria.

65.• Tharp MD: Chronic urticaria: pathophysiology and treatment approaches. *J Allergy Clin Immunol* 1996, 98:325–330.
This paper discusses mechanisms and possible therapies in chronic urticaria.

66.• Toubi E, Blant A, Kessel A, Golan TD: Low-dose cyclosporin A in the treatment of severe chronic idiopathic urticaria. *Allergy* 1997, 52:312–316.
The investigators conduct a study exploring the use of the immunosuppressive cyclosporin A in the treatment of severe chronic urticaria. Their findings reveal benefit, although limited in patients requiring high doses of corticosteroids or with longstanding disease.

67. Gelfand JA, Shermis RJ, Alling DW, Frank MM: Treatment of hereditary angioedema with danazol: reversal of the clinical and biochemical abnormalities. *N Engl J Med* 1976, 2195:1444–1448.

68. Sheffer AL, Fearon DT, Austen KF: Clinical and biochemical effects of stanazolol therapy for hereditary angioedema. *J Allergy Clin Immunol* 1981, 68:181–187.

69.• Waytes AT, Rosen F, Frank M: Treatment of hereditary angioedema with a vapor-heated C1-inhibitor concentraate. *N Engl J Med* 1996, 334:1630–1634.
Report of studies demonstrating that the C1-inhibitor concentrate was safe and effective for the prophylaxis and treatment of attacks of angioedema in patients with hereditary angioedema.

CHAPTER 15

"Allergic" Dermatoses

Vincent S. Beltrani

Many abnormalities of the skin or of its appendages are often erroneously labeled "allergic," both by physicians and by the lay public. The overt disregard of the precise definition of the term *allergy*—namely, that the adverse (inflammatory) reaction must be immunologically activated, and then confounded by clinically similar inflammatory reactions initiated by nonimmunologic (or "pseudoallergic") mechanisms—results in these semantic misconceptions.

An elucidation of the term *allergy* was made in 1957, when Gell and Coombs [1] defined four immunologic mechanisms to which clinical entities can be relevantly assigned. When a specific "trigger" is identifiable, the term *allergy* is more easily applicable, but when the stimulus that incites an immunologic reaction is yet to be identified, the understanding of *allergy* becomes nebulous.

The skin, with its potentially proinflammatory structural cells (*eg*, keratinocytes, dendritic cells (Langerhans' cells), endothelium, dermal mast cells, fibroblasts, and (T-cell) lymphocytes, which have been referred to as skin-associated lymphoid tissue [SALT]), is now recognized as the "peripheral arm of our immune system" [2••]. Obviously, it becomes a very accessible organ for observing allergic, or, more accurately, immunologic reactions. Essentially, all inflammatory skin diseases are manifestations of complex interactions between resident cells and infiltrating inflammatory cells, activated by cytokine-driven cell–cell interactions [2••]. In this chapter, those dermatologic conditions ascribed to immunologic mechanisms (Table 15-1) are discussed and, wherever applicable, differentiated from clinically similar but nonimmunologic dermatoses.

URTICARIA (HIVES)

No other dermatologic symptom suggests an "allergic etiology" more often than the clinical appearance of hives. Although a cause for the short-lived, episodic urticaria is often identifiable, this is rarely the case for the patient with chronic urticaria. The arbitrary assignation determined by duration (*ie*, less than 6 weeks' time being called "acute," and more than 6 weeks labeled "chronic") may deter from the relevant understanding and appropriate management of what is often a frustrating problem.

Urticaria must be appreciated as the result of resident mast cell or summoned (late-phase) basophil degranulation; it is the cause of vasodilation (erythema), increased vascular permeability (producing the wheal), and pruritus, known as the Triple Response of Lewis. This

Table 15-1. CLASSIFICATION OF IMMUNOLOGIC MECHANISMS UNDERLYING ALLERGIC DERMATOSES

Dermatosis	Target cell	Stimulus	Latency	Mediators

Urticaria
  Acute
  Chronic
	Mast cell (tryptase/
	  chymase type)
	Basophil
	Eosinophil
		IgE complement (C3a, C5a)
		Substance P
		IgG
			Seconds to minutes	Histamine
				Leukotrienes
				Prostaglandins
				Bradykinin
				Platelet activating factor
				Adenosine
				Chemotactics
				Cytokines

Bullous disease
  Pemphigus
  Pemphigoid
  Dermatitis
  Herpetiformis
	Keratinocytes
	Basement membrane
		Circulating IgG or IgM
		  antibodies
			Hours to days	Complement

Autoimmune disease
  Vasculitides
    Systemic lupus erythematosus,
    rheumatoid arthritis
  Dermatomyositis
  Serum sickness
		"Immune complexes"	Hours to days	Complement

"Eczemas"
  Contact dermatitis
  Atopic dermatitis
	T cells	Haptens	Days to weeks	Lymphokines
				Cytokines

Adapted from *Gell and Coombs [1]; with permission.*

response is the result of histamine, the predominant "preformed" mediator released from activated mast cells. The reaction can be imitated by "prick testing" or skin testing with histamine. To confuse matters, there are other inflammatory mediators that can produce some (but not all) of the clinical manifestations of the Triple Response of Lewis. Accordingly, the clinical presentations of urticaria, which are tainted with mediators besides histamine, are subtly different (Fig. 15-1). As a result, we can also conclude that pruritus without urticaria is most likely *not* due to histamine (and therefore, antihistamines would be of little value). The pruritogenic mediators for urticaria are listed in Table 15-2 [3].

The immunologic triggers (or secretagogues) of both mast cell and basophil degranulation activate those cells by attaching to specific receptors on their cell surfaces. A threshold number of stimulated receptors are required to initiate the release of the mediators. The best-studied secretagogue is IgE. All mast cells and basophils possess IgE receptors. These cells are the protagonists for the classic "immediate" (type I) reaction (Fig. 15-2). Although IgE-induced reactions can occur in any individual, the atopic population seems to be more prone to experiencing these IgE-type reactions due to a genetic predisposition to 1)

produce increased amounts of IgE, and 2) possess "hyperreleasable" mast cells.

Other immunologic secretagogues include cytokines, such as histamine-releasing factors (HRF), which can be released from mast cells, basophils, eosinophils, T cells, and platelets as well as neuropeptides (especially substance P), C3a, C5a, IgG4, basic polypeptides, major basic protein, gastrin, platelet activating factors, and bacterial lectins. These secretagogues are all receptor specific. Most recently, "autoimmune" IgG antibody directed to the high-affinity IgE receptor on the mast cell and basophil has been identified [4]. This antibody can induce degranulation (in up to 30% of the chronic urticaria patients under study), introducing the concept of autoimmunity as a possible cause of chronic idiopathic urticaria.

We now distinguish human mast cells as a heterogeneous group of multifunctional tissue-dwelling cells with roles in conditions as diverse as allergy, parasite infestation, inflammation, angiogenesis, and tissue remodeling. The mast cells containing tryptase and chymase (MC_{TC}) are found in the connective tissue, and the mast cell containing only tryptase (MC_T) are found predominantly at mucosal surfaces. However, variable

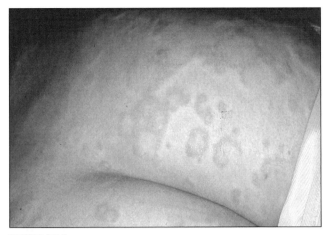

FIGURE 15-1.
Chronic idiopathic urticaria. The wheal and erythema indicate a clinical presentation different from that of skin testing with histamine (as the sole mediator). Incomplete response to antihistamines reflects the presence of other mediators.

Table 15-2. PRURITOGENIC MEDIATORS FOR URTICARIA

Amines
    Histamine—most abundant pruritogen
    Serotonin
Peptides
    Bradykinin—most potent pruritogen
    Substance P
    Vasoactive intestinal polypeptide
    Endorphins
    Neurotensin
    Secretin
Cytokines
    Interleukins 1–4
    Tumor necrosis factor
Proteases
    Trypsin
    Chymase
    Kallikrein
Arachidonic acid products
    Prostaglandins—potentiates itch
    Leukotrienes
    Platelet activating factor
Opiates
    Act as a pruritogen and cause histamine release
        from mast cells

From *Wahlgren [3]; with permission.*

amounts of both mast cell subtypes are present within any given tissue; their relative number varies with need (*eg*, in allergy or fibrosis) [5]. Thus, it is not surprising that there is also a functional heterogeneity between mast cells of different tissues. It has been shown that only the mast cells in the skin (MC$_{tc}$ type) express receptors for C3a and C5a, allowing them to be activated in complement-mediated disease; (hence, the urticarial phases of bullous pemphigoid and of immune-complex diseases as discussed later in the chapter). In addition, the MC$_{tc}$ mast cells alone respond to a variety of non-immunologic secretagogues including drugs, such as opiates and muscle relaxants. The response to these drugs explains the flushing reactions observed in sensitive individuals in the absence of overt rhinorrhea or bronchoconstriction, which require MC$_T$ mast cells.

Each secretagogue, after causing the release of pre-formed mediators, produces a different concoction of "newly formed" mediators [6]. Thus, the variable clinical presentations can be explained despite the presence of immunocytochemically identical mast cells. The different secretagogues also have different latent periods from excitation to mediator release. Substance P has the shortest duration (2 to 3 minutes), IgE has a somewhat longer duration (8 to 15 minutes), and immune complexes (C3a and C5a) may take days. IgE is also the secretagogue releasing the greatest amount of histamine. Thus the term *anaphylaxis*, the multisystem manifestation of massive mast cell degranulation, is reserved for the IgE-induced and most catastrophic immunologic reactions, whereas *anaphylactoid* reactions are not IgE-induced and are less often fatal [7]. The more sudden (explosive) and generalized the urticarial episode, the more foreboding the event. Relying on the presence of

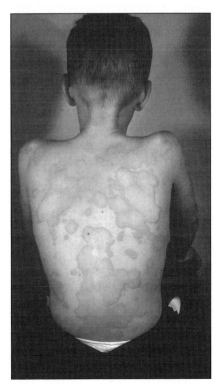

FIGURE 15-2.
"Acute" penicillin-induced urticaria. Generalized hives appearing within 20 minutes of an injection with penicillin G. Subsequently noted to be prick-test–positive to penicillin. Clinical urticaria is predominantly histamine-induced but still different from the histamine prick test. These are usually more, but rarely completely, responsive to antihistamines.

urticaria to recognize impending anaphylaxis may be foolhardy, because 12% of anaphylactic reactions are reported to occur without urticaria. Itchy palms, soles, genitals, and soft palate, with or without flushing, can be the only cutaneous manifestations of a fatal anaphylactic reaction [8].

The tissue reactions occurring after immunologic mast cell activation can be biphasic, consisting of an early and a late phase. Early-phase reactions in the skin result from the release of the pre-formed mediators (histamine, tryptase, kinins, and chemotactic factors) solely from mast cells. This response is recognized in the skin as a wheal and erythema with pruritus (Triple Response of Lewis) that develops within minutes. Late-phase reactions involve the later release of "newly formed" mediators (leukotrienes, prostaglandins, and platelet activating factor), plus the influx of inflammatory cells, especially the basophil and eosinophil with the release of their respective mediators. This response is recognized in the skin as a deep, tender, red induration that develops within 4 to 6 hours after the early reaction. Elicitation of late-phase reactions usually requires higher concentrations of secretagogues than for immediate reactivity [9]. The nonimmunologic or pseudoallergic triggers for mast cell degranulation are listed in Table 15-3 [10–13].

There is extensive literature regarding the role of the psyche or "nerves" causing urticaria [14,15]. Patients with chronic urticaria have been psychometrically described as unstable, sensitive, cyclothymic, and more neurotic than control subjects. With our present knowledge of neuropeptides and their effect on mast cells, it is conceivable that in patients who experience a neuropeptide release, neuropeptides can immunologically affect the vasculature, or the "twitchy mast cells," resulting in an exacerbation of urticaria.

An important distinction between immunologic and nonimmunologic secretagogues is that many of the former require prior sensitization, whereas the nonimmunologic-triggered reactions can occur with the first exposure to the agent. Intradermal, prick, or radioallergosorbent testing (RAST) are only of value for the IgE-induced reaction; thus, testing for radio contrast media, opiates, aspirin, and nonsteroidal anti-inflammatory drugs (NSAIDs) is of no value. Interestingly, lobster can act both as an immunologic or a nonimmunologic secretagogue, as can penicillin (which most often causes IgE-induced reactions, but can at other times be an ionophore, ie, force Ca+ into the mast cell, a requisite for mast cell degranulation). Although many patients report being allergic to strawberries, positive IgE results are extremely rare. Strawberry peptides are suspected of having a "direct" effect on the mast cell.

Flushing and urticarial-like reactions may occur with the ingestion of histamine-containing foods, especially

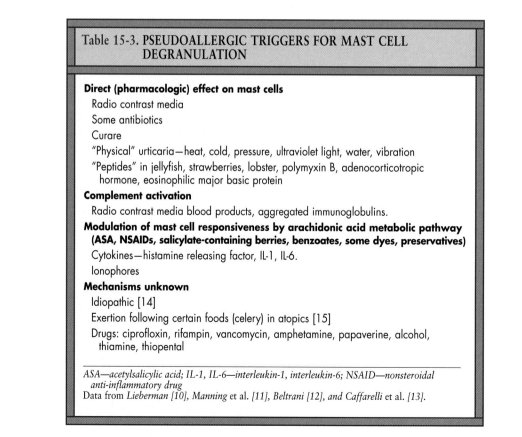

Table 15-3. PSEUDOALLERGIC TRIGGERS FOR MAST CELL DEGRANULATION

Direct (pharmacologic) effect on mast cells
Radio contrast media
Some antibiotics
Curare
"Physical" urticaria—heat, cold, pressure, ultraviolet light, water, vibration
"Peptides" in jellyfish, strawberries, lobster, polymyxin B, adenocorticotropic hormone, eosinophilic major basic protein

Complement activation
Radio contrast media blood products, aggregated immunoglobulins.

Modulation of mast cell responsiveness by arachidonic acid metabolic pathway (ASA, NSAIDs, salicylate-containing berries, benzoates, some dyes, preservatives)
Cytokines—histamine releasing factor, IL-1, IL-6.
Ionophores

Mechanisms unknown
Idiopathic [14]
Exertion following certain foods (celery) in atopics [15]
Drugs: ciprofloxin, rifampin, vancomycin, amphetamine, papaverine, alcohol, thiamine, thiopental

ASA—acetylsalicylic acid; IL-1, IL-6—interleukin-1, interleukin-6; NSAID—nonsteroidal anti-inflammatory drug
Data from Lieberman [10], Manning et al. [11], Beltrani [12], and Caffarelli et al. [13].

some raw fish eaten as sushi (*eg*, tuna, mahi-mahi, and mackerel, when spoiled), red wines (especially Chianti), yeast, aged cheeses (blue cheese, gorgonzola), tomatoes, eggs, and spinach.

Evaluating patients with urticaria

"Chronic" urticaria, or patients who experience almost daily hives for long periods of time, does not routinely warrant an extensive laboratory or "allergy" work-up with skin or RAST testing, because urticaria is *never* the sole symptom of an underlying disease.

Of patients with chronic hives, 50% will also report episodes of angioedema, 40% do not experience angioedema, and 10% of patients only experience angioedema without urticaria. Patients with chronic urticaria (with or without angioedema) have "twitchy" mast cells, and by obtaining a detailed history, one can usually identify several secretagogues, both immunologic and nonimmunologic, or signs and symptoms of underlying pathology (if present). Most intriguing is the incidence of "autoimmune-induced" urticaria occurring in patients with other autoimmune diseases, *eg*, thyroiditis, Crohn's disease, vitiligo, and alopecia areata. Quaranta *et al.* [16] and others have demonstrated the futility of any routine battery of tests for patients with chronic urticaria and no sign or symptom of underlying disease (Table 15-4).

A 2-mm skin biopsy is indicated if 1) individual urticarial lesions persist for more than 24 hours; 2) the hives are "less" pruritic; and 3) response is minimal to adequate antihistamine (H_1 plus H_2) therapy. Increased numbers of mast cells are noted in both lesional and uninvolved skin of all types of urticaria [17]. Dermal edema and dilated lymphatic and vascular capillaries are seen almost exclusively in involved skin. Should the perivascular inflammatory infiltrate show a significantly increased number of neutrophils, a therapeutic trial of colchicine or dapsone may be warranted. Thus, biopsies are of greater value to identify leukocytoclastic vasculitis differentiating urticarial vasculitis from urticaria [18]. It is strongly recommended that all skin biopsies be read by a dermatopathologist.

Management of patients with urticaria

Identifying and eliminating the trigger causing mast cell or basophil degranulation is the decisive goal of the urticaria patient's management. Although this can be fairly easy in some patients (especially in the sporadic, short-lived episodes), it is rarely attainable for chronic urticaria patients. The natural history of chronic urticaria patients has been reported as the duration of each chronic episode: 50% resolve spontaneously within 3 to 12 months, 20% resolve spontaneously within 12 to 36 months, 20% resolve spontaneously within 36 to 60 months, and 1.5% last up to 25 years.

Table 15-4. LABORATORY EVALUATION OF 86 PATIENTS WITH CHRONIC URTICARIA

Test	Patients tested, *n*	Positive, %
Complete blood count/ differential	57	0
Chemical panel	54	0
Erythrocyte sedimentation rate	37	0
Rheumatoid factor	6	0
Complement levels	22	0
Urinalysis	42	0
Antinuclear antibodies	32	0
IgE level	4	0
Immune complexes	16	0
Thyroid functions	7	0
Hepatitis antigen	1	0
Skin tests	22	59

When angioedema accompanies urticaria, 75% of the patients have symptoms for more than 1 year and up to 20% for more than 20 years. Of patients with "chronic" urticaria, 40% have recurrent episodes.

Symptom relief should be the realistic goal for the management of patients with chronic urticaria. This is usually achieved with the proper administration of H_1 (and occasionally H_2) antagonists. The pharmacologic effects of H_1 antagonists derive primarily from inhibition of histamine action at H_1-receptors; the antagonists act by binding to H_1-receptors [19]. Because they do not displace histamine from an H_1 receptor, they are most effective if administered prior to the attachment of histamine. Thus, antihistamines should be administered "around-the-clock," not just as needed when the hives appear. Available pharmacokinetic and clinical pharmacology information about H_1-receptor antagonists enables us to make a rational choice of which preparation to use in the various clinical circumstances. A limiting factor of the first-generation "older, sedating" antihistamines is their short half-life, thus requiring frequent administration. Although second-generation, nonsedating antihistamines may be slightly more effective H_1-antagonists, their longer half-life, which requires administration only once or twice a day, is decidedly advantageous. However, in addition to being pharmacologic antagonists to histamine, many of the second generation H_1 antihistamines have properties besides receptor blockade, *eg*, they decrease mediator and interleukin (IL)-1 synthesis and release and Ca^+ mobilization and also inhibit eosinophil migration [20]. Selection of particular H_1 antihistamines must be made on an individual basis and tailored to each situation. It is usually based on side effects and additional antiallergic properties rather than on antihistaminic efficacy alone, because most H_1 antagonists will reduce symptoms of urticaria (especially the pruritus) to some degree.

Current experience with first-generation antihistamines in the treatment of chronic urticaria suggests that they are only mildly effective in the recommended dosages. Hydroxyzine is probably the agent most frequently used for the treatment of chronic urticaria, and as an antihistamine it has been shown to be 88 times more effective (in vitro) than diphenhydramine and is also a serotonin antagonist. An added advantage of the newer, "nonsedating" antihistamines is that they possess additional antiallergic properties that may be of value [21]. Simons *et al.* [22] performed a single-dose, placebo-controlled, double-blind, cross-over comparative study of the antihistaminic effects on the "wheal and flare reaction" of the second-generation H_1 antihistamines. Overall, cetirizine was found to be superior to terfenadine, astemizole, loratadine, chlorpheniramine, and placebo.

Tricyclic antidepressants

Tricyclic antidepressants (doxepin and amitriptyline) have been shown to possess potent H_1 and H_2 blocking activities. Their in-vitro H_1-antihistaminic effect is approximately 779 times greater than that of diphenhydramine and 56 times greater than hydroxyzine; their H_2-antihistaminic effect is seven times greater than cimetidine [23]. A recent in-vivo relative antihistaminic potency comparison of doxepin 25 mg and hydroxyzine 25 mg showed that it took 2.85 times more histamine to produce the same size wheal after hydroxyzine than after doxepin [24]. However, doxepin has been used successfully in chronic urticaria patients who were resistant to the conventional H_1-antihistamines. The addition of H_2 antihistamines has been more helpful when the patient with chronic urticaria demonstrates flushing, angioedema, or dermatographism [25,26]. The addition of oral β-agonists (albuterol) has been of help in some patients with urticaria, whereas aerosolized epinephrine can be life-saving for some patients with airway obstruction resulting from angioedema [27]. There are two reports suggesting the use of calcium channel blockers (nifedipine) for patients with urticaria [28,29]. Dapsone and colchicine have been effective as immunosuppressants, especially for patients with urticarial vasculitis or for those patients whose biopsy reveals a predominantly neutrophilic infiltrate [30]. Anabolic agents (danazol, stanozolol) are indicated for the treatment of hereditary angioedema by increasing the serum levels of C_1-esterase inhibitor. NSAIDs are recommended for the treatment of pressure urticaria. However, this family of drugs are also recognized secretagogues for mast cell degranulation, releasing several leukotrienes. An effec-

tive treatment for aspirin-induced asthma and angioedema/urticaria is the use of anti-leukotriene therapy. Excellent response with zileuton (Zyflo; Abbott Laboratories, Abbott Park, IL [600 mg every 6 to 12 hours]), a 5-lipoxygenase inhibitor, added to doxepin (10 to 100 mg daily) for the management of "idiopathic" angioedema with or without urticaria has been noted by the author in several patients.

Corticosteroids

Corticosteroids only provide symptomatic relief of urticaria, serum sickness, and pressure urticaria. They have no place in the "routine" therapy of chronic urticaria. Their anti-inflammatory and immunosuppressant activities do not effect cutaneous mast cell degranulation [31]. They have been very useful when administered as a "pulse dose" (0.5 to 1.0 mg/k/d) to help break the cycle of a persistent episode [32]. Corticosteroids are occasionally indicated for patients with persistent chronic urticaria minimally responsive to maximum doses of H_1 and H_2 antihistamines (and trials of β-adrenergics, the anti-leukotriene zileuton). Kaplan's [31] schedule of prednisone administration is recommended with the goal of maintaining the patient (able to function at work and at home) on the lowest-dose alternate-day regimen. Cyclosporine A (3 to 6 mg/k/d) has been used successfully to control chronic urticaria in small series of patients [33]. Cyclosporine A inhibits cytokine release from T cells, decreases antibody production, and may act as a mast cell stabilizer. However, its administration requires close monitoring of the patient's blood pressure and renal status.

BULLOUS DISEASE AND AUTOIMMUNE DISEASES

When the immune system fails to differentiate self from non-self, the deregulated immune mechanisms are activated to remove or destroy the autologous "trigger." The immune mechanisms most often reacting in this way are the type II (or cytotoxic) and type III (or immune complex) reactions. The cutaneous manifestations of these reactions are noted as "bullous diseases" and "connective tissue or rheumatic diseases."

The human epidermis and dermal–epidermal junction are highly complex biochemically. They contain proteins, glycoproteins, and proteoglycans that have the potential to act as antigens, which may be recognized as foreign by the patient's immune system, resulting in a bullous disease. The autoantibodies (usually IgG or IgA) bind to specific tissue sites and fix complement. Mast cells are then attracted and release one or more chemical mediators (C3 and C5 are immunologic secretagogues), producing clinical urticaria, seen as the "urticarial phase" of bullous pemphigoid or urticarial vasculitis of systemic lupus erythematosus. Clinically, the lesions of urticarial vasculitis are less pruritic; the individual lesions last longer than 24 hours and often demonstrate an ecchymotic or a petechial character.

The terms *bullous diseases* and *autoimmune connective tissue diseases* refer to 1) groups of immune-mediated cutaneous diseases that are characterized by the development of intraepidermal or subepidermal blisters; or 2) extremely heterogeneous clinical entities involving the skin alone or in combination with one or more internal organs.

ECZEMA

Eczema is a symptom, not a disease. From the Greek *ek zein*, it means "boiling over." Clinically, "boiling over" is recognized as tiny bubbles or vesicles in the skin. The disease entity causing the eczema can produce a spectrum of clinical presentations (Table 15-5) varying from microscopic intercellular (between keratinocytes) edema, which is labeled spongiosis as seen in dermatophytoses; to bulla formation, as seen in acute contact dermatitis (poison ivy); or to the thickened, dry, scaly plaques of chronic atopic dermatitis (AD). This spectrum of clinical manifestations is chronologically subdivided into three, frequently overlapping stages: acute, subacute, and chronic.

The common denominator of eczemas is the dermal infiltration of T-helper (T_H) cells. All eczemas are histologically similar; thus, biopsy is not specifically diagnostic but can be helpful in ruling out clinically similar eruptions, such as psoriasiform dermatitis, cutaneous T-cell lymphoma, and perivascular dermatitis.

T-helper cells play a central role in all eczematous eruptions. Like the mast cell, there are many secretagogues, both immunologic and nonimmunologic, that result in the release of chemical mediators causing a generic intercellular edema (spongiosis). In immunogenic eczemas, clones of sensitized T cells have the unique ability to "home" to the site of "insult." The resulting varied clinical presentations are affected by the varied mixture of T-cell mediators that are released and by the cytokinal milieu in which the T cell habitates. In this chapter, the emphasis is placed on eczematous eruptions with identifiable extrinsic immunologic "triggers."

Contact dermatitis

The spectrum of "contact" dermatitis comprises all adverse cutaneous reactions resulting from the direct contact of an exogenous agent (a "foreign" molecule, ultraviolet light, temperature) to the epidermis [34•]. The offending stimulus may initiate an immunologic response (Fig. 15-3) [35], nonimmunologic response, or both. Allergic contact dermatitis (ACD) is recognized as the prototypic cutaneous delayed-hypersensitivity immunologic reaction. Irritant contact dermatitis (ICD) is conceived to be a nonimmunologic reaction, caused by direct tissue damage. Despite their dissimilar pathogeneses, at times ACD and ICD are clinically and histologically indistinguishable (Tables 15-6 and 15-7) [36,37]. These two eczematous entities are the most common skin problems requiring medical intervention, and are also the leading causes of occupational disease [38].

Allergic contact dermatitis

The diagnosis of ACD is made by associating exposure of the involved skin to a potential allergenic substance. Thus, the exposed areas of skin (hands and face) are more likely to develop ACD. Patch testing is the gold standard for identification of a contact allergen. The paradox of patch testing lies in its deceptive simplicity. Although the application of antigens for patch testing is rather simple, antigen selection and patch test interpretation require some expertise. The basic battery of commercially available standard antigens is helpful in the great majority (80%) of cases. The most common cause of ACD is poison ivy, and its antigen is not included in any patch test tray. Nickel, a very common sensitizer, is included in all standard patch test trays. Rubber allergy, another common cause of ACD, is evaluated with a battery of rubber mixes containing many of the chemicals involved in rubber manufacturing. Sensitivity to natural rubber latex has been recognized to be a cause of either a delayed-type contact dermatitis or an immediate-type reaction, especially among health-care workers [39]. Deaths have been reported, and many have occurred during surgical (and dental) procedures. RAST and skin-prick testing (rather than patch testing) are required for evaluation of the immediate-type sensitive patient, who is usually atopic and often also sensitive to avocados, bananas, figs, kiwis, and several other fruits [40••].

Irritant contact dermatitis

Irritant contact dermatitis cannot be defined as a single clinical entity, but rather a spectrum of diseases [41,42]. The different types of ICD have been described as acute, acute delayed, irritant reaction, cumulative, traumatic, pustular and acneiform, nonerythematous, and subjective. The clinical manifestations of the ICD syndromes are modified by external factors (type of irritant, duration of exposure, environmental factors such as pressure, temperature, and humidity) and on predisposing characteristics of the individual (age, gender, preexisting skin condition, especially atopic diathesis). Most irritants are thought to cause symptoms and signs within minutes to hours, whereas contact allergens take days. The morphologic, histologic, and immunologic overlap between irritant and allergic reactions puts into perspective the difficulty of assessing the nature of the dermatitis on any given patient. A substance is believed to be an irritant when the reaction cannot be explained by a positive patch test to a known allergen [43].

Table 15-5. CLINICAL DIFFERENTIAL DIAGNOSIS OF ECZEMATOUS RASHES

Disorder	Lesion	Common sites	Onset	Pruritus	Other features
ACD	Erythema, papulovesicles, oozing or crusted bulla	Exposed skin	Any age	+++ to +	Must be suspect for all chronic persistent eczematous eruptions; rashes largely correspond to area of antigen exposure
ICD	Erythema, papulovesicles (can be necrotic)	Site of contact	Any age	0 to ++	Clinical spectrum; most common is "eczema"
Seborrheic dermatitis	Macular erythema with a greasy scale; dandruff	Scalp, nasolabial fold presternum, axilla, inguinal, gluteal folds	<2 mo; puberty; >30 y	±, 0, + to ++	Chronic, remitting-relapsing, stress-related; prevalent in CNS and immunologic diseases (HIV)
AD	Erythematous papulovesicles, scaly, lichenified plaques; usually excoriated	Early infancy—extensor surfaces, face, and scalp; late—flexural areas; can generalize	From birth to puberty; rarely past 20s	+++ to +	Associated with family or personal history of asthma or hay fever and dry skin; may be localized on palms, soles, or eyelids
Nummular eczema	Single or several coin-shaped papulovesicular erythematous plaques Early—oozy or crusted Late—dry and scaly	Extremities, occasionally on trunk	Rarely prepuberty; adulthood	++	Related to dry skin and low humidity (improves in summer); possibly associated with atopy, especially as ICD in workplace
Stasis dermatitis	Erythema, possibly scaly, circumferential, associated with edema and nutmeg hyperpigmentation	Ankles	Adulthood	+ to ++	Multiple etiologies associated with peripheral edema; leg ulcers common
Dyshidrosis	Macrovesicles with or without erythema; late—lichenified and scaly	Palms and soles; especially along sides of digits	Adulthood usually, except children with AD	++ to +++	Usually symmetrical; typically exacerbates and remits spontaneously; secondarily infected at times
Lichen simplex chronicus	Lichenified, papular, scaly plaques	Areas accessible to scratching or rubbing	Any age	++ to +++	Reported pleasure from scratching; common cause of pruritus vulva or ani
Autosensitization or "Id"	Symmetrical papulovesicles, minimally scaly	Generalized, especially palms and soles	Any age	+++	Follows localized contact; fungal or bacterial eruption
Dermatophytosis (tinea)	Circular, sharply demarcated, raised, scaly border; single or multiple lesions; central resolution produces "ring"	Exposed skin, scalp, groin, buttocks, nails	Any age (except tinea pedis, which is rare prepubertally)	+ to ++	Recurs in patients with T-cell defects (atopics, diabetics; KOH exam or culture confirms diagnosis)
Pityriasis rosea	Discrete oval, dull pink maculopapules, with fine, grey, marginal collarette of scale; "herald" patch is largest and first lesion	Truncal, proximal extremities, with distinctive dermatomal distribution	Any age, but predominantly 10–35 y	0 to ++	Resolves spontaneously in 6–8 wk; rarely recurs
Photoallergic and photocontact dermatitis	Macular erythema with or without papulovesicles; confined to sun-exposed skin only	Sun-exposed skin	Any age	++ to +++	Requires confirmation by photopatch testing
Polymorphous light eruption	Nonspecific, photodistributed erythematous papules; occur after first significant sun exposure of season	Sun-exposed skin	Females, 20–40 y	+++	Seasonal (spring and summer); requires phototesting for definitive confirmation; biopsy may show perivascular dermatitis
Drug-induced eczema	Round, sharply demarcated, scaly plaques; may appear lichenoid	Symmetrical, generalized	Adults	+++	Rare; most common after gold, dilantin, or bleomycin
Wiskott-Aldrich syndrome	"Classic" AD	Face, scalp, arms, legs; usually spares trunk	Early childhood	+++	Eczema, immunodeficiency
Acrodermatitis enteropathica	Persistent, localized, vesiculobullous, erosive, crusty plaques	Periorificial; acral	Infancy	0/+	Alopecia, diarrhea, and apathy; dramatically responsive
Hyper-IgE syndrome	Generalized chronic eczema	Generalized, symmetric	Early childhood	+ to ++	Job's syndrome—rare recurrent bacterial infections of skin and sinuses; IgE >2000 IU

ACD—allergic contact dermatitis; AD—atopic dermatitis; CNS—central nervous system; ICD—irritant contact dermatitis; KOH—potassium hydroxide.

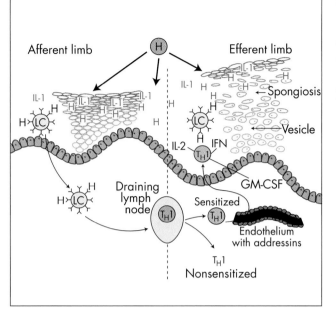

FIGURE 15-3.

Pathogenesis of allergic contact dermatitis. Afferent limb: a hapten (H) gains entrance to the epidermis, activating keratinocytes, which release inflammatory cytokines. Haptenated Langerhans' cells then migrate to a draining lymph node (within 24 hours). The hapten is then presented to T_H0-cells in the lymph node, producing a clone of hapten-specific T_H1-cells. Efferent limb: The "sensitized" T_H1-cells, with their skin-specific homing receptors home to the hapten-provoked skin site, where they release T_H1 cytokines resulting in spongiosis (within 36 hours). GM-CSF—granulocyte-macrophage colony-stimulating factor; IFN—interferon; IL—interleukin; LC—Langerhans' cells; T_H—T-helper cells; TNF—tumor necrosis factor. (*From* Beltrani and Beltrani [35]; with permission.)

Table 15-6. DISTINGUISHING FEATURES OF IRRITANT VERSUS ALLERGIC CONTACT DERMATITIS

Features	Irritant contact dermatitis	Allergic contact dermatitis
Frequency	80%	20%
Common causes	Water	Cosmetics (fragrance and preservative ingredients)
	Soaps	Metallic salts (*eg*, nickel, chromium, cobalt)
	Detergents	Germicides (*eg*, formaldehyde, formaldehyde releasers)
	"Wet work"	Plants
	Solvents	Rubber additives (*eg*, latex)
	Greases	Plastic resins (*eg*, epoxy, acrylic)
	Acids and alkalis	Rosin (*eg*, colophony)
	Fiberglass	Topical medications
	Particulate dusts	
Concentration of agent	More critical	Less critical
Mechanism/trigger	Nonimmune; sensitization not required; damage to keratinocytes	Immune; sensitization required; interaction of antigens with primed T cells
Atopic predisposition	Increased	Decreased
Diagnostic test	None	Patch test

Adapted from *Marks and DeLeo [36] and Nicol* et al. *[37]; with permission.*

Table 15-7. CLINICAL FEATURES OF IRRITANT VERSUS ALLERGIC CONTACT DERMATITIS		
Feature	Irritant	Allergic
Reaction delay after contact	Usually within 48 hours	Many hours to 5 to 6 days
Sharp demarcation	Often typical	May occur
Time for clinical resolution	Frequently diminished by 96 hours	Many days

Management of contact dermatitis

The ideal therapy for all contact dermatitides is the identification and subsequent elimination or avoidance of the offending substance from the patients skin. Once the offending substance is identified, the patient must be instructed as to where it may be encountered and should be advised as to available substitutes whenever necessary and if possible. Screening for predisposing factors to develop contact dermatitis, *eg*, atopy or history of prior reactions to contactants, is a most appropriate preventative measure in the workplace. Barrier creams have been inconsistently effective and often disappointing. Hyposensitization for delayed hypersensitivity reactions have never been successfully attained; thus, despite the prevalent lay misconception, there is no effective poison ivy pill or shot.

Pharmacotherapy for all eczematous eruptions is virtually the same. The more acute (vesicular) the process, the more aggressive the treatment. Cold compresses applied to oozing lesions offer gratifying relief. Lack of available antagonists for T-cell mediators compels us to rely on generic immunosuppressants for management (not a cure). Thus, corticosteroids remain the most effective and safest medication for T-cell diseases. Topical steroids are useful for the more chronic lesions, or for acute lesions involving limited areas of the body. Mid-potency corticosteroids are often adequate for the more chronic or lichenified lesions. When the lesions are most acute (bullous) or involve more than 20% of the body, systemic prednisone (0.5 to 1.0 mg/k/d) is justified. Knowledge of the natural history of acute ACD, such as poison ivy, determines the duration of therapy. With or without treatment, these rashes usually resolve spontaneously within 21 days, so relief of symptoms with prednisone may be necessary for that period of time. Slow weaning from corticosteroids at the suggested doses for the duration indicated by the natural history of ACD is not warranted. Although the lesions are frequently coated with a yellow, sticky crust (dry serum), antibiotics are rarely required unless symptoms of infection (rubor, calor, tumor, and dolor) are present. Because neither mast cells nor basophils, the source of histamine, are instrumental in delayed hypersensitivity, antihistamines are virtually useless in the management of contact dermatitis.

Irritant contact dermatitis may require a more varied algorithm for management. Prompt removal of the offending substance is essential, with rinsing or neutralization. The amount of tissue damage may preclude the use of corticosteroids, and antibiotics may be required.

Atopic dermatitis

Atopic dermatitis is well recognized as the third component of the "atopic triad" [44••]. Although allergens are universally considered to be triggers causing asthma and rhinitis, their role in AD remains a source of contention. Patients with asthma and rhinitis are properly advised of their hyperreactive airways and are usually fully aware of exposure to triggers other than allergens, which can cause wheezing or sneezing. It must be emphasized that patients with the atopic diathesis should be made aware that they may also have hyperreactive skin. Thus, allergens should not be regarded as the sole cause of respiratory cutaneous symptoms in these patients. No doubt, allergens play a more prominent role for respiratory problems; however, few can deny that there is a subset of patients who can experience an exacerbation of AD following the ingestion of allergenic foods or inhalation of an aeroallergen. Unfortunately, allergists have a tendency to proselytize aeroallergens as the cause of AD, and dermatologists tend to deny it [45]. Fortunately, neither specialty can deny the immunopathogenesis of AD (Fig. 15-4) [46].

Atopics have a genetic predisposition to producing excessive amounts of IgE antibodies to allergens and having excessive T_H2-cell activation [47]. The atopic patient's monocyte/T-cell interaction enhances development of a T_H2-dominant cytokine system whose IL-4 and IL-5 expression augments the noted T_H2/T_H1 imbalance and eosinophil infiltration [48,49].

Diagnosis of atopic dermatitis

The diagnosis of AD can be made by fulfilling the criteria established by Hanifin and Rajka [50], which include the presence of three major signs and symptoms and of three or more minor signs or symptoms. The major signs

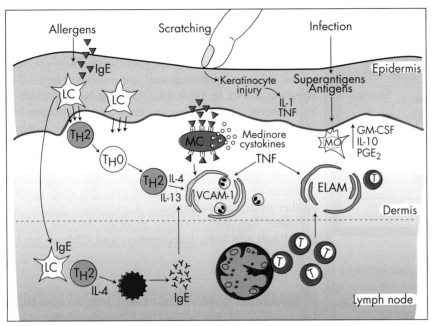

FIGURE 15-4.
Pathogenesis of atopic dermatitis. The immunologic cellular and cytokine interactions involved in the pathogenesis of atopic dermatitis. ELAM—endothelial cell leukocyte adhesion molecule; GM-CSF—granulocyte-macrophage colony-stimulating factor; IL—interleukin; LC—Langerhan's cell; MC—mast cell; MO—monocyte; PGE_2—prostaglandin E_2; T—T cells; T_H—T-helper cells; TNF—tumor necrosis factor; VCAM—vascular cellular adhesion molecule. (*From* Leung [46]; with permission.)

or symptoms are 1) personal or family history of atopy; 2) history of pruritus; and 3) eczema (spongiotic dermatitis). The minor signs or symptoms are frequently associated with the atopic diathesis, but their presence is not exclusive to the atopic state. They include allergic shiners, Dennie-Morgan lines, xerosis, keratosis pilaris, white dermatographism, defective cell-mediated immunity, palmar or plantar hyperlinearity, anterior neck fold, vernal conjunctivitis, and keratoconus.

Atopic dermatitis without atopy would be an oxymoron. Atopy can be detected from the familial or personal incidence of hay fever, wheezing, or eczema in approximately 90% of patients with AD [51]. The genetic predisposition to mount an IgE response to allergens can be used as an objective marker of atopy. The highest levels of IgE have been reported in AD; however, elevated levels of IgE are not always present in these patients, nor are the levels indicative of the severity of involvement [52]. Positive skin or RAST tests indicate the presence of IgE antibodies to an allergen but do not confirm a cause and effect relationship, because the positive results are almost always false-positives, merely representing the afferent limb of the immunologic response.

"The diagnosis of AD cannot be made if there is no history of itching!" exclaimed Dr. George Rajka (Personal communication, 1993). The fact that pruritus is the primary event in AD is widely accepted [53]. Although itching is a central phenomenon in AD, knowledge of its pathogenesis is poorly understood. The itchy skin of atopics best resembles hyperalgesia and has been termed *alloknesis*. This term implies that once itching is initiated, it causes the surrounding skin to react to the lightest stimulus with itching. Itchy skin is not the same

as a lowered threshold, which implies that pruritus is evoked by milder pruritogenic stimuli [54].

As Wahlgren [55] has reported, the most common itch provokers are those cited in Table 15-8, to which I [56] added dust mites (33%, but in selected cases up to 77% [57]). Despite reports of more mast cells and histamine in the skin of patients with AD [58,59], recent studies claim that other mediators besides histamine may be responsible for the development of the acute eczematous and pruritic skin reactions [60]. Because several itching dermatoses, such as AD, contact dermatitis, and lichen planus, are characterized by mononuclear (T-cell) infiltrates, the possibility that cytokines act as the pruritogenic factor in those diseases has been considered.

Supporting this theory is the observation that cyclosporin A, a drug that inhibits cytokines effectively, reduces the itch of AD [61–63] and other T-cell–induced diseases, whereas (nonsedating) antihistamines offer a clinically small decrease of itch in patients with those diseases [64].

The (Koebnerized) eczema of AD, which is histologically indistinguishable from all the other eczematous eruptions, is the result of mediators released by the infiltrating mononuclear cells. But the characteristic preponderance of allergen-specific T_H2 cells in AD instead of T_H1 cells as in contact dermatitis introduces another set of triggers and an alternative pathway causing the eczema. Recent evidence supports cytokines, which are produced in situ by the T_H cells and contribute to the generation and maintenance of the skin lesions of AD [65,66]. The cytokinal profile of the infiltrating T_H2 cells of AD revealed a preponderance of IL-4 and IL-5, which induce IgE production and attract eosinophils,

adults. Patients with the atopic diathesis (allergic rhinitis, allergic asthma, or AD) have a higher risk for the expression of acute anaphylaxis (and death from same). Patients with documented nonurticarial eruptions to drugs are at no greater risk of subsequent anaphylaxis to the same drug than the general population.

Diagnosis of drug allergy

The diagnosis of all drug reactions is based on the history and physical examination. Most often, the patient is on multiple medications and virtually any drug the patient is taking can be the culprit. The *Drug Eruption Reference Manual* [81] is an outstanding reference book and a must have for any practitioner who evaluates possible drug eruptions. Fortunately, the great majority of reactions occur within the first or second week of administration, occasionally later than the second week, and rarely after the drug is discontinued. Most severe reactions occur from intramuscular or intravenous administration; although the oral route is the most common cause of systemic reactions, they are generally less severe. While considering prescription drugs as causes of drug reactions, always bear in mind the possibility of dyes and additives, over-the-counter and illicit recreational drugs, and drugs that are inserted, inhaled, injected, or taken by other means. Bear in mind the basic pharmacologic tenet that all chemically related drugs cross-react, *eg*, the penicillin family of drugs cross-reacts with first-generation cephalosporin, (but probably not with third-generation cephalosporins) and sulfonamides may cross-react with sulfonylureas, thiazides, or furosemide.

There is no gold standard for diagnosing a drug allergy. Intradermal or RAST tests, which should be attempted only by experienced physicians, are only of value for the urticarial or IgE-mediated immune reactions, and there are but a handful of acceptable standardized antigens (*eg*, major and minor determinants of penicillin, tetanus toxoid, and insulin). Although a rechallenge with the drug can be the only definite diagnostic procedure, it is much too risky for IgE potentially anaphylactic type reactions. Several studies have determined the frequency of drug eruptions resulting from a variety of drugs (Table 15-12) [82,83].

Treatment of drug reactions

Be prepared for anaphylaxis when the patient presents with a sudden, explosive, generalized pruritus, with or without urticaria. An important sign of impending disaster is itching of the scalp, soft palate, palms, and genitalia. These patients require immediate epinephrine, plus an H_1 and H_2 antagonist (doxepin, 10 to 25 mg), and cardiopulmonary monitoring. Intravenous corticosteroids are required for aborting the late-phase reaction, and they have no effect on the early massive mast cell

Table 15-12. LIKELIHOOD OF DRUG ERUPTIONS

Top offenders	
Morbilliform and urticarial	Toxic epidermal necrolysis
Amoxicillin	Sulfonamides
Trimethoprim-sulfamethoxazole	Barbiturates
Ampicillin	Oxyphenbutazone
Penicillin G	NSAIDs
Synthetic penicillins	Allopurinol
Cephalosporins (first generation)	
Blood products	

Drugs unlikely to cause eruptions	
Digoxin	Nitroglycerin
Antacids	Meperidine
Promethazine hydrochloride	Aminophylline
Acetaminophen	Propranolol
Spironolactone	Prednisolone

NSAID—nonsteroidal anti-inflammatory drug.
Adapted from *Bigby* et al. *[82] and Guillaume* et al. *[83];
with permission.)*

degranulation; thus, they should be administered after the patient has been stabilized to prevent that late-phase reaction.

All drug reactions demand that the suspected drug or drugs be discontinued. The non-IgE–induced reactions are treated for symptom relief. The basis of that treatment is corticosteroids, preferably topically, but systemic administration is often required for comfort until the reaction resolves.

Adverse drug reactions are prevented by judicious use of any medication. A precise personal or family drug history is essential, with a complete knowledge of drug cross-reactivity.

REFERENCES AND RECOMMENDED READING

Recently published papers of particular interest have been highlighted as:
• 	Of interest
•• 	Of outstanding interest

1. 	Gell PCH, Coombs RRH, eds: *Clinical Aspects of Immunology* edn 2. Oxford: Blackwell Scientific; 1968.

2.•• 	Beck L, Charlesworth EN: The skin as an immune organ. In *Cutaneous Allergy*. Edited by Charlesworth EN. Cambridge: Blackwell Science; 1996: 1–33.
This is an excellent, current understanding of the skin as the peripheral arm of our immune system. Both authors are dermatologists with special interests in recognizing the skin as an accessible structure manifesting the complex relationships of various immune mechanisms.

3. Wahlgren CF: Pathophysiology of itching in urticaria and atopic dermatitis. *Allergy* 1992, 47:66–75.

4. LiJuan Tong, Balakrishnan G, Kochen JP, *et al.*: Assessment of autoimmunity in patients with chronic urticaria. *J Allergy Clin Immunol* 1997, 99:461–465.

5. Church MK, Levi-Schaffer F: The human mast cell. *J Allergy Clin Immunol* 1997, 99:155–160.

6. Soter NA: Biology of the dermis and pathophysiology of urticaria/angioedema and cutaneous necrotizing venulitis. In *Pathophysiology of Dermatologic Diseases*, edn 2. Edited by Soter NA, Baden HP. New York: McGraw-Hill; 1991:329–348.

7. Herrera AM, deShazo RD: Current concepts in anaphylaxis: pathophysiology, diagnosis and treatment. *Immunol Allergy Clin* 1992, 12:517–534.

8. deShazo RD: Anaphylaxis and/or anaphylactoid reactions. Workshop at American College of Allergy. Atlanta, GA; November 1993.

9. Mathews KP: Chronic urticaria. In *Clinical Management of Urticaria and Anaphylaxis*. Edited by Schocket E. New York: Marcel Dekker; 1993:21–68.

10. Lieberman P: Anaphylactoid reactions to radiocontrast material. *Immunol Allergy Clin* 1992, 12:649–670.

11. Manning ME, Stevenson DD, Mathison DA: Reactions to aspirin and other nonsteroidal anti-inflammatory drugs. *Immunol Allergy Clin* 1992, 12:611–632.

12. Beltrani VS: Current therapy: urticaria and angioedema. *Dermatol Clin* 1996, 14:171–198.

13. Caffarelli C, Cataldi R, Giordano S, Cavagni G: Anaphylaxis induced by exercise and related to multiple food intake. *Allergy Asthma Proc* 1997, 18:245–248.

14. Sibbald RG, Cheema AS, Lozinski A, *et al.*: Chronic urticaria: evaluation of the role of physical, immunologic and other contributory factors. *Int J Dermatol* 1991, 30:381–386.

15. Shertzer CL, Lookingbill DP: Effects of relaxation therapy and hypnotizability in chronic urticaria. *Arch Dermatol* 1987, 123:913–916.

16. Quaranta JH, Rohr AS, Rachelefsky, *et al.*: The natural history and response to therapy of chronic urticaria and angioedema. *Ann Allergy* 1989, 62:421–424.

17. Haas N, Toppe E, Henz BM: Microscopic morphology of different types of urticaria. *Arch Dermatol* 1998, 134:41–46.

18. Kano Y, Orihara M, Shiohara T: Cellular and molecular dynamics in exercise-induced urticarial vasculitis lesions. *Arch Dermatol* 1998, 134:62–67.

19. Bousquet J, Campbell AM, Canonica CW: H_1-receptor antagonists: structure and classification. In *Histamine and H_1-receptor Antagonists in Allergic Disease*. Edited by Simons FER. New York: Marcel Dekker; 1996:91–116.

20. Simons FER, Simons KJ: The pharmacology and use of H_1-receptor-antagonist drugs. *N Engl J Med* 1994, 330:1663–1670.

21. Sim TC, Grant JA: H_1-receptor antagonists in chronic urticaria. In *Histamine and H_1-receptor Antagonists in Allergic Disease*. Edited by Simons FER. New York: Marcel Dekker; 1996:273–296.

22. Simons FER, McMillan JL, Simons KJ: A double-blind, single dose, cross-over comparison of cetirizine, terfenadine, loratidine, astemizole, and chlorpheniramine versus placebo: suppressive effects on histamine induced wheals and flares during 24 hours in normal subjects. *J Allergy Clin Immunol* 1990, 86:540–547.

23. Gupta MA, Gupta AK, Ellis CN: Antidepressant drugs in dermatology. *Arch Dermatol* 1987, 113:647–652.

24. Foster M, Kottler WF, Hendeles L: Relative antihistaminic potency of doxepin and hydroxyzine. *J Clin Dermatol* 1998:7–10.

25. Mansfield LE, Smith JA, Nelson HS: Greater inhibition of dermatographia with a combination of H_1 and H_2 antagonists. *Ann Allergy* 1983, 50:264–270.

26. Bleehen SS, Thomas SE, Greaves MW, *et al.*: Cimetidine and chlorpheniramine in the treatment of chronic idiopathic urticaria: a multicenter, randomized, double-blind study. *Br J Dermatol* 1987, 117:81–91.

27. Heilborn H, Hjemdahl HH, Daleskog M, *et al.*: Comparison of subcutaneous injection and high-dose inhalation of epinephrine-implications for self-treatment to prevent anaphylaxis. *J Allergy Clin Immunol* 1986, 78:1174–1179.

28. Bressler RB, Sowell K, Huston DP: Therapy of chronic idiopathic urticaria with nifedipine: Demonstration of beneficial effect in a double-blinded, placebo-control cross-over trial. *J Allergy Clin Immunol* 1989, 83:756–763.

29. Liu HN, Pan LN, Hwang SC, *et al.*: Nifedipine for the treatment of chronic urticaria: a double-blind crossover study. *J Dermatol Treatment* 1990, 1:187–189.

30. Muramatsu C, Tanabe E: Urticarial vasculitis: response to dapsone and colchicine [letter]. *J Am Acad Derm* 1985, 13:1055.

31. Kaplan AP: Urticaria and angioedema. In *Allergy*. New York: Churchill Livingstone; 1985:439–471.

32. Monroe EW: Treatment of urticaria. *Dermatol Clin* 1985, 4:51–55.

33. Fradin MS, Ellis CN, Goldfarb MT, Voorhees JJ: Cyclosporin A for chronic urticaria. *J Am Acad Dermatol* 1991, 25:1065–1067.

34.• Beltrani VS, Beltrani VP: Contact dermatitis. *Ann Allergy Asthma Immunol* 1997, 78:160–175.
This review article was written specifically for the nondermatologist who wants to diagnose and treat contact dermatitis.

35. Beltrani VS, Beltrani VP: Contact dermatitis. *Ann Allergy Asthma Immunol* 1997, 79:1–30.

36. Marks JG, DeLeo VA: *Contact and Occupational Dermatology*. St. Louis: Mosby Yearbook; 1992.

37. Nicol NH, Ruszkowski AM, Moore JA: Contact dermatitis and the role of patch testing in its diagnosis and management. *Dermatol Nurs* 1995(suppl):5–10.

38. Marrakachi S, Maibach HI: What is occupational contact dermatitis? *Dermatol Clin* 1994, 12:477–479.

39. Sussman GL, Tarlo S, Dolovich J: The spectrum of IgE-mediated response to latex. *JAMA* 1991, 265:844–847.

40.•• Hamann CP, Sullivan KM: *Cutaneous Allergy*. Edited by Charlesworth EN. Cambridge: Blackwell Science; 1996.
There is no better source for any information regarding latex and its many reactions. This is a reference which can be quoted with the utmost reliable authority.

41. Beltrani VS: Contact dermatitis: irritant and allergic. *Immunol Allergy Clin* 1997.

42. Iliev D, Elsner P: Clinical irritant contact dermatitis syndromes. *Immunol Allergy Clin* 1997, 17:365–375.

43. Rietschel RL: Comparison of allergic and irritant contact dermatitis. *Immunol Allergy Clin* 1997, 3:359–364.

44.•• Leung DYM, ed: *Atopic Dermatitis: From Pathogenesis to Treatment*. Austin: RG Landes Co; 1996.
This textbook updating AD reflects Dr. Leung's astute expertise and emphasizes a significant understanding of this perplexing affliction. Each contributor brings with them an extensive personal experience with their assigned topic.

45. Halbert AR, Weston WL, Morelli JG: Atopic dermatitis: is it an allergic disease? *J Am Acad Dermatol* 1995, 33:1008–1018.

46. Leung DYM: Atopic dermatitis: the skin as a window into the pathogenesis of chronic allergic disease. *J Allergy Clin Immunol* 1995, 96:302–319.

47. Zachary CB, Allen MH, MacDonald DM: In situ quantification of T-lymphocyte subsets and Langerhans cells in the inflammatory infiltrate of atopic eczema. *Br J Dermatol* 1985, 112:149–156.

48. Hanifin J, Chan SC: Diagnosis and treatment of atopic dermatitis. *Dermatol Ther* 1996, 1:9–18.

49. Lewis JC, Yiannias JA: Eosinophilia-related syndromes. In *Cutaneous Allergy*. Edited by Charlesworth EN. Cambridge: Blackwell Science; 1996:35–90.

50. Hanifin JM, Rajka G: Diagnostic features of atopic dermatitis. *Acta Dermatovener (Stockh)* 1980, 92(suppl):44–47.

51. Hanifin JM: Immunologic aspects of atopic dermatitis. *Dermatol Clin* 1990, 4:747–750.

52. Svensson A: *Diagnosis of Atopic Skin Disease Based on Clinical Criteria*. Kristianstad; 1989.

53. Bernhard JD: Pruritus in skin diseases. In *Itch: Mechanisms and Management of Pruritus*. Edited by Bernhard JD. New York: McGraw-Hill; 1994:37–67.

54. Hagermark O, Wahlgren CF: Itch in atopic dermatitis: the role of histamine and other mediators and the failure of antihistamine therapy. *Dermatol Therapy* 1996, 1:7555–7582.

55. Wahlgren CF: Itch and atopic dermatitis: clinical and experimental studies. *Acta Derm Venerol* 1991, 165(suppl):1–53.

56. Beltrani VS: The role of dust mites in atopic dermatitis. *Immunol Allergy Clin* 1997, 3:431–441.

57. Ring J, Darsow U, Abeck D: The atopy patch test as a method of studying aeroallergens as triggering factors in atopic eczema. *Dermatol Ther* 1996, 1:51–60.

58. Mihm MC, Soter NA, Dvorak HF, Austen KF: The structure of normal skin and the morphology of atopic eczema. *J Invest Dermatol* 1976, 67:305–312.

59. Ring J, Thomas P: Histamine and atopic eczema. *Acta Venereol Suppl (Stockh)* 1989:70–77.

60. Amon U, Menz U, Wolff HH: Investigations on plasma levels of mast cell mediators in acute atopic dermatitis. *J Dermatol Sci* 1994, 7:63–67.

61. Wahlgren CE, Scheumois A, Hagermark O: Antipruritic effect of oral cyclosporine A in atopic dermatitis. *Acta Derm Venereol (Stockh)* 1990, 70:323–329.

62. Ross JS, Camp RDR: Cyclosporine A in atopic dermatitis. *Br J Dermatol* 1990, 122(suppl 36):41–45.

63. Munro CS, Higgins EM, Marks JM, *et al.*: Cyclosporine A in atopic dermatitis: therapeutic response is dissociated from effects on allergic reactions. *Br J Dermatol* 1991, 124:43–8.

64. Doherty V, Sylvester DGH, Kennedy CTC, *et al.*: Treatment of itching in atopic eczema with antihistamines with a low sedative profile. *Br Med J* 1989, 298:6–10.

65. Grewe M, Walter S, Gyufko K, *et al.*: Analysis of the cytokine pattern expressed in situ in inhalant allergen patch test reactions of atopic dermatitis patients. *J Invest Dermatol* 1995, 105:407–410.

66. Hamid Q, Boguniewicz M, Leung DYM: Differential in situ cytokine gene expression in acute versus chronic atopic dermatitis. *J Clin Invest* 1994, 94:870–876.

67. Hanifin JM, Schneider LC, Leung DYM, *et al.*: Recombinant interferon-γ therapy for atopic dermatitis. *J Am Acad Dermatol* 1993, 28:189–197.

68. Reinhold U, Kukel S, Brzoska J, Kreysel HW: Systemic interferon-γ treatment in severe atopic dermatitis. *J Am Acad Dermatol* 1993, 29:58–63.

69. Wüthlich B: Epidemiology and natural history of atopic dermatitis. *Allergy Clin Immunol Int* 1996, 8:77–82.

70.• Borkowski TA, Sampson HA: A combined dermatology and allergy approach to the management of suspected food allergy. *Dermatol Ther* 1996, 1:38–50.
The experience of the authors is readily appreciated concerning this frequently suspected etiologic problem. Emotion is miniaturized by the "facts."

71. Fuenmayor MC, Champion RH: Specific hyposensitization in atopic dermatitis. *Br J Dermatol* 1979, 101:697–700.

72. Zacheariaea H, Cramers M, Herlin T, *et al.*: Nonspecific immunotherapy and specific hyposensitization in sever atopic dermatitis. *Acta Derm Venereol Suppl (Stockh)* 1985, 1140:48–54.

73. Pacor ML, Biasi D, Maleknia T: The efficacy of long-term specific immunotherapy for *D. pteronyssinus* in patients with atopic dermatitis. *Recenti Prog Med* 1994, 85:273–277.

74. Ruzicka T, Bieber T, Schopf E, *et al.*: A short-term trial of tacrolimus for atopic dermatitis. *N Eng J Med* 1997, 337:816–821.

75. Hanifin JM, Schneider LC, Leung DYM, *et al.*: Recombinant interferon-γ therapy for atopic dermatitis. *J Am Acad Dermatol* 1993, 28:189–197.

76. Rustin MH, Poulter L: Chinese herbal therapy in atopic dermatitis. *Dermatol Ther* 1996, 1:83–93.

77.•• Beltrani VS: Dermatologic manifestations of adverse drug reactions. *Allergy Immunol Clin* 1998, in press.
As both an allergist and dermatologist, I have reviewed the significant literature of both specialties, and have presented an overview of "all" adverse reactions due to drugs.

78. Bork K, ed: Etiologic reaction patterns in drug intolerance. *Cutaneous Side Effects of Drugs*. Philadelphia: WB Saunders; 1988:5–26.

79. Wood AJJ: Adverse reactions to drugs. In *Harrison's Principles of Internal Medicine* edn 13. Edited by Isselbacher KJ, Braunwald E, Wilson JD, *et al.* New York: McGraw-Hill; 1994:407–411.

80. Goldstein SM, Wintroub BU: *Adverse Cutaneous Reactions to Medication: Roche Dermatologics*. New York: CoMedica; 1994.

81. Litt JZ, Pawlak WA: *Drug Eruption Reference Manual*. Cleveland: The Parthenon Publishing Group; 1997.

82. Bigby M, Jick S, Jick H, *et al.*: Drug-induced cutaneous reactions: a report from the Boston collaborative drug surveillance program on 15,438 consecutive inpatients, 1975 to 1982. *JAMA* 1986, 256:3358–3363.

83. Guillaume JC, Roujeau JC, Revuz J, *et al.*: The culprit drugs in 87 cases of toxic epidermal necrolysis (Lyell's Disease). *Arch Dermatol* 1987, 123:1166–1170.

CHAPTER 16

Food Allergy

Marianne Frieri

Food allergy or food hypersensitivity is the result of abnormal immune reaction to certain food allergens mediated by IgE or non-IgE mechanisms [1•]. In contrast, food intolerance due to host or food factors is an abnormal physiologic response to either a food or an additive. The most common foods eliciting reactions, especially in children, include milk, eggs, peanuts, wheat, soy, nuts, and fish. In adults, nuts, peanuts, fish and shellfish are the major offenders. Table 16-1 illustrates several of these reactions, which develop within several minutes to hours of ingestion. These may include involvement of the oropharynx, skin , upper or lower airway, gastrointestinal tract or systemic involvement with life-threatening anaphylaxis. Thus, the clinical manifestations can range from palate, tongue, throat or lip pruritus or swelling, throat tightness or hoarseness, urticaria and angioedema, rhinoconjunctivitis, nasal congestion, pruritus, rhinorrhea, sneezing, asthmatic symptoms, nausea, abdominal cramping, vomiting, diarrhea, or cardiovascular collapse. Severe life-threatening reactions in children and adolescents are usually associated with seafood, nuts, and peanuts.

The highest prevalence of food allergy occurs in early life, with approximately 6% of children under 3 years of age exhibiting food allergy. About 2% of the general population has been reported to have food allergy, with 30% of atopic children with atopic dermatitis and 10% with asthma having concomitant food allergy. The true prevalence in children and adults is much less than surveys have suggested, which is about 25% of the population [2,3]. A study on the public's perception of food allergy indicated that, although confirmed food allergy is uncommon, perceived food allergy is a widespread and persistent international problem with significant consequences [4].

PATHOPHYSIOLOGIC MECHANISMS

Several food antigens have been characterized by sequencing with isolation and cloning of complementary DNA (Table 16-2). Food proteins are mostly glycoproteins that have molecular weights between 10,000 and 60,000.

Current biotechnology can produce new varieties of plants with desirable attributes such as insect resistance or reduced expression of certain allergenic proteins. Careful approaches have been recommended to the food industry in order to avoid transfer of known allergens to the modified food form, as occurred when Brazil nuts were engineered into soybean [5] and to screen modified plants for unexpected allergens (Fig. 16-1) [6–8].

or maintenance [17]. Hypothetical mechanisms and events in food allergic diseases are illustrated in Figure 16-3 [17]. Food proteins reach the gut-associated lymphoid tissue (GALT) after luminal intracellular digestion and processing. In a normal situation, this process would induce clinical tolerance. The immune response can be directed under conditions that reduce the normal inductive process that leads to tolerance, such as occurs with a biparental history of atopy or with intercurrent inflammatory reactions in the gut interfering with the normal antigen-presenting pathway, with and without an increased uptake of antigen [17].

CD4+ T helper cells (T_H) can be functionally divided on the basis of their cytokine secretion pattern after activation. T_H1 effector cells predominantly secrete

interferon (IFN)-γ and interleukin (IL)-2, which trigger delayed hypersensitivity responses. T_H2 lymphocytes predominantly secrete IL-4, IL-5, and IL-10 and are not only involved in regulating IgE production but also may down-regulate T_H1 lymphocyte responses. T_H0 cells lack a particular specialization and are able to secrete cytokines of either cell type (T_H1 or T_H2). T_H1 immunity is more likely to induce cell-mediated damage to the mucosa. T_H2 responses preferentially lead to IgE-mediated immunity, which could, in turn, affect intestinal physiology [17].

Antigen encounter preferentially induces T_H2 T lymphocyte type IL-4, IL-5 or IL-10 responses in the gut [18,19]. The basic regulatory mechanisms of oral tolerance have been shown to involve suppressive cytokines such as transforming growth factor (TGF)-β–secreting CD8+ cells, which can then act on other immune cells that are naive to the antigen and suppress their reactivity (Fig. 16-4) [20].

After passing through the mucosa and being processed by antigen-presenting cells, the antigen is presented to lymphocytes for subsequent reactions. Selected presentation in association with class I antigens could lead to specific CD8+ T suppressor cell activation, whereas class II antigens will activate CD4+ T cells and lead to memory induction. Thus, a regulatory interaction between CD4+ and CD8+ T cells is possible [20]. Activated CD8+ T cells can also provide a negative signal to autoreactive cells in affected target organs. A negative signal could be provided by TGF-β. In the absence of a co-stimulatory signal (eg, through CD28-CD8+ [B7 family]), T-cell anergy or tolerance could be induced [20]. Other regulatory pathways are possible, and the role of CD8+ and CD4+ cells in suppressing unwanted immune responses

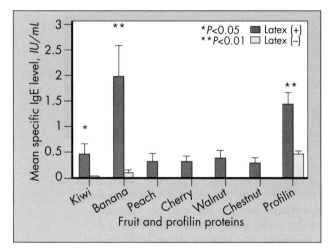

FIGURE 16-2.
Specific IgE levels to fruits and profilin in latex-positive and latex-negative patients. (*From* Tillah *et al.* [13]; with permission.)

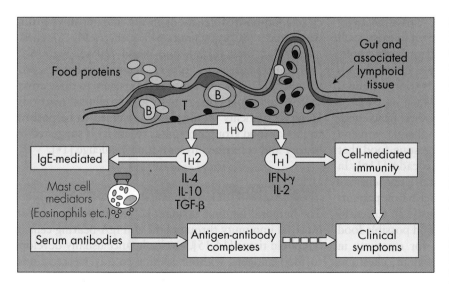

FIGURE 16-3.
Hypothetical mechanisms and events in food allergic diseases. Food proteins are shown reaching the gut-associated lymphoid tissue (GALT), leading to clinical tolerance. CD4+ T-helper (T_H) cells can be functionally divided on the basis of their cytokine secretion pattern after activation. The effector cells predominantly secrete interferon (IFN)-γ and interleukin (IL)-2, whereas T_H2 lymphocytes predominantly secrete IL-4, IL-5, and IL-10 involved in regulating IgE production and down-regulating T_H1 lymphocyte responses. T_H0 cells lack a particular specialization and are able to secrete cytokines of either cell type (T_H1 or T_H2). T_H1 immunity is more likely to induce cell-mediated damage to the mucosa. T_H2 responses preferentially lead to IgE-mediated immunity, which could in turn affect the intestinal physiology. B—B cells; T—T cells. (*From* Strobel [17]; with permission.)

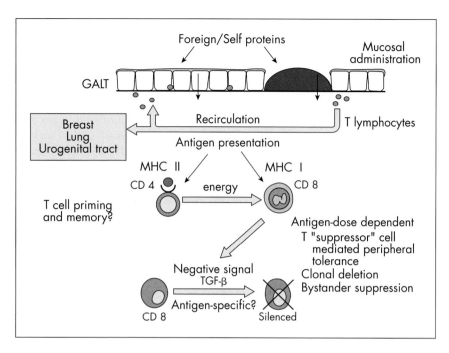

FIGURE 16-4.
A hypothesis of immune deviation after administration of food and self-protein. Antigen is presented in connection with class I and class II molecules after passage through the mucosa and processing by gut-associated lymphoid tissue (GALT). Preferential presentation, in association with class I antigens, could lead to activation of specific CD8+ T cells and can also provide a negative signal to auto reactive cells provided by transforming growth factor (TGF)-β. In the absence of a co-stimulatory signal (*eg*, through CD28-CD8+ [B7 family]), T-cell anergy (tolerance) could be induced. MHC—major histocompatibility complex. (*From* Strobel [17]; with permission.)

requires more study. The antigen dose dependency and the exact requirements remain unknown. Interestingly, neither type of CD4+ lymphocytes are absolutely necessary for oral tolerance induction (Fig. 16-4) [20].

Cellular immunity and cytokines have been suggested to play some roles in the pathophysiology of food hypersensitivity [15]. Several in vitro studies have demonstrated increased lymphocyte proliferation after stimulation with food protein [21]. In one study, combining cord blood lymphocytes with food antigens appeared to be useful for the prediction of allergic disorders [22]. Induction of IL-2 responsiveness is necessary for antigen-activated T cells to induce cell-mediated immunity.

One study of immunologic reactivity to foods involved 15 atopic children and adult patients, aged 20 months to 42 years, who had allergic rhinitis, asthma, atopic dermatitis, or urticaria. A history of food hypersensitivity and milk- or egg-protein positivity through skin test or specific IgE test were examined. Milk- or egg-specific IL-2–triggered T-cell proliferation was demonstrated [23]. The food-specific T-cell proliferation was shown to decline in several patients after elimination diets.

Two studies, a 3-week milk elimination diet in 11 children and a 3-week to 2-month elimination diet in several adult patients who had undergone a careful clinical evaluation and confirming skin-prick or in-vitro specific IgE testing, were performed. Diet diaries were assessed for clinical improvement. Diet modification improved cutaneous and gastrointestinal symptoms, and all patients had decreased serum IL-4 levels [23]. This preliminary data requires more investigation with double-blind placebo-controlled food challenges. Cytokine involvement through IL-4, which promotes the growth

of mast cells and IgE production, may contribute to the complex immediate and delayed-type mechanisms in food-allergic individuals [23].

We further investigated the role of cellular and serum IFN-γ, serum IL-4, and IgE levels in several patients with atopic dermatitis [24]. In mitogen- or antigen-stimulated cell cultures, IL-4 levels were detected in a few patients, but decreased levels of IFN-γ were noted compared to normal controls. Thus, cellular and humoral IL-4 and IFN-γ production can be dysregulated in certain patients with atopic dermatitis [24].

Nakazawa *et al.* [25] evaluated the predominance of type-2 cytokine-producing CD4+ and CD8+ cells in 45 patients with atopic dermatitis and 24 healthy controls. The frequency of IL-4–producing CD4+ cells and CD8+ cells from patients was significantly higher ($P < 0.001$) compared to controls, whereas the frequency of IFN-γ–producing CD4+ and CD8+ cells was decreased ($P < 0.01$) [25]. The frequency of type-2 cytokine-producing cells correlated well with the severity of atopic dermatitis.

Beyer *et al.* [26•] noted that severe allergic reactions to foods are predicted by increases of CD4+ CD45RO+ T cells and loss of L-selectin expression.

Peripheral blood mononuclear cells were prepared from 19 children with atopic dermatitis and stimulated in vitro with the suspected allergen (cow's milk, hen's egg), tetanus toxoid, and pokeweed mitogen. After 14 days in culture, quantitative and qualitative distribution of cell surface marker expression was assessed by flow cytometry, and results were compared with the clinical outcome of a subsequent oral food challenge [26•]. After stimulation with the allergen, a significant increase of CD4+ CD45RO+ T cells ($P < 0.05$) was detected selectively for patients showing severe clinical reactions. This increase was not detected for patients with mild or no clinical reactions or in six nonatopic control subjects. Increased expression of CD45RO+ was paralleled by a significant decrease in L-selectin expression ($P < 0.05$) for the same patient group. The combined assessment of CD4+ CD45RO+ and CD4+ L-selectin expression on T cells was more sensitive for the prediction of the clinical outcome of the food challenge ($P < 0.01$) than was measurement of cytokines or immunoglobulins in cell culture supernatants. These data indicate that a shift in lymphocyte functions may predict the development of severe allergic reactions in food-sensitized children with atopic dermatitis [26•].

HYPERSENSITIVITY REACTIONS

Four types of immune-mediated food hypersensitivity reactions exist. Food protein allergens stimulate mucosal type I reactions through mast cells or basophils releasing potent mediators (Table 16-3) [27]. Activated mast cells can lead to local immunosuppression of lymphocyte function [28] and generate cytokines and growth factors such as IL-2, IL-3, IL-4, IL-5, IL-6, IFN-γ, tumor necrosis factor (TNF)-α, and endothelin-1 [27]. Type II cytotoxic reactions have been suggested to occur in a few incidences with cow's milk allergy and antibody-dependent thrombocytopenia. Type III or immune complex reactions have been suggested to play a possible role in celiac disease or food protein enterocolitis disorders. Antigen-antibody immune complexes also occur in the serum of normal subjects in addition to those with food hypersensitivity [1•]. Intact antigenic macromolecules from food protein can traverse the epithelium of the gastrointestinal tract, and generate the active secretion of IgA with subsequent immune complex formation [14,15]. IgG1 antibodies are more effective in activating complement and both IgG and IgG1 antibodies to the cytoskeletal protein, tropomyosin, in lamina propria cells have been demonstrated in patients with ulcerative colitis [29]. Some investigators have argued that inflammatory bowel diseases, such as ulcerative colitis and Crohn's disease, are due to an immune response to a dietary constituent.

Although IgG4 has been implicated as an anaphylactic antibody in animal models of food allergy [27], there is little evidence that IgG4 contributes to food-related immediate-type hypersensitivity reactions. Rafei *et al.* [30] evaluated IgG4 levels in food-allergic subjects and suggested a slight correlation between early- and late-challenge responses and the presence of IgE and IgG. Frieri *et al.* [31,32] investigated IgE, IgG4 and cellular immune food responses in patients with food allergy and Crohn's disease. It was felt that IgG4 did not play a pathogenic role in Crohn's disease but the presence of increased levels of IgG4 may indicate a greater antigen load or a genetic predisposition to an immune response

to a specific food [32]. An animal study that examined intestinal inflammation induced during cow's-milk protein sensitization revealed a larger degree of sensitization through specific IgE and IgG antibodies [33]. Thus, intestinal inflammation can increase gut permeability, enhancing the sensitization process.

The involvement of IL-4, which can enhance the production of IgG4 from purified human B cells, has been demonstrated in spontaneous in vitro IgE synthesis in patients with atopic dermatitis [34]. In preliminary studies in several patients with atopic dermatitis and a history of food hypersensitivity to milk antigen, we demonstrated B-cell growth factor in peripheral blood mononuclear cells stimulated with milk protein [35].

Type IV or cell-mediated immune reactions have been reported in food-allergic subjects [23,24,32,35]. Although in-vitro T-cell responses are commonly reported in normal subjects [21], studies suggest that activation of food antigen–specific lymphocytes in milk-induced eczema leads to a preferential homing of lymphocytes to specific target organs [36].

Peripheral blood mononuclear cells from a group of children with eczema and type I milk hypersensitivity

Table 16-3. MAST CELL AND BASOPHIL MEDIATORS

Substances rapidly eluted from the granule under physiologic conditions
  Histamine
  5-Hydroxytryptamine (rodents)
  Chemotactic factors
  Exoglycosidases
  Activators of kinin, complement and clotting systems
  Vasoactive intestinal polypeptide analogues
Substances remaining granule-associated after activation
  Proteoglycans
  Proteinases (tryptase, chymase)
  Peroxidase
  Superoxide dismutase
Secondary mediators synthesized upon activation
  Prostaglandins
  Leukotrienes
  Platelet activating factor
Mediators whose release requires protein synthesis
  IL-2, IL-3, IL-4, IL-5, IL-6
  IFN-γ
  TNF-α*
  Endothelin-1

Some TNF-α may also be stored within mast cells and rapidly released upon activation.
IFN—interferon; IL—interleukin; TNF—tumor necrosis factor.
From Barrett [27]; with permission.

stimulated with the milk protein casein resulted in T-cell proliferation. The T cells in this study expressed the cutaneous lymphocyte antigen (CLA) but no CLA+ expression was noted in milk sensitive children with asthma or gastrointestinal allergy [36]. Further studies indicated that antigen-stimulated peripheral-blood T cells expressed mostly IL-5 and IL-13. In food-sensitive children with eczema, proliferative responses to food antigens and specific IgE antibodies were also evaluated with respect to age [37]. As previously shown, proliferative responses to peripheral-blood mononuclear cells to food antigens decreased rapidly after patients were placed on elimination diets [22]. The authors proposed that such diets may trigger a reduction in the responsiveness of food-sensitive CD4+ cells, with possible oral tolerance or development of fewer gastrointestinal absorptive functions, inducing these immunologic changes [37]. Type I and type IV reactions are thought to account for the majority of food-hypersensitive reactions (Fig. 16-3) [1•,17].

CLINICAL EVALUATION OF FOOD ALLERGY

The clinical signs and symptoms related to type I hypersensitivity are listed in Table 16-4 [38]. These consist of generalized, cutaneous, respiratory and gastrointestinal reactions with manifestations as listed in the introduction to this chapter. Systemic reactions have also been reported after eating cross-reactive foods in latex-allergic subjects [39] or after ingestion of food after exercise [40]. A recent review on the clinical methods and challenge procedures of the food-allergic patient has been reported by Assad [41]. Evaluation of the patient involves a detailed history, physical examination, skin-prick or in-vitro diagnostic testing, diet diaries, and single- and double-blind challenges. In other disorders, such as malabsorption syndromes or eosinophilic gastroenteropathy, endoscopy and biopsy may be indicated.

The oral allergy syndrome with symptoms of oral pruritis, irritation, swelling of the lip, tongue, palate, and throat with oral mucosal blistering was described in patients with ragweed and birch pollinosis reacting to fresh melon, bananas, apples, and hazelnuts [42]. In a more recent study on the oral allergy syndrome, one of the most frequent clusters of associations in Italy was fruit hypersensitivity in the prunoideae subfamily (cross-reactivity between peach, cherry, apricot and plum) [43]. No association between allergy to peach, cherry, apricot, or plum and any type of pollinosis was found, although fruit and vegetable hypersensitivity are reported to be clinically associated with allergic rhinitis caused by pollens, such as grasses, mugwort, and birch [11•,14,42,44,45]. The most recent report on the oral allergy syndrome has been reviewed by Pastorello and Ortolani [46]. Allergenic cross-reactivity of foods was recently reviewed and characterization of food allergens and extracts described by Bernhisel-Broadbent [47].

Non-IgE–mediated food hypersensitivity include cutaneous, respiratory, gastrointestinal, and neurologic reactions (Table 16-1) [1•]. History, physical examination and selected laboratory tests are the methods for evaluating IgE-mediated disorders [38,41]. The differential diagnosis of food hypersensitivity is listed in Table 16-5 [38]. In infants, several gastrointestinal disorders and enzyme deficiencies may mimic food hypersensitivity with vomiting, diarrhea, and abdominal pain. Several gastrointestinal disorders associated with infectious or structural defects can occur, as listed in Table 16-5. Additives, chemicals, and toxins can produce similar symptoms. Scombroid poisoning from fish due to elevated histamine levels can occur with ingestion of improperly processed tuna or mackerel, and ciguatera poisoning from Caribbean fish can lead to many gastrointestinal and constitutional symptoms. Various foodstuffs can be contaminated, and amines, alcohol, or xanthines can cause headaches, nervousness, or tachycardia. Foods may also be contaminated by materials or other foods [10••]. Hidden allergic reactions to milk-contaminated hot dogs, ice cream, and tuna have been reported [48]. Hidden seeds and nuts in desserts can lead to severe allergic reactions. Peanut butter hidden in a chili dinner resulted in one fatal and one near-fatal event [49], and a severe anaphylactic reaction developed to mustard masked in chicken dips and to the dust mite *Dermatophagoides farinae* in beignets [50,51]. Storage-

---

Table 16-4. PRESUMED IMMUNOGLOBULIN E-MEDIATED FOOD-HYPERSENSITIVITY REACTIONS REPORTED IN BLIND CHALLENGES

Generalized reactions
  Anaphylaxis
  Food-dependent, exercise-induced anaphylaxis
Cutaneous reactions
  Urticaria/angioedema
  Food-dependent, exercise-induced urticaria/angioedema
  Atopic dermatitis
Respiratory reactions
  Rhinoconjunctivitis
  Laryngeal edema
  Asthma
Gastrointestinal reactions
  Gastrointestinal anaphylaxis (abdominal pain, nausea, vomiting, and diarrhea)
  Colic
  Allergic eosinophilic gastroenteritis (with gastroesophageal reflux)

From *Sampson* [38]; *with permission.*

Table 16-5. DIFFERENTIAL DIAGNOSIS OF FOOD HYPERSENSITIVITY

Enzyme deficiencies
Transient fructose/sorbitol malabsorption
Lactase deficiency
Sucrase deficiency
Phenylketonuria

Gastrointestinal disease
Postinfectious malabsorption
　Viral, bacterial, parasitic
Hiatal hernia
Peptic ulcer
Gallbladder disease
Postsurgical dumping syndrome
Neoplasia
Inflammatory bowel disease
Pancreatic insufficiency

Additives and contaminants
Dyes
　Tartrazine
Exogenous chemicals
　Nitrates and nitrites
　Monosodium glutamate
　Sulfiting agents
　Antibiotics

Endogenous chemicals
Caffeine
Histamine
Tyramine
Phenylethylamine
Alcohol
Theobromine
Tryptamine

Toxins
Bacterial toxins
　Aflatoxin
　Botulism
　Ergot
　Fungi
　Staphylococcal toxin
　Toxigenic *Escherichia coli*
　　Vibrio cholerae
Endogenous toxins
　Certain mushrooms (α-amanitine)
　Shellfish (saxitoxin)
Psychological reactions
　Bulimia
　Anorexia nervosa

From *Sampson [38]; with permission.*

mite reactivity was also noted in a patient with chronic urticaria [52]. Sanchez-Borges *et al.* [53•] evaluated 30 atopic subjects for reactions to mite-contaminated wheat flour. These authors felt this problem may be more prevalent in tropical and subtropical countries than previously recognized [53•].

In taking history prior to a food challenge, the presumed incriminated food, quantity, state of rawness or cooking, length of time between ingestion and prior reactions, and other factors, such as concomitant exercise should be noted [1•,41]. Diet diaries can be useful in detecting a correlation and elimination diets can be used in both the diagnosis and the management of reactions [1•,23,41]. With a positive history, type I or IgE-mediated hypersensitivity can be confirmed with a positive in-vivo skin test or in-vitro radioallergosorbent test (RAST) that determines the presence of specific IgE antibodies. However, 60% of positive skin-prick tests do not reflect symptomatic food allergy. The skin test is a good negative predictor, because skin test results are rarely negative in subjects with provocation-proven type-I reactions. Fresh food materials rather than allergenic extracts have been shown in European studies to reflect a greater predictive value. Because the in-vitro

RAST tests have been modified and improved, they can provide similar information to the skin prick tests in good-quality laboratories [1•]. There are no other screening laboratory tests that can be useful in differentiating immunologic mechanisms. A review of in-vitro testing has been reported by Murali [54]. Open or single-blind challenges can be used to screen suspected food proteins, but these must be confirmed by a double-blind challenge [1•]. It is rare for patients to have multiple sensitivities, and overrestriction of foods can lead to nutritional deficiencies. Therefore, it is important to validate clinical reactions to foods. If the open challenge is negative, foods can be reintroduced and other causes of symptoms should be considered. In an open challenge study in food-hypersensitive adult patients, our division demonstrated that both serum and food antigen–stimulated IL-4 levels decline after dietary restriction [55] as previously reported in egg- and milk-sensitive children for IL-2– and IL-4–induced lymphocyte proliferation [23]. Thus, an objective measure was identified as a possible biomarker for food allergy.

The double-blind, placebo-controlled food challenge (DBPCFC) is the gold standard for the absolute diagnosis of food hypersensitivity in a clinic hospital setting [56].

However, it may not be as practical as once thought. Foods must be eliminated from the diet 10 to 14 days prior to the challenge. Subjects with positive skin tests and a definite history of severe anaphylaxis should not be challenged [1•]. The challenge usually starts with 125 to 500 mg of dry, powdered food, and the amount is doubled every 15 to 60 minutes for 2 to 4 hours. Type-I immediate hypersensitivity is excluded after 10 g of powdered food is administered in blinded capsules or liquid. Following a negative challenge, the food is then administered openly to exclude the rare false-negative challenge [1•].

Currently, there is no clinical evidence for diagnosis using in-vitro–specific IgG or IgG4 levels, lymphocyte activation markers or proliferation, food immune complex assays, or sublingual provocation.

TREATMENT

Strict elimination of the incriminated food allergen is the only proven therapy. Food labels must be carefully read and patient information literature can be obtained from the Food Allergy Network (1-800-929-4040). When reading food labels, other names indicating the presence of a food must be identified. Be careful to note changes in ingredients or vague labeling. Other patient resources including milk, egg, and corn-free diets, and hypoallergenic formulas can be found in the appendix of *Food Hypersensitivity and Adverse Reactions: A Practical Guide for Diagnosis and Management* [10].

Premedication with H_1 and H_2 antihistamines, oral cromolyn, or ketotifen can alter symptoms but generally have minimal efficacy [1•]. The use of immunotherapy, oral desensitization, neutralization, or subcutaneous provocation have not been proven.

Therapy for anaphylaxis should involve the immediate use of epinephrine followed by observation in an emergency room setting. Patients with food allergy should carry injectable epinephrine and wear a Medi-Alert bracelet. Family members should be educated about hidden food allergens and the immediate use of epinephrine if a reaction occurs.

REFERENCES AND RECOMMENDED READING

Recently published papers of particular interest have been highlighted as:
- •   Of interest
- ••   Of outstanding interest

1.• Sampson HA: Food allergy. In *Primer on Allergic and Immunologic Diseases* edn 4. Edited by Baker JR. *JAMA* 1997, 278:1888–1894.
This is an excellent, recent review of food allergy in general, which covers prevalence, pathophysiology, types of reactions, clinical manifestations, diagnosis, therapy, and future directions.

2. Bock SA: Prospective appraisal of complaints of adverse reactions to foods in children during the first 3 years of life. *Pediatrics* 1987, 79:683–688.

3. Young E, Stoneham MD, Petruckevitch A, *et al.*: A population study of food intolerance. *Lancet* 1994, 343:1127–1130.

4. Altman DR, Chiaramonte LT: Public perception of food allergy. *J Allergy Clin Immunol* 1996, 97:1247–1251.

5. Townsend JJ, Thomas LA, Kullisek ES, *et al.*: Improving the quality of seed proteins in soybean. In *Proceedings of the 4th Bienniel Conference of Molecular Biology of Soybean.* Ames: Iowa State University 1992:4.

6. Metcalfe DD, Astwood JD, Townsend R, *et al.*: Assessment of the allergenic potential of foods derived from genetically engineered crop plants. *Crit Rev Food Sci Nutr* 1996, 36(suppl):S186–S265.

7. Astwood JD, Leach JN, Fuchs RL: Stability of food allergens to digestion in vitro. *Nature Biotech* 1996, 14:1269–1273.

8. Astwood JD, Fuchs RL, Lavrik PB: Food allergy: adverse reactions to foods and food additives. In *Food Biotechnology and Genetic Engineering* edn 2. Edited by Metcalfe DD, Sampson HA, Simon RA. Massachusetts: Blackwell Science; 1997:65–92.

9. Ahlroth M, Alenius H, Turjanmaa K, *et al.*: Cross-reacting allergens in natural rubber latex and avocado. *J Allergy Clin Immunol* 1995, 96:167–173.

10.•• Frieri M: Cross-reactive and hidden food allergies. In *Food Hypersensitivity and Adverse Reactions: A Practical Guide for Diagnosis and Management.* Edited by Frieri M, Kettelhut B. New York: Marcel Dekker; 1998: in press.
This is an important article addressing cross-reactive and hidden food allergies.

11.• Therattil J, Frieri M: Systemic anaphylaxis to a hidden cross-reactive food in a surgical resident with latex hypersensitivity. *Ped Allergy Asthma and Immunol* 1997, 11:141–146.
This is an interesting case report and brief article on systemic anaphylaxis to a hidden cross-reactive food in a health-care worker with latex allergy. This is an increasing and important problem in which food proteins, such as avocado, kiwi, and other fruits, can trigger severe allergic reactions in certain risk populations.

12. Fitzgerald D, Chavarria V, Cosachov J, Frieri M: Evaluation and counseling of latex-allergic subjects. *J Allergy Clin Immunol* 1994, 93:7a.

13. Tillah F, Therattil J, Mitrache I, *et al.*: Latex allergy and food cross-reactivity in an outpatient setting. *Ann Allergy Asthma Immunol* 1998, 80:A.

14. Frieri M: IgE/IgA-bearing cells in gut lymphoid tissue with special emphasis on food allergy. In *Food Allergy: A Practical Approach to Diagnosis and Management.* Edited by Chiaramonte L, Schneider A, Lifshitz F. New York: Marcel Dekker; 1988:45–70.

15. Frieri M: Humoral and cellular immunity. In *Food Hypersensitivity and Adverse Reactions: A Practical Guide for Diagnosis and Management.* Edited by Frieri M, Kettelhut B. New York: Marcel Dekker; 1998: in press.

16. Hanson DG, Vaz N, Maia L, *et al.*: Inhibition of specific immune responses by feeding protein antigen. *Int Arch Allergy Appl Immunol* 1977, 55:1518–1524.

17. Strobel S: Oral tolerance: immune responses to food antigens. In *Food Allergy: Adverse Reactions to Foods and Food Additives* edn 2. Edited by Metcalfe DD, Sampson HA, Simon RA. Massachusetts: Blackwell Science; 1997:107–135.

18. Garside P, Stell M, Worthey EA, *et al.*: T helper 2 cells are subject to high-dose oral tolerance and are not essential for its induction. *J Immunol* 1994, 154:5649–5655.

19. Aroeisa LS, Cardilla F, de Albuquerque DA, *et al.*: Anti–IL-10 treatment does not block either the induction or the maintenance of orally induced tolerance to OVA. *Scand J Immunol* 1995, 41:319–323.

20. Miller A, Lider O, Weiner HL: Antigen-driven bystander suppression after oral administration of antigens. *J Exp Med* 1991, 174:791–798.

21. Hoffman K, Ho D, Sampson H: Evaluation of the usefulness of lymphocyte proliferation assays in the diagnosis of cow milk allergy. *J Allergy Clin Immunol* 1997, 99:360–366.

22. Kobayashi Y, Konda N, Shinoda S, *et al.*: Predictive values of cord blood IgE and cord blood lymphocyte responses to food antigens in allergic disorders during infancy. *J Allergy Clin Immunol* 1994, 94:907–916.

23. Frieri M, Martinez S, Agarwal K, *et al.*: A preliminary study of interleukin-4 detection in atopic pediatric and adult patients: effect of dietary modification. *Ped Asthma Allergy Immunol* 1993, 7:27–35.

24. Knapik M, Frieri M: Altered cytokine production in atopic dermatitis: a preliminary study. *Ped Asthma Allergy and Immunol* 1993, 7:127–133.

25. Nakazawa M, Sugi N, Kawaguchi H, *et al.*: Predominance of type-2 cytokine-producing CD4+ and CD8+ cells in patients with atopic dermatitis. *J Allergy Clin Immunol* 1997, 99:673–682.

26.• Beyer KE, Niggemann B, Nasert S, *et al.*: Severe allergic reactions to foods are predicted by increased of CD4+ CD45RO+ T cells and loss of L-selection expression. *J Allergy Clin Immunol* 1997, 99:522–529.
This is an interesting article suggesting that certain T-cell phenotypic markers and other inflammatory molecules, such as L-selectin, may predict more severe allergic reactions to foods.

27. Barrett KE: Mast cells, basophils and immunoglobulin E. In *Food Allergy: Adverse Reactions to Foods and Food Additives* edn 2. Edited by Metcalfe DD, Sampson HA, Simon RA. Massachusetts: Blackwell Science; 1997:27–48.

28. Frieri M, Metcalfe DD: Analysis of the effect of mast cell granules in lymphocyte blastogenesis: identification of heparin as a granule-associated suppressor factor. *J Immunol* 1983, 131:1942–1949.

29. Biancone L, Mandal A, Yang H, *et al.*: Production of IgG, IgG1 antibodies to cytoskeletal protein by lamina propria cells in ulcerative colitis. *Gastrointest* 1995, 109:3–12.

30. Rafei AE, Peters SM, Harris N, Bellanti JA: Diagnostic value of IgG4 measurements in patients with food allergy. *Ann Allergy* 1989, 62:91–93.

31. Frieri M, Bhat B, Zitt M, *et al.*: Specific immunoglobulin G4 and E levels in food-sensitive patients. *Immunol Allergy Pract* 1988, 10:9–16.

32. Frieri M, Claus M, Boris M, Harris N: Preliminary investigation on humoral and cellular immune responses to selected food proteins in patients with Crohn's disease. *Ann Allergy* 1990, 64:345–351.

33. Fargeas MJ, Theodorou V, Mare J, *et al.*: Boosted systemic immune and local responsiveness after intestinal inflammation in orally sensitized guinea pigs. *Gastroenterology* 1995, 109:53–62.

34. Vollenweider S, Saurat JH, Rochen M, Hauser C: Evidence suggesting involvement of interleukin-4 production in spontaneous in-vitro IgE synthesis in patients with atopic dermatitis. *J Allergy Clin Immunol* 1991, 87:1088–1095.

35. Frieri M: Preliminary investigation of interleukin-4 for food hypersensitivity in atopic patients. *Clin Res* 1990, 38:486a.

36. Abernathy-Carcer K, Sampson H, Pickei L, Leung D: Milk-induced eczema is associated with the expansion of T cells expressing cutaneous lymphocyte antigen. *J Clin Invest* 1995, 95:913–918.

37. Iida S, Kondo N, Agata H, *et al.*: Differences in lymphocyte proliferative responses to food antigens and specific IgE antibodies to foods with age among food-sensitive patients with atopic dermatis. *Ann Allergy Asthma Immunol* 1995, 74:334–340.

38. Sampson HA: Immediate reactions to foods in infants and children. In *Food Allergy: Adverse Reactions to Foods and Food Additives* edn 2. Edited by Metcalfe DD, Sampson HA, Simon RA. Massachusetts: Blackwell Science; 1997:169–182.

39. Frieri M: Latex allergy in health care workers: Nassau County Medical Center Proceedings. 1997, 24:1–6.

40. Romano A, Forso M, Giuffreda F, *et al.*: Diagnostic work-up for food-dependent exercise-induced anaphylaxis. *Allergy* 1995, 50:817–824.

41. Assad A: Clinical methods and challenge procedures. In *Food Hypersensitivity and Adverse Reactions: A Practical Guide for Diagnosis and Management*. Edited by Frieri M, Kettlehut B. New York: Marcel Dekker; 1998: in press.

42. Ortolani C, Ispano M, Pastorello, *et al.*: The oral allergy syndrome. *Ann Allergy* 1988, 61:47–52.

43. Pastorello EA, Ortolani C, Farioli L, *et al.*: Allergenic cross-reactivity among peach, apricot, plum, and cherry in patients with oral allergy syndrome: an in-vivo and in-vitro study. *J Allergy Clin Immunol* 1994, 94:699–707.

44. Pauli G, Bessot JC, Dietemann-Molard A, *et al.*: Celery sensitivity: clinical and immunological correlations with pollen allergy. *Clin Allergy* 1985, 15:273–279.

45. Ebner C, Birkner T, Valenta R, *et al.*: Common epitopes of birch pollen and apples. Studies by Western and Northern blot. *J Allergy Clin Immunol* 1991, 88:588–595.

46. Pastorello EA, Ortolani C: In *Food Allergy: Adverse Reactions to Foods and Food Additives* edn 2. Edited by Metcalfe DD, Sampson HA, Simon RA. Massachusetts: Blackwell Science; 1997:221–233.

47. Bernhisel-Broadbent J: Allergenic cross-reactivity of foods and characterization of food allergens and extracts. *Ann Allergy Asthma Immunol* 1995, 75:295–303.

48. Gern JE, Yang E, Evrard HM, Sampson HA: Allergic reactions to milk-contaminated "non-dairy" products. *N Engl J Med* 1991, 324:976.

49. FDA Ad Hoc Committee on Hypersensitivity to Food Constituents: Report. Washington DC: US Food and Drug Administration; 1986.

50. Kanny G, Fremont S, Talhouarne G, *et al.*: Anaphylaxis to mustard as a masked allergen in chicken dips. *Ann Allergy Asthma Immunol* 1995, 75:340.

51. Erken A, Rodriques JL, McCullough J, *et al.*: Anaphylaxis following ingestion of *D. farinae*–contaminated beignet. *J Allergy Clin Immunol* 1992:208a.

52. Frieri M, Madden J: Chronic steroid-resistant urticaria. *Ann Allergy* 1993, 70:1–7.

53.• Sanchez-Borges M, Capriles-Hulett A, Fernandez-Caldas E, *et al.*: Mite-contaminated foods as a cause of anaphylaxis. *J Allergy Clin Immunol* 1997, 99:738–743.
This is an important article because hidden contaminants and allergens in foods, such as dust mite–containing wheat flour, can lead to anaphylaxis, which may be more common in tropical climates.

54. Murali M: Immunologic methods for evaluation. In *Food Hypersensitivity and Adverse Reactions: A Practical Guide for Diagnosis and Management*. Edited by Frieri M, Kettlehut B. New York: Marcel Dekker; 1988: in press.

55. Chavarria V, Young R, Zitt M, *et al.*: Interleukin-4 and plasma histamine levels in challenged food-hypersensitive patients. *Ann Allergy* 1994, 72:57a.

56. Bock Sa, Sampson HA, Atkins FM, *et al.*: Double-blind, placebo-controlled food challenge (DBPCFC) as an office procedure: a manual. *J Allergy Clin Immunol* 1988, 82:986–997.

CHAPTER 17

Conjunctivitis and Allergic Eye Diseases

Tina C. Zecca

Leonard Bielory

The eye can often be viewed as a common target of allergic and immunologic disorders. Primary care physicians are usually the first to correlate ocular diagnosis with systemic findings in a patient and formulate a treatment plan.

Ocular inflammation often presents itself in the form of a "red eye." The most common etiologies include allergic or infectious agents. In the majority of cases, a thorough history and physical examination focusing on signs and symptoms will yield a presumptive diagnosis. Other etiologies will need to be considered in patients with atypical clinical signs and symptoms and in patients who do not respond to standard therapy. This chapter reviews conjunctivitis in its many different forms as well as other allergic ocular disorders.

CATEGORIES OF OCULAR INFLAMMATION AND OCULAR MAST CELLS

The eye is a complex organ usually involved in allergic and immunologic disorders. The conjunctiva is often described as the most immunologically active tissue of the external eye [1••]. Histologically, it is divided into two layers—the epithelial and substantia propria. Mast cells, Langerhans' cells, CD3+ lymphocytes, cytotoxic antibodies, and immune complexes are all involved in the ocular immunological hypersensitivity reactions (Table 17-1) [2•].

Mast cells are the principal cell type that initiates inflammatory responses, which are associated with immediate hypersensitivity reactions. Histamine, leukotrienes, prostaglandins, proteoglycans, and neutral proteases (tryptase, chymase) are all pre-formed mediators that are released by mast cells upon activation. Two different types of mast cells exist, based on their tryptase-chymase content. Ocular mast cells are normally of the tryptase-positive, chymase-positive type, which is commonly designated as the connective tissue type mast cell. We currently have strong evidence for the role of the mast cell in chronic inflammatory diseases of the eye because examination of conjunctival tissue reveals invasion by mast cells with release of mast cell mediators in tear fluid [3••]. Vernal conjunctivitis, giant papillary conjunctivitis (GPC), and atopic keratoconjunctivitis are disorders in which increased concentrations of mast cells have been reported [3••,4••].

HISTORY AND PHYSICAL EXAMINATION

Obtaining an accurate and detailed history is by far the key element in making a differential diagnosis between allergic and nonallergic dis-

Table 17-1. CATEGORIES OF OCULAR INFLAMMATION

Category	Recognition component	Cellular response	Associated disease
IgE/mast cell	IgE	Eosinophils	Allergic conjunctivitis
		Neutrophils	Anaphylaxis
		Basophils	Atopic keratoconjunctivitis
Cytotoxic antibody	IgG	Neutrophil	Vernal keratoconjunctivitis
	IgM	Macrophage	Mooren's ulcer
			Pemphigus
			Pemphigoid
Immune complex	IgG	Neutrophils	Corneal immune rings
	IgM	Eosinophils, lymphocytes	Serum sickness
			Lens-induced uveitis
			Behçet's syndrome
Delayed hypersensitivity	T lymphocytes	Lymphocytes	Vaculitis
	Monocytes	Monocytes	Corneal allograft rejection
		Eosinophils	Sympathetic ophthalmia
		Basophils	Sarcoid-induced uveitis

eases of the eye. Patients may reveal recent exposure to individuals with upper respiratory tract illnesses or conjunctivitis, either at home or at the workplace. Obtaining a sexual history may further reveal clues to suggest chlamydial or neisserial infection. A complete past medical history may give the clinician clues to associated ocular conditions, such as in rheumatoid arthritis or other collagen vascular disorders. Patients will often present to a physician with ocular symptoms consisting of low-grade ocular and periocular itching, tearing, burning, stinging, photophobia, and watery discharge. Patients most commonly complain of a red and itchy eye. Symptoms tend to be better during cool and rainy weather and are generally worse when the weather is warm and dry. Symptoms, such as tearing, irritation, stinging, burning, and photophobia, tend to be nonspecific. Pruritus is an essential element of allergic conjunctivitis. It is, by far, the most important feature distinguishing allergic from nonallergic eye disorders. Patients should point out the location of itching in order to distinguish conjunctival versus itching of the eyelid skin. Itching related to eyelid skin may be related to a contact allergy affecting both the skin and conjunctiva. Discharge may also be present in patients complaining of a red and itchy eye. The discharge can be variably described from watery (serous) to purulent. A purulent discharge with morning crusting indicates an infectious etiology. A stringy, ropy discharge is usually present in allergic disorders.

Environmental allergens commonly affect both eyes simultaneously. Ocular pain is not usually associated with allergic disorders and should be referred to an ophthalmologist to rule out other causes.

A thorough examination of the eye is necessary to confirm a diagnosis. One need not be an experienced ophthalmologist in order to perform a routine ocular examination. Evidence of eyelid involvement including blepharitis, dermatitis, swelling, discoloration, and ptosis should be noted. Conjunctival involvement may take the form of chemosis, hyperemia, palpebral and bulbar papillae, cicatrization, and presence or absence of secretions (Fig. 17-1). A funduscopic evaluation will reveal evidence of uveitis, which is an inflammation commonly seen in collagen vascular and autoimmune disorders or cataracts, that may be associated with atopic dermatitis or chronic steroid use [3••].

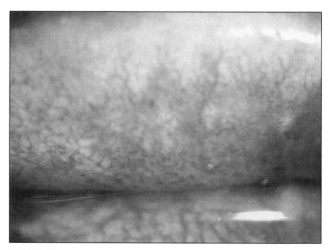

FIGURE 17-1.

Chemosis, injection, and papillae of the lower conjunctiva. (*Courtesy of* Marc Dinowitz, Newark, NJ)

The conjunctiva should be thoroughly examined. To examine the bulbar conjunctiva, ask the patient to look up and down while gently retracting the opposite lid. Examine the palpebral (tarsal) conjunctiva by grasping the upper lid at its base with a cotton swab on the upper portion of the lid while the patient looks down, and the lower tarsal conjunctiva by everting the lower eyelid while placing a finger near the lid margins and drawing downward. If a beefy, red conjunctiva as well as purulent discharge is present, a bacterial etiology is indicated. If edema is present and severe, patients will usually exhibit periorbital edema, which is more prominent around the lower lids secondary to gravity. Allergic shiners, which are ecchymotic areas thought to result from impaired venous return from the skin and subcutaneous tissues, have also been described in allergic patients.

The superior limbus and superior tarsal conjunctiva should also be examined, because these are the areas where Trantas' dots and giant papillae form in more severe ocular allergies.

OPHTHALMIC EXAMINATION

In addition to a thorough history and physical examination, an ophthalmic examination should be performed to help determine the presence of ocular allergic disease. The examination will help to differentiate between viral and bacterial conjunctivitis as well as allergic ocular disorders versus a more serious ocular disease (Table 17-2).

Thorough observation of a patient should be done prior to any hands-on assessment. This approach can often help the physician or health-care provider determine the appropriate examination and testing techniques needed for diagnosis [5]. Facial features may reveal forehead and eyelid vesicular eruptions often seen in ophthalmic zoster. A clue to a diagnosis of systemic lupus erythematosus may be a malar rash. Proptosis and lid lag is often seen in Graves' ophthalmopathy. Sjögren's syndrome is associated with enlarged parotid glands and extreme dryness of the mouth and lips. A patient's extremities should also be examined for signs of flexor contracture deformities, which may be seen in rheumatoid arthritis, or of Raynaud's phenomenon, which is seen in scleroderma.

The next step in the examination is the formal ocular examination. A patient's visual acuity should be assessed using a Snellen chart. The chart is usually placed 20 feet from the patient under appropriate lighting. Normal visual acuity is expressed as 20/20.

In examining patients for ocular allergy, the eyelids and lashes are assessed first, followed by the sclera and conjunctiva. The cornea and precorneal tear film are assessed last. Illumination and magnification are essential for appropriate examination; use a penlight, pocket flashlight, or a hand-held magnifying lens. A direct ophthalmoscope (Welch-Allyn; Tycos, Arden, NC) combines the essentials of both illumination and magnification [6]. This instrument is basically a light source connected to a magnified viewing system. Magnification is produced by a series of built-in "plus" and "minus" lenses, which are selected by moving the dial of the Kekoss disk found on the sides of the ophthalmoscope head piece. "Plus" lenses are color-coded with green numbers, whereas "minus" lenses are coded with red numbers. Larger images can be produced with the more powerful "plus" lens or higher green number used. A "plus 10" lens or greater is used frequently to examine external ocular disease or ocular allergy.

Proper positioning is very important in an ophthalmologic examination. Typically, direct ophthalmoscopy is performed with the eye that corresponds to the patient eye being examined. The eyelids and eyelashes are examined under the maximal intensity of light that can be tolerated by the patient. The superficial lid structures are examined by moving the ophthalmoscope light beam from the lateral to the medial canthus.

The examination of the conjunctiva includes examination of the palpebral, limbal, and bulbar conjunctiva.

Table 17-2. DIFFERENTIAL DIAGNOSIS OF CONJUNCTIVAL INFLAMMATORY DISORDERS

Disorder	Seasonal	Itching	Tearing	Discharge	Bilateral	Cell type	Cobblestoning
Allergic conjunctivitis	+	+++	++	Mucoid	Yes	Mast cell; eosinophil	-
Bacterial conjunctivitis	No	No	±	Mucopurulent	Variable	PMN	-
Viral conjunctivitis	Variable	No	+/++	Watery; clear mucoid	Yes	PMN, lymphocyte, monocyte	±
Vernal conjunctivitis	Yes	+++	++	Stringy mucoid	Yes	Lymphocyte, eosinophil	++
Giant papillary conjunctivitis	Variable	++	++	Clear white	Variable	Lymphocyte, eosinophil	++

PMN—polymorphonuclear neutrophil.

The palpebral conjunctiva is examined after lid eversion [7]. This procedure is performed by asking the patient to look down while gently pressing the skin below the lower lid with a cotton-tipped applicator and pulling downward. The upper conjunctiva is assessed by gently pulling the upper lid margin away from the globe by grasping the eyelashes while the patient looks down. A cotton-tipped applicator is placed at the upper lid crease. The upper eyelid is gently pulled down and out while the applicator stick is lightly dragged downward against the upper eyelid. This will give a good view of the upper conjunctiva. After completion of this examination, release the upper eyelid and ask the patient to look up.

The limbal and bulbar conjunctiva are examined under diffuse illumination. Fluorescein and rose bengal can be used to evaluate denuded and damaged epithelial cells of the conjunctiva. Fluorescein pools in surface irregularities of the cornea and conjunctiva. Rose bengal stains dead and degenerating epithelium and evaluates the ocular surface. Direct ophthalmoscopy can be used to evaluate abnormalities of the cornea. For optimal viewing, the ophthalmoscope light beam should be held near the temporal limbus and shined across the front of the eye toward the nose.

The precorneal tear film is evaluated after instillation of fluorescein. After the patient blinks several times (this allows a uniform spread of fluorescein over the corneal surface), the cobalt blue filter is used to measure the tear film breakup time (TBUT). The TBUT is a measure of tear film stability and is determined as the period between the opening of the eyes and the first appearance of a defect (black spot) in the green fluorescein layer. The average normal TBUT is 20 seconds, with a normal range between 15 to 35 seconds. An abnormal TBUT is less than 10 seconds [8]. A glossary of ophthalmologic terms used in this chapter is given in Table 17-3.

CONJUNCTIVITIS

Conjunctivitis can be defined as a broad group of ocular clinical disorders involving inflammation of the conjunctiva. It can often result from viral or bacterial infections that involve the eyelids, cornea, or conjunctivae, or from ocular allergy.

Bacterial conjunctivitis

Patients with bacterial conjunctivitis usually do not follow a seasonal pattern. Ocular itching is usually not present in this disorder. Ocular inflammation and its degree often correlate with the causative pathogen. Certain systemic diseases often manifest as conjunctivitis. Examples include Kawasaki disease and infectious mononucleosis.

Common signs and symptoms that tend to lead to a diagnosis of bacterial conjunctivitis include morning crusting with difficulty opening the eyelid, as well as ocular stinging or burning and purulent secretions. *Streptococcus* or *Haemophilus* species commonly produce acute catarrhal conjunctivitis in children. A mucopurulent discharge, as well as irritation and redness of the conjunctiva, is often present (Fig. 17-2). In the newborn period, conjunctivitis caused by *Neisseria gonorrhoeae* should always be included in the differential diagnosis. It often produces a profuse and purulent discharge. Chronic bacterial conjunctivitis can usually be attributed to *Staphylococcus* or *Moraxella* species.

Ocular conjunctivitis caused by a bacterial organism is seen in both adults and children, although the etiologies between the two groups differ. *Streptococcus pneumoniae* and *Haemophilus influenzae* are common pathogens seen in the pediatric population. Adults frequently encounter *Staphylococcus* species as the main etiologic organism.

The treatment of bacterial conjunctivitis is aimed at preventing patient discomfort, reducing infection, and

Table 17-3. GLOSSARY OF OPHTHALMIC TERMS

Term	Definition
Blepharitis	Inflammation of eyelid margins, which may have an infectious or inflammatory etiology. Clinical features include telangiectasia, lash collars and rosettes, thickening, crusting, and ulceration of eyelid margin.
Chemosis	Edema of the conjunctiva due to transudate leaking though fenestrated conjunctival capillaries.
Keratitis	Inflammation and infection of the corneal surface, stroma, and endothelium, with numerous causes.
Papillae	Large, hard, polygonal, flat-topped excrescences of the conjunctiva seen in many inflammatory and allergic ocular conditions.
Photophobia	Extreme sensitivity of the eye to light.
Proptosis	Forward protrusion of the eye or eyes.
Ptosis	Drooping of the eyelid, which may have neurogenic, muscular, or congenital causes. Conditions specific to the eyelid that may cause a ptotic lid include chalazia, tumors, and preseptal cellulitis.
Trantas' dots	Pale, grayish-red, uneven nodules with a gelatinous composition seen at the limbal conjunctiva in vernal conjunctivitis.

preventing the spread to others. Several antimicrobial ophthalmic preparations are available. Treatment is typically empirical, because cultures are often not obtained in acute cases of conjunctivitis. Broad spectrum antimicrobial preparations are often used in the treatment of bacterial conjunctivitis. These agents include trimethoprim-polymyxin B, bacitracin-neomycin, sulfacetamide, tobramycin, fluoroquinolones, and erythromycin. Topical corticosteroid and antibiotic-corticosteroid combinations should be avoided. Trimethoprim sulfate and polymyxin B combination is often well tolerated and provides excellent coverage for both gram-positive and gram-negative organisms. Agents such as tobramycin should be limited to use in more serious infections. Topical fluoroquinolones have also become available for use in severe cases of bacterial conjunctivitis.

Viral conjunctivitis

Viral conjunctivitis often presents itself with redness, itching, and, occasionally, a nonpurulent, serous discharge in one or both eyes. In examining the eye, one may note follicular hypertrophy and preauricular lymphadenopathy (Fig. 17-3). Adenovirus types 8, 19, and 37 are the likely etiologies of viral conjunctivitis in school-age children. Adenovirus types 3, 4, and 7 often produce a triad of symptoms including pharyngitis, conjunctivitis, and fever, which is often referred to as the PCF triad. Infection is usually self-limited and dissipates in 7 to 10 days. Subconjunctival hemorrhages, which are commonly benign (ie, they look worse than they are), can also be seen with viral conjunctivitis. Enterovirus species commonly cause acute hemorrhagic conjunctivitis. Treatment for viral conjunctivitis is primarily symptomatic.

Allergic conjunctivitis

Allergic conjunctivitis is a common clinical problem affecting approximately 25% of the general population

[3••]. The mast cell plays an important role in allergic conjunctivitis because millions of mast cells are contained in the conjunctiva. Seasonal and perennial allergic conjunctivitis are commonly seen, and cases of seasonal outweigh perennial allergic conjunctivitis. Grass pollen has been found to produce ocular symptoms, especially during the spring season. Common signs and symptoms include itchy or burning eyes with a watery discharge that may become stringy in the chronic form. Papillary hypertrophy of the tarsal conjunctiva can be seen in severe cases (Fig. 17-4). Signs and symptoms are commonly bilateral and recurrent in nature. Photophobia or visual disturbances are not often seen in allergic conjunctivitis. On physical examination, injection of the conjunctival surface with chemosis may be noted (Fig. 17-5). Lid edema may occur as well. If conjunctival scrapings and Giemsa stain were performed, eosinophil infiltration would be seen in 25% of patients with allergic conjunctivitis [9]. Tear-fluid IgE is present in almost all (96%) of the tear fluid samples [3••,10]. Interestingly, recent studies have shown that the nervous system may have a role in the inflammatory process in allergic conjunctivitis, because elevated levels of substance P have been found in tears of patients with allergic conjunctivitis [11].

As the name implies, perennial allergic conjunctivitis persists throughout the year. Dust mites, animal dander, and feathers are often the etiologic allergens. Like seasonal allergic conjunctivitis, mast cell–mediated hypersensitivity occurs. Both seasonal and perennial allergic conjunctivitis are similar with reference to age range and length of history.

Treatment of allergic conjunctivitis includes the use of antihistamine vasoconstrictor eye drops. Antihistamines relieve ocular itching that is often seen in allergic conjunctivitis. Most antihistamines are used four times a day and are effective in whitening the eye through the

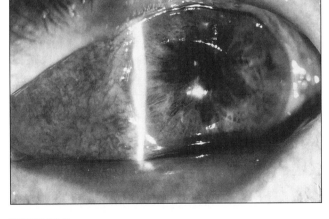

FIGURE 17-2.
Patient with conjunctivitis. A mucopurulent discharge, irritation, and redness of the conjunctiva are present. (*Courtesy of* Marc Dinowitz, MD, Newark, NJ.)

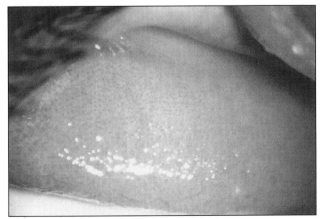

FIGURE 17-3.
Follicular reaction of the lower conjuctiva. Follicular hypertrophy and preauricular lymphadenopathy are apparent. (*Courtesy of* Marc Dinowitz, MD, Newark, NJ.)

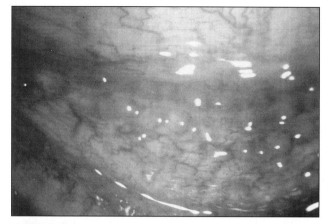

FIGURE 17-4.
Papillary hypertrophy. Everted lid revealing papillary hypertrophy of the tarsal conjunctiva. (*Courtesy of* Marc Dinowitz, MD, Newark, NJ.)

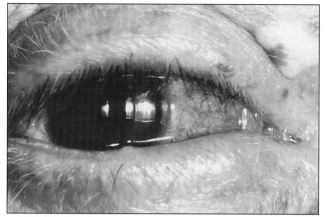

FIGURE 17-5.
Patient with allergic conjunctivitis. Injection of the conjunctival surface with chemosis is noticeable. (*Courtesy of* Marc Dinowitz, MD, Newark, NJ.)

constriction of the conjunctival blood vessels. Mast cell stabilizers are also effective for treatment, although a longer course of therapy (usually 10 to 14 days) is needed before relief is obtained.

More recently, two new antiallergic ophthalmic solutions have been added to the armamentarium of eye drops. Ketorolac tromethamine 5% (Acular; Allergan, Irvine, CA) is a nonsteroidal anti-inflammatory drug (NSAID) that has been shown to relieve itching and reduce levels of prostaglandin E_2 in tears [3••]. The only drawbacks to its use are a sensation of burning upon installation of the drops and the limited duration of use. Levocabastine hydrochloride (Livostin; CiBA Vision Ophthalmics, Duluth, GA) is an antihistamine that blocks the H_1 histamine receptor. This product, too, relieves ocular itching and is highly potent with few known irritation effects. Olopatadine (Patanol; Alcon, Fort Worth, TX) is one of the newer ophthalmic solutions which belongs to the antihistamine/mast cell stabilizer family. It prevents ocular itching associated with allergic conjunctivitis. The usual dosage for patients above the age of 3 years is one to two drops in the affected eye(s) twice daily at 6 to 8 hour intervals. The use of topical corticosteroids should be reserved for use by an ophthalmologist because the associated complications of these agents far outweigh their benefit for use in allergic conjunctivitis.

Vernal conjunctivitis

Vernal conjunctivitis is a perennial disorder that has a noticeable increase in spring. Symptoms include bilateral itching, tearing, photophobia, and mucus discharge. The disorder is a childhood disease that affects prepubertal males more than females. The disease has been linked to gender-related influences, and studies have shown that tarsal and bulbar conjunctival biopsy specimens stain

positive for estrogen and progesterone receptors. Therefore, hormones may possibly influence eosinophilic activity in patients with vernal conjunctivitis [12]. The pruritus seen in vernal conjunctivitis seems to be exacerbated by time, wind, bright light, hot weather, or physical exertion. Photophobia and lacrimation are also seen. On physical examination, conjunctival hyperemia with papillary hypertrophy ("cobblestoning") on the superior tarsal conjunctiva is seen. A thin, copious, milk-white, fibrinous secretion is usually composed of eosinophils, epithelial cells, and Charcot-Leyden granules. Conjunctival or limbal "yellow-white points," also known as Horner's points and Trantas' dots, can be present. In severe cases, the epithelium can break down and form corneal ulcerations, which are more common in children and can cause severe visual disturbances if scarring should result. Follicles are usually not present in this disorder. The disease is self-limited for the great majority of patients. Medical therapy includes antihistamines, vasoconstrictors, mast cell stabilizers, and NSAIDs. Corticosteroids can be considered for short-term management in resistant cases but only under the supervision of an ophthalmologist. Surgical measures should also be considered in resistant cases [13••]. Therapy using laser phototherapeutic keratectomy is beneficial in removing superficial corneal scars. Vernal plaques may be removed using superficial keratectomy in the hope that reepithelialization of the cornea occurs.

Giant papillary conjunctivitis

Giant papillary conjunctivitis is a syndrome that has been directly linked to contact lens use or use of other foreign materials, such as sutures or ocular prosthetics. A mast cell-mediated as well as a lymphocyte-mediated process has been implicated [14•]. Symptoms usually include decreased lens tolerance, mucus production upon awakening that chronically becomes thick and stringy, redness, burning, and itching. On physical examination, inflammation and papules can be seen, mainly on the upper tarsal conjunctiva. Patients may also develop Trantas' dots, limbal infiltration, and bulbar conjunctival hyperemia and edema.

Giant papillary conjunctivitis may develop from wearing any type of contact lens; after insertion in the eye, contact lenses develop a coating often seen in GPC. The cause of GPC and whether it is purely an immunologic disorder or result of mechanical trauma are unknown. It has been hypothesized that the coating on the contact lens stimulates an inflammatory reaction that results in GPC [14•].

The treatment of GPC consists of contact lens discontinuation in severe cases. Other modalities are aimed at contact lens care, including daily cleaning, weekly enzymatic treatment, and daily-wear lenses. Cromolyn sodium has been used with great success in treating GPC, and NSAIDs have also been reported to be effective. In a recent study done on patients with contact lens–associated GPC, the use of loteprednol etabonate was found to have a rapid therapeutic response [15]. Again, the use of topical steroids should be reserved for use by experienced ophthalmologists.

REFERENCES AND RECOMMENDED READING

Recently published papers of particular interest have been highlighted as:
• Of interest
•• Of outstanding interest

1.•• Bielory L, Wagner RS: Allergic and immunologic pediatric disorders of the eye. *J Invest Allergol Clin Immunol* 1995, 5:309–317.
This is an excellent article giving a general review of the anatomy of the eye, related allergic disorders of the eye, and a few pediatric immunologic ocular disorders.

2.• Irani AA: Ocular mast cells and mediators. *Immunol Allergy Clin North Am* 1997, 17:1–13.
This article focuses on mast cells and their mediators as they relate to ocular disorders. The different types of mast cells and their significance to ocular disorders are reviewed.

3.•• Bielory L, Friedlaender MH: Allergic conjunctivitis. *Immunol Allergy Clin North Am* 1997, 17:19–31.
This is a comprehensive review of allergic conjunctivitis. It includes an excellent discussion on treatment options in allergic conjunctivitis and a detailed discussion on history and physical examination as they pertain to allergic conjunctivitis.

4.•• Friedlaender MH: A review of the causes and treatment of bacterial and allergic conjunctivitis. *Clin Ther* 1995, 17:800–809.
This article summarizes important differences between allergic and bacterial conjunctivitis, and gives important clinical clues in distinguishing between the two disorders.

5. Wilson FM: *Practical Ophthalmology: A Manual for Beginning Residents.* San Francisco: American Academy of Ophthalmology; 1996.

6. Luff A, Elkington A: Better use of the ophthalmoscope. *Practitioner* 1992, 236:161–165.

7. Knoop K, Trott A: Ophthalmologic procedures in the emergency department part 3: slit lamp use and foreign bodies. *Acad Emerg Med* 1995, 2:224–230.

8. Toda I, Shimazaki J, Tsubota K: Dry eye with only decreased tear, but is sometimes associated with allergic conjunctivitis. *Ophthalmology* 1995, 102:302–309.

9. Abelson MB, Madiwale N, Weston JH: Conjunctival eosinophils in allergic ocular disease. *Arch Ophthalmol* 1983, 101:555.

10. Hoffmann-Sommergruber K, Ferreira ED, Ebner C, *et al.*: Detection of allergen-specific IgE in tears of grass pollen–allergic patients with allergic rhinoconjunctivitis. *Clin Exp Allergy* 1996, 26:79–87.

11. Fujishima H, Takeyama M, Takeuchi T, *et al.*: Elevated levels of substance P in tears of patients with allergic conjunctivitis and vernal keratoconjunctivitis. *Clin Exp Allergy* 1997, 27:372–378.

12. Bonini S, Lambiase A, Schiavone M, *et al.*: Estrogen and progesterone receptors in vernal keratoconjunctivitis. *Ophthalmology* 1995, 102:1374–1379.

13.•• Lee Y, Raizman M: Vernal conjunctivitis. *Immunol Allergy Clin North Am* 1997, 17:33–51.
This article gives a comprehensive review of vernal conjunctivitis, including clinical signs and symptoms, pathogenesis, differential diagnosis, laboratory evaluation, and treatment options. The article ends with an excellent discussion on individual therapeutic treatment options used in treating ocular allergies.

14.• Donshik P, Ehlers WH: Giant papillary conjunctivitis. *Immunol Allergy Clin North Am* 1997, 17:53–73.
This is a detailed article on GPC that includes descriptions of different stages of GPC and an interesting discussion on epidemiology. The article gives treatment options based on the different stages of GPC.

15. Bartlett JD, Howes JF, Ghormley NR, *et al.*: Safety and efficacy of loteprednol etabonate for treatment of papillae in contact lens–associated giant papillary conjunctivitis. *Curr Eye Res* 1993, 12:313–321.

CHAPTER 18

Drug Allergy

John A. Anderson

Recent advances in the diagnosis and management of true allergic (IgE-mediated) immunologic reactions and allergic-like reactions to drugs focus on published information relating to reactions with β-lactam antibiotics, other antibiotics (*eg*, sulfa), aspirin, other nonsteroidal anti-inflammatory drugs (NSAIDs), local anesthetics, radio contrast media (RCM), and angiotensin-converting enzyme inhibitor (ACEI) anti-hypertensive medications. Allergy skin tests are key to the evaluation of the patient with a history of β-lactam allergy. However, because all skin test reagents are not commercially available, patients with a history of severe reaction, regardless of a negative penicillin skin test, should be challenged. Incremental oral challenge is the only way to verify allergic-like reactions to other antibiotics. Desensitization is possible for both β-lactam antibiotic allergy and sulfa reactions if these medications are required for therapy. Reactions to the β-lactam side chain are unusual in the United States, but may be more common in other countries. Patients with penicillin allergies are probably not more likely to develop reactions to other antibiotics than the general population. Isolated periorbital edema may be a new aspirin/NSAID allergic-like syndrome. Repeated reactions to RCM dye may be effectively managed with a steroid-antihistamine pretreatment, and the use of low-osmol, nonionic RCM. Reactions to human insulin are possible but uncommon, and adverse reactions to endogenous insulin are rare. Allergic-like reactions, such as angioedema or cough to ACEI, are a definite problem and may occur late (months or years) into therapy.

CLASSIFICATION OF ADVERSE REACTIONS TO MEDICATIONS

An *adverse drug reaction* in a patient is an unwanted, often unexpected effect of medication that differs from the intended therapeutic purpose of that medication. The mechanisms of most adverse drug reactions have not been well defined, but few are thought to result from changes in the immune system. An allergic reaction implies an immunologic mechanism. When describing drug allergies, the allergist or immunologist usually discusses those reactions that are either known to be caused by an immunologic mechanism (a true allergic reaction) or other drug reactions that have clinical features suggestive of an allergic reaction (an allergic-like reaction). It is difficult to classify all of the known types of adverse drug reactions in a simple framework. In 1987, Anderson and Adkinson [1] classified drug reactions as either drug intolerances (unknown and nonimmunologic mechanism) or drug allergies (immunologic mechanism) (Table 18-1). Drug allergies were further classified as type I (IgE mediated), type II (antitissue antibody mediated), type III (immune complex and complement mediated), or type IV (cell mediated).

Anderson [2] used a broader classification based on three types of reactions: organ specific, generalized, or pseudoallergic. deShazo and Kemp [3••] used a simplified classification: type A (common and predictable) and type B (uncommon and unpredictable). Allergic reactions to β-lactam antibiotics, such as anaphylaxis, and reactions to RCM are categorized as type B reaction under the subclassification of "Hypersensitivity" (Table 18-1). The many clinical manifestations of adverse drug reactions were then further classified by deShazo and Kemp as either a multiple organ system pattern or one of six organ-specific patterns. Over the past decade, although the classification of adverse drug reactions has changed somewhat, the number and variety of different clinical manifestations of these reactions has not changed. Adverse drug reactions, referred to as *drug allergies*, are still defined as reactions proven or suspected to be caused by an immunologic event. When the clinical manifestations of the reaction are similar to those usually found in allergic diseases, the reaction is referred to as an *allergic-like* reaction.

β-LACTAM ANTIBIOTICS

Allergy to the β-lactam antibiotic penicillin and allergy to insulin protein represent two of the best-studied and best-defined examples of IgE-mediated immunologic

drug reactions. In the case of penicillin and other β-lactam antibiotics, such as amoxicillin and cephalosporin, reactions are the most frequently reported, compared with allergic-type reactions reported to other medications [2]. The prevalence of β-lactam antibiotics is 2%. It is estimated that as many as 400 to 800 deaths due to anaphylaxis to this group of medications occur annually [3••]. If use of penicillin/amoxicillin to treat common respiratory illnesses is reduced in the future, in favor of other antibiotics less likely to cause anaphylaxis, these death rates are likely to decrease. Today, however, β-lactam antibiotics are frequently used in different forms—especially amoxicillin, as demonstrated in statistics from a large health maintenance organization in the United States [4,5••].

IMMUNOGLOBULIN E ANTIBODIES DIRECTED TOWARD THE β-LACTAM RING VERSUS THE ANTIBIOTIC SIDE CHAIN

The four-member β-lactam chemical ring is found in all penicillins, cephalosporins, monobactams, carbapenems, oxacephems, and clavams. [4]. IgE antibodies are usually directed against this chemical structure and are responsible for most cases of β-lactam antibiotic allergy. In addition to the β-lactam ring, these antibiotics have side chains (and, in most cases, other unique chemical ring structures). In a few rare cases, individuals have been found to react to other epitopes in the antibiotic rather than the β-lactam ring, evidenced by tolerance to other β-lactam antibiotics containing this ring [6]. Although most of these latter cases are thought to react to the side chain of the antibiotic, recent studies

Table 18-1. CLASSIFICATION OF ADVERSE DRUG REACTIONS OVER A DECADE, BY STUDY

Anderson and Adkinson [1]	Anderson [2]	deShazo and Kemp [3••]
Drug intolerance Unknown or nonimmunologic mechanism Drug Allergy Type I (IgE-mediated) Type II (antitissue Ab-mediated) Type III (immune-complex– and complement-mediated) Type IV (cell-mediated)	Organ-specific reactions Skin, blood, lung, liver, heart, gastrointestinal system Generalized reactions Mast cell–mediated (anaphylaxis, urticaria) Serum sickness Drug fever Autoimmune Vasculitis Pseudoallergic Mediator-related Other allergic-like reactions (RCM and aspirin sensitivity)	Type A (common and predictable) Overdose Adverse Secondary/indirect Drug interactions Type B (uncommon and unpredictable) Intolerance Idiopathic Hypersensitivity (immunologic plus anaphylactoid, eg, RCM and aspirin sensivitity) Organ-specific patterns of reactions Multiorgan, dermatologic, hepatic, renal, hematologic, neurologic

RCM—radio contrast media

have presented evidence that IgE antibodies also can be directed against other components of the chemical structure of the antibiotic [7,8].

A group of patients allergic to ampicillin/amoxicillin who tolerated penicillin was identified in Spain [6]. Recently, a Canadian woman aged 33 years who developed systemic anaphylaxis after intravenous cefazolin was identified as skin-test positive to cefazolin only. She tested negative on penicillin/ampicillin skin test and negative to penicillin/amoxicillin and four other cephalosporins on oral challenge [9••]. This rare case was discovered after 9 years of study among 1000 patients referred for possible β-lactam antibiotic allergy. The only similar type of reaction to cephalosporin side chain in North America reported in the literature involves four other patients given cefazolin [10]. A single case was reported in the United States in 1996, involving a child who developed a late-onset maculopapular rash associated with a delayed (5 to 8 hours) but not immediate amoxicillin skin test [11]. The relationship of these findings to IgE-mediated β-lactam allergy is unknown.

Recently, selective side-chain allergic reactions to ampicillin in patients who were skin-test negative to the β-lactam ring were studied in two countries, Spain and Italy [12••]. In both countries, 93% of the patients presenting with a reaction to ampicillin/amoxicillin were skin-test positive to the β-lactam ring. Selective sensitivity to ampicillin/amoxicillin side chains in Spain was identified six times more often than it was in Italy where this type of reaction was considered very uncommon. These observations confirm that almost all true allergic reactions to β-lactam antibiotics are the result of IgE antibodies directed against the β-lactam ring. Reactions to the side chain or to other chemical structures in the antibiotic are rare—except in certain areas of the world, where they seem to be more prevalent for unknown reasons.

DIAGNOSIS AND MANAGEMENT OF PATIENTS WITH SUSPECTED ALLERGY TO β-LACTAM ANTIBIOTICS

If the patient develops an adverse reaction compatible with anaphylaxis while taking a β-lactam antibiotic, such as a rash or systemic sign, the antibiotic should be discontinued immediately and a substitute antibiotic outside the β-lactam class should be given, if necessary, to treat the remaining infection [12••,13]. Appropriate management of the rash or systemic reaction should also be instituted immediately.

If the patient has a history of allergy to β-lactam antibiotics or has recovered fully, for two weeks, from an acute reaction, he or she should be evaluated by an allergy/immunology specialist before reinstituting β-lactam antibiotics of any type.

PENICILLIN-ALLERGY SKIN TESTING

Allergy skin tests to penicillin and its drug metabolites are key to the evaluating patients with suspected allergy to any β-lactam antibiotics. In-vitro tests to confirm penicillin allergy by measuring IgE antibodies to various penicillin metabolites are not reliable in ruling out penicillin allergy at this time [14].

Elective penicillin-allergy skin testing is safe and should be promoted [2,3••,5••,15]. In a large outpatient study of children with a history reactions to β-lactam antibiotics, the risk of sensitization after skin testing and subsequent β-lactam antibiotic administration in a patient who was skin-test negative, was found to be 1% [15]. In a recent study involving a small number of adults with a history of penicillin sensitivity who test negative on penicillin skin tests, the risk of subsequent positive skin-test reactions or clinical reactions when challenged with penicillin was found to be approximately 5% [16].

In a large allergy outpatient clinic, where penicillin skin tests are routine, a 30-year period of experience has shown that only 10% of children and 20% of adults who present for elective skin testing, based on a history of adverse reactions to β-lactam antibiotics, will have a positive skin test [2].

When penicillin is metabolized, 95% results in a penicilloyl hapten. This major determinate of penicillin has been coupled to a carrier protein, polylysine, to create a commercially available skin testing agent, Pre-Pen (Akron Manufacturing, Decatur, IL). The remaining 5% of penicillin metabolites (minor determinants of penicillin) are a group of chemicals, including penicilloate and penilloate. At present, there is no commercially available penicillin minor determinate "mix" available in the United States [5••].

Table 18-2 demonstrates how suspicion of β-lactam antibiotic allergy can be confirmed through skin testing. Skin tests (intracutaneous or, if necessary, intradermal) can be done safely in most allergy and immunology specialists' offices using penicillin products, such as Pre-Pen and freshly prepared (up to 1 week) penicillin G, from stock medications available through the pharmacy. This latter agent only tests for some of the penicillin minor determinants.

Although not commercially available, some allergy and immunology specialists have developed a penicillin minor determinate mix (Table 18-2) as a skin-test reagent [5••,17]. This type of skin-test reagent, if properly prepared, measures most of the allergy sensitivity to the minor penicillin metabolites [5••].

Skin testing to all three antigens (Pre-Pen, benzyl penicillin G, and penicillin minor determinate mix) will identify 92% or more of all patients with a history of penicillin allergy. On the this basis, most patients, if negative to all three tests, may then take β-lactam

Table 18-2. β-LACTAM ANTIBIOTIC SKIN TESTING

Skin-test reagent	Dilution	Route of administration	Test dose
Pre-Pen* injection, USP	Penicilloyl-polylysine single test dose	Intracutaneous	One drop
		Intradermal‡	0.02 mL
Potassium/penicillin G	10,000 units/mL	Intracutaneous	One drop
		Intradermal‡	0.02 mL
Penicillin minor determinant mix†	Individually prepared, containing penicilloate and penilloate, ≤ 0.01 mol/L	Intracutaneous	One drop
		Intradermal‡	0.02 mL
Other β-lactam antibiotics†	Individually prepared, 0.05, 0.1, 0.5, 1.0 mg/mL	Intracutaneous‡	One drop
		Intradermal‡	0.02 mL

Akron Manufacturing, Decatur IL
† Additional skin test if available or necessary
‡ Serial skin testing; lower concentrations may be necessary in very-sensitive patients.

antibiotics safely [3••,18,19]. In a 1997 study involving patients with a history of reactions to β-lactam antibiotics who had a negative skin test to all three anitgen tests, 5% of patients reacted when challenged [5••]. All of these reactions were thought to be minor in nature and occurred within an hour.

A positive skin test to Pre-Pen tends to correlate with patients who have a dermal-type reaction (a rash) while taking a β-lactam antibiotic. A positive skin test to the penicillin minor determinate mix tends to identify those patients who have developed systemic, life-threatening reactions to the β-lactam. In recent studies, 20% of a series of patients who reacted to positive-allergy skin testing reacted to the penicillin minor determinant [5••]. Based on these results, a skin test of only two antigens (Pre-Pen and benzyl penicillin G) could be expected to identify only 70% of truly penicillin-allergic patients (Table 18-2). This is the situation that most practicing allergist/immunologists find themselves in today, because most do not have a penicillin minor determinant mixture at their disposal as a skin test reagent.

ORAL CHALLENGE WITH A β-LACTAM ANTIBIOTIC

Patients presenting with a reaction to penicillin that is only a rash and is not life threatening should be skin tested with the three penicillin antigens (if the allergist or immunologist has the reagents available to him, including the minor determinate mix). If those skin tests are clearly negative, most allergy and immunology specialists would advise the referring physician that it is safe for the patient to receive β-lactams in the future. This test is at least 92% reliable (Table 18-3). However, if the reaction is systemic (eg, asthma, rhinitis, angioedema, or shock plus urticaria or rash), a negative skin test with the three antigens does not ensure safety

for subsequent β-lactam administration. The next step in these circumstances is to challenge the patient with an oral β-lactam antibiotic (Table 18-4).

Usually, amoxicillin is used in the challenge procedure; however, any specific β-lactam antibiotic could be used [5••]. Using an oral suspension of the antibiotic allows more precise measurement of the dose. Typically, the total challenge necessary amounts to the usual single therapeutic dose of that drug adjusted by age. Thus, 150 mg and 300 mg of amoxicillin would be the usual challenge doses for a child or adult, respectively. The patient may be given an incremental increase in the amount, such as 16% to 33% to 50% of the cumulative dose at 15 to 20 minute intervals under close observation. If no reactions occur, further observation may be completed in the waiting area for up to a total of 2 hours. Adjustments in the dose, time intervals of administration, and waiting location should be appropriate for the individual clinical situation.

If the three penicillin-reagent skin tests are equivocal, an oral β-lactam challenge is advised (Table 18-3). If the allergy/immunology specialist has only two penicillin skin-test reagents and does not have the minor determinate mix, it is safest in almost all situations to advise a subsequent incremental penicillin β-lactam antibiotic challenge. Information gained from skin-test reagents alone gives a predictability of safety of only 70%.

CROSS-REACTIONS BETWEEN β-LACTAM ANTIBIOTICS

Although most patients allergic to a β-lactam antibiotic react to the β-lactam chemical ring structure found in all penicillins, cephalosporins, carbapens, and monobactams, the chances of cross-reacting when sensitive to one agent vary with the type of drug. Thus, the

Table 18-3. ALLERGY CONSULTANTS' APPROACH TO PATIENTS SUSPECTED OF ALLERGY TO β-LACTAM ANTIBIOTICS

Clinical situation	Penicillin skin tests	Oral challenge	Consultants' report
Rash	Battery of 3*: negative	Not necessary	Not allergic Skin test 92% or more reliable Possible minor rash on subsequent administration Not allergic if both skin test and challenge negative‡ Risk of subsequent allergy on administration: child 1%, adult 5%
Systemic anaphylaxis (asthma, shock, laryngeal edema)	Battery of 3*: negative	Yes	Not allergic if both skin test and challenge negative‡ Risk of subsequent allergy on administration: child 1%, adult 5%
Any reaction	Skin test: equivalent	Repeat skin test or oral challenge	
Any reaction	Battery of 2†: negative	Yes or No: Yes in all severe cases	Skin test alone only 70% reliable Greater risk if challenge not done Not allergic if both skin test and challenge negative‡

* Pre-Pen (Akron Manufacturing, Decatur, IL), penicillin G, and penicillin minor determinant mix
† Pre-Pen and penicillin G
‡ Only reliable for next course of β-lactam antibiotic

Table 18-4. ORAL CHALLENGE OF β-LACTAM ANTIBIOTICS FOLLOWING NEGATIVE PENICILLIN SKIN TESTS*

Drug†	Time interval‡	Dose§	
		Volume, mL	Milligrams, mg
Amoxicillin suspension 125 mg per 5 mL (or other β-lactam antibiotic)	Initial	1 to 2	25 to 50
	15 to 30 min	2 to 4	50 to 100
	15 to 30 min	3 to 6	75 to 150
		Total¶	150 to 300

* Time of waiting in office: 2 hours after last challenge.
† Use only if allergic skin test to penicillin or other β-lactams is negative or equivocal.
‡ Longer time intervals should be used with more clinically sensitive patients.
§ Incremental doses should be adjusted according to patient age.
¶ Total cumulative dosage should be equivalent to one average daily dose (eg, daily dose = 125 mg three times daily, challenge dose = 150 mg)

estimates of reaction in a patient proven sensitive to penicillin when given a first-generation cephalosporin are 10%, and only 3% when given a third-generation cephalosporin [3••,4]. The immunologic cross-reactivity between penicillin and the carbapens is high; the cross-reactivity between penicillin and the monobactams is quite low. However, it is important to remember that if the patient is proven to be allergic to penicillin, the risk for that patient to react at any subsequent time to any type of β-lactam antibiotic is 100%, and therefore, all β-lactams should be avoided [2].

If allergic to a β-lactam antibiotic, the patient's chances of having that IgE antibody directed toward epitopes—other than the β-lactam ring—in the chemical structure of the antibiotic are remote [9••,10]. Therefore, skin testing to individual β-lactam antibiotics is not necessary except in unusual cases [2]. The only validated β-lactam skin test involves penicillin and its metabolites as shown in Table 18-2 [2,19]. Skin tests to other individual β-lactam antibiotics are possible in selected cases; however, the results are less reliable.

MULTIPLE-ANTIBIOTIC SENSITIVITY IN PATIENTS ALLERGIC TO PENICILLIN

Since 1966, reports have been published indicating that patients, either proven or presumed allergic to penicillin, were three to nine times more likely to develop a reaction to a non–β-lactam antibiotic than the nonallergic population [20,21]. Recently, Koury and Warrington [22••] studied 44 consecutive penicillin-allergy skin-test histories and skin-test–positive patients compared to 44 age-matched control patients (penicillin allergy-history positive but penicillin skin-test negative) and 44 patients with nonallergic rhinitis (penicillin-history and skin-test negative). In contrast to previous reports, there was no difference in the frequency or type of allergic reaction to non–β- lactam drugs in patients with a past history of a reaction to β-lactams who are now either skin-test positive or negative to penicillin compared to patients in the control group (no penicillin-allergy or allergic rhinitis). Although this study is limited in numbers, involves mostly women, and is retrospective, it is better controlled and of the same size as previous studies. Only a larger, prospective, well-controlled study can provide a clear-cut answer to this question of the risk potential of a reaction to another antibiotic after becoming penicillin allergic.

MANAGEMENT OF PATIENTS PROVEN ALLERGIC TO β-LACTAM ANTIBIOTICS

In most clinical situations, β-lactam antibiotics can be avoided, and safe, alternative, non–cross-reactive agents are available. Over time, it has been estimated that β-lactam sensitivity declines at a rate of approximately 10% per year [2,3••]. In 1996, a prospective study of 48 penicillin-allergic patients demonstrated that (in 58% of patients) the β-lactam skin test became progressively negative after six years of strict allergy avoidance [23]. Therefore, even in proven β-lactam–allergic patients, repeat skin tests should be performed, especially if alternative drugs for these patients are not optimal and some time has elapsed since the initial allergic diagnosis was made.

In cases where there are no appropriate substitutes for a β-lactam, desensitization may be considered. This process eliminates the acquired reactivity or sensitivity through cautiously administering progressively larger incremental doses of the drug until the patient tolerates a therapeutic level of medication [24]. Although desensitization had been best-studied and best-proven to be successful in IgE-mediated drug reactions, such as with β-lactam antibiotics (penicillin allergy and insulin allergy), it has also been applied to some cases of nonimmunologic reactions to drugs, especially with antimicrobial agents, such as sulfa medications.

Desensitization is a potentially dangerous procedure and should only be performed under controlled conditions and with patient consent [24]. The exact method for preparing for this procedure varies with the clinical situation; however, model protocols exist to guide the practitioner [2,24,25•]. Although the published series of patients undergoing β-lactam antibiotic desensitization are small, analysis of cumulative data would indicate that both the oral and intravenous route of drug administration in this situation are safe [24].

MANAGEMENT OF ALLERGIC-LIKE REACTIONS TO ANTIMICROBIAL AGENTS OTHER THAN β-LACTAM ANTIBIOTICS

The most common manifestation of an adverse drug reaction to an antibiotic is a rash. If the rash involves urticaria, with or without angioedema, and systemic symptoms, especially those resembling anaphylaxis (anaphylactoid reaction), drug allergy is often suspected. As a confirmation test, the only type of skin test available for antibiotic sensitivity are those to β-lactam antibiotics.

Therefore, for identification of an antibiotic that can be safely administered in a clinical situation when there is a history of allergic-like reaction, the only test is an incremental drug challenge [2,24]. This has been termed as "test dosing" by some authors [13]. A model protocol that can be used for incremental drug challenge is shown in Table 18-5. The use of drugs in suspension form rather in pills or capsules offers more flexible dosing. It should be noted that, in patients who have had a more serious clinical reaction, the starting dose should be small, the dosing interval should be relatively long, and the incremental dose should be small. All such challenges can be done in an office setting if the physician and staff are prepared to manage any adverse effect. The patient should be prepared to wait 1 to 2 hours after the challenge is completed.

In a situation where the reaction to the non–β-lactam antibiotic is systemic in nature, incremental drug challenge should be avoided in favor of drug desensitization—if this latter procedure has been proved to be helpful for the specific condition.

If the history of the original reaction to the antibiotic was either an erythema multiform type of rash or Stevens-Johnson syndrome, both drug challenge and desensitization should be avoided because further contact with the drug may result in a potentially-life threatening situation.

REACTIONS TO SULFA ANTIBIOTICS IN PATIENTS WITH HUMAN IMMUNODEFICIENCY VIRUS INFECTIONS

Adverse reactions to sulfonamides usually involve a maculopapular, urticaria, or simple erythema multiform rash. Systemic and more serious reactions, such as drug fever,

Table 18-5. INCREMENTAL ORAL DRUG CHALLENGE PROTOCOL* FOR NON–β-LACTAM ANTIBIOTIC SENSITIVITY

Drug concentration[†], mg/mL	Child	Adult
	125/5	250/5
	25/1	50/1

Time interval[‡]	Dose, mg/mL	
	Child	Adult
Initial		
15 to 30 min	2.5/0.1	5/0.1
15 to 30 min	12.5/0.5	25/0.5
15 to 30 min	25/1	50/1
15 to 30 min	37.5/1.5	75/1.5
	50/2	100/2
	Total[§] = 127.5 mg	Total[§] = 255 mg

Time of waiting in office: 2 hours after last challenge dose
* This protocol is suggested as a model for a graded drug challenge in a controlled situation. Schedule should be adjusted to meet the clinical situation.
† Drug concentration should be adjusted to age. In very-sensitive patients, the initial dose may be lower (eg, 1 mg) and the dose increments should be smaller.
‡ Longer time between challenge doses should be allowed in clinically sensitive patients.
§ Total cumulative dose should be equivalent to one average daily dose (eg, daily dose = 250 mg 3 times a day, total challenge dose = 255 mg)

Stevens-Johnson syndrome, toxic epidermal necrolysis, thrombocytopenia, or neutropenia, may occur, but are less frequent [3••]. The prevalence of drug reactions is increased in the AIDS population. The increase is related partly to the degree of T-cell deficiency. For example, in the general population, the degree of rash due to trimethopin sulfunethoxal (TSM) is 3%. This reaction rate increases to 12% in T-cell–deficient HIV-negative patients, and 29% to 70% in patients with AIDS [2].

Although IgE antibodies may develop during some sulfonamide reactions, no reliable skin test or in-vitro test is available to confirm or otherwise help in the management of patients who have had an adverse reaction in the past but require a sulfonamide [3••]. This is of particular importance in patients who have AIDS, where *Pneumocystis carinii* infections are frequent and TSM is the preferred treatment and prophylactic medication.

In the patient who develops a rash to a sulfa antimicrobial agent, avoidance of the agent and use of an alternative antimicrobial drug are advised. If the patient requires a sulfa drug and only has a rash, an incremental drug challenge (Table 18-5) should be safe. In the AIDS patient, desensitization usually is advised for patients who had a rash with or without a fever because the consequences of direct drug challenge have been found to be unpredictable [3••,25•]. An important exception are those patients with Stevens-Johnson syndrome or thrombocytopenia, where re-exposure to sulfa medication is contraindicated [2].

Several different protocols for TSM and other sulfa desensitization are available in the literature. [2,13,25•,26•]. These protocols range in time from 8 hours to 30 days. Beal et al. [25•] provide a good, current discussion of management options with this condition. Unfortunately, there is often too little data to judge the reliability of any of these desensitization protocols based on outcomes. However, Caumes et al. [26•] recently reported on the outcome of 48 AIDS patients who were desensitized with TSM over 2 days on an outpatient basis and then followed for a median of 16 months (range, 5 to 24 months). Of the patients studied, 37 tolerated the procedure and were still taking the TSM. Of the 11 reactions, eight occurred during the desensitization procedure and two others occurred within 2 weeks of the procedure. Predictors of desensitization failure included a relatively high CD4 and CD4/CD8 cell ratio in the HIV-infected patients.

ALLERGIC-LIKE REACTIONS TO ASPIRIN AND NONSTEROIDAL ANTI-INFLAMMATORY DRUGS

Aspirin and NSAIDs are associated with several types of adverse drug reactions including gastrointestinal bleeding, hepatotoxicity, and renal insufficiency, as well as allergic-like reactions [3••]. There are three well-described groups of patients who manifest allergic-like reactions: 1) rhinitis-polyps-asthma triad; 2) urticaria with angioedema; and 3) anaphylactoid reactions. In the group with respiratory reactions, patients typically have the aspirin triad of rhinitis, nasal polyps, and severe asthma. These patients usually are adults and have long histories of perennial nonallergic rhinitis, sinusitis, or polyps and steroid-dependent asthma. The asthma in this condition is at least partially induced by a defect in cyclo-oxygenase pathway. Aspirin desensitization after a positive oral challenge has proved to be efficacious in improving the ability to management of these patients long term.

In a 1996 report, Stevenson et al. [27•] described 65 aspirin-sensitive patients with asthma who were positive to aspirin challenge and were then desensitized and kept on daily aspirin over a period of 1 to 6 years (median, 3.1 years). The outcome of this management technique demonstrated a significant reduction in the need for systemic steroid in asthma control and in the number of acute episodes of sinusitis. A protocol for aspirin challenge and desensitization can be found in the papers by deShazo and Kemp [3••] and Anderson [24]. It should be noted that the mechanism of aspirin desensitization is not completely understood, but the procedure renders the patient tolerant to all NSAIDs [3••].

Aspirin and other NSAIDs may induce urticaria with angioedema, and are the most common type of drugs—after β-lactam antibiotics—to be associated with this type of skin reaction in adults worldwide [2]. Use of aspirin and other NSAIDs can also worsen chronic idiopathic urticaria and acute urticaria from other causes; thus, this type of medication should be avoided in all cases of urticaria with angioedema. Aspirin desensitization does not usually improve chronic urticaria with angioedema, and therefore, this technique is not usually recommended for this allergic-like reaction [3••]. However, antidotal experience has demonstrated that, in some patients with a cutaneous reaction to aspirin or NSAIDs, aspirin desensitization up to 75 mg may be successful. This technique may be attempted in those patients who require this medication on a daily basis (one baby aspirin) as a blood thinner.

Aspirin-induced anaphylactoid reactions (urticaria with angioedema plus asthma and shock) are usually the result of sensitivity to aspirin itself or a single type of NSAID [3••,28••]. This type of sensitivity resembles IgE allergy, although no IgE antibodies to drug epitopes have been isolated. Recently, Quiralte et al. [28••], in Spain, challenged 240 patients with a history of aspirin or NSAID drug reactions with a battery of different forms of these medications under controlled conditions. In 18 patients with systemic anaphylactoid reactions, no reactions to other NSAIDs (except the one type that produced the original reaction) were found.

In 1993, Katz et al. [29] described two cases of isolated periorbital angioedema due to aspirin sensitivity. This was thought to be a relatively unusual manifestation of aspirin sensitivity. However, in the recent series of patients challenged in Spain [28••], 52 of the 98 patients with positive challenges had isolated periorbital edema as the single clinical manifestation of an allergic-like reaction. This group was significantly younger than other groups of aspirin-sensitive patients (mean age, 21 years). The patients with isolated periorbital edema also tended to be allergic and to have hay fever or bronchial asthma. All (100%) of these patients were atopic, versus the urticaria groups, where atopy was only 14%. When challenged with a battery of NSAIDs, 50 of the 52 patients reacted to several types rather than a single agent. Isolated periorbital edema represents a fourth clinical manifestation of allergic-like reactions to aspirin and NSAIDs.

ALLERGIC-LIKE REACTIONS TO LOCAL ANESTHETICS
Allergic or allergic-like reactions to injectable local anesthetics are rare. Although IgE skin-prick and intradermal skin tests have been advocated for many years in patients presenting with allergic-like symptoms to local anesthetics, only a few cases have been reported with positive skin tests [30••].

In a 1996 report from Germany by Gall et al. [30••], 177 patients with alleged allergic reactions to a variety of local anesthetics were seen over a period of 10 years. Patients were skin tested both by the prick and intradermal methods to either the causative agent or a battery of unrelated local anesthetics. Each patient was then challenged by subcutaneous injection of increasing amounts of both the causative agent and other local anesthetics to a cumulative dose of 3.8 mL. Three patients reacted with objective signs (2%). None developed objective reactions to other local anesthetics or preservatives. Of the patients who reacted, one proved by biopsy and patch test to be a type-IV delayed cellular immune reaction. The other two patients developed local urticaria and angioedema at the time of the sucutaneous injection, but the hives resolved spontaneously within 2 hours for unknown reasons.

Most adverse reactions to local anesthetics can be attributed to dose-related toxic events due to large amounts of local anesthetics, cardiac/vasostatic effect of epinephrine added to the local anesthetic, or direct intravascular injection of a bolus of the local anesthetic with or without the epinephrine. They can also be attributed to psychomotor reactions (anxiety/vasovagal) or unrelated allergy reactions, such as to natural rubber latex sensitivity [30••]. Although the preservatives in the local anesthetics (eg, methylparaben) have been accused as the agents responsible for these reactions, this has rarely been confirmed. In the study of Gall et al. [30••], the investigators could not find any cases where, on challenge, these symptoms were caused by preservatives in the local anesthetics.

In most situations, skin testing and incremental challenge with local anesthetic is advised [2,24]. Although it is very rare that a skin test would be positive, it is a safe way to screen for sensitivity to several types of local anesthetics, with or without preservatives, including the local anesthetic suspected as the causative agent in the original reaction. The subsequent incremental subcutaneous challenge with the local anesthetic, however, is the most helpful test when dealing with this situation [2,3••,24,30••]. Most experts suggest challenging with a different local anesthetic than that allegedly involved in the original reaction [2,3••,24]. Protocols for these challenges are generally available; however, the doses are usually administered at 15- to 30-minute intervals beginning at 0.1 mL of 1:100, 0.1 mL of 1:10, 0.1 mL of full-strength local anesthetic, and 0.5 mL and 1.0 mL full-strength material. Higher dose challenges (eg, 2.0 mL) are advised by some [2,30••]. It is important to use only local anesthetics (skin test or challenge) that are free of epinephrine. It is also important to point out to the referring physician or dentist that even if the skin test and challenge are negative, subsequent use of the same local anesthetic in a surgical or dental practice with epinephrine and at higher doses of local anesthetics could result in a subsequent toxic, vascular, or psychotropic reaction.

ANAPHYLACTOID REACTIONS TO RADIO CONTRAST MEDIA

One of the more common clinical situations involving individuals with a drug sensitivity other than reactions to β-lactam, other antibiotics, or aspirin/NSAIDs, are the history of reactions to conventional RCM. Adverse reactions are reported to be as common as 4% to 13 % [31•]. Most of these reactions are not severe, but 0.04% to 0.4% may experience generalized, life-threatening anaphylactoid reactions. Re-exposure to conventional RCM in patients with a history of reaction can result in another reaction in up to 30% of patients. Although the exact cause of these reactions is unknown, increased mediator release by the conventional/ionic RCM diagnostic material is thought to be involved [31•]. An immune reaction involving IgE antibodies is not thought to be involved in the pathogenesis of RCM reactions.

Use of newer, lower-osmol, or nonionic RCM diagnostic agents have reduced the overall incidence of adverse reactions to less than 3% and those involving a generalized anaphylactoid reaction to less than 0.04% [31•].

There is no way to predict an adverse reaction to RCM. However, there is an increased risk of anaphylactoid RCM reactions in patients who take a β-adrenergic blocking agent or who are asthmatic [32,33]. Because allergy is not the cause of RCM reactions, prior exposure or sensitization is not necessary. The allergy type of antibody skin tests or in-vitro assays are not helpful in predicting or verifying sensitivity. It is estimated that 15% to 30% of patients who develop an anaphylactoid reaction to RCM upon re-exposure are at increased risk of another reaction [2,3••,31•,32].

The potential risk of a severe RCM reaction can be significantly reduced by the universal use of low-osmol or non-ionic RCM in all patients [31•]. However, the cost of such a universal policy outweighs the safety issue, because at least 87% of all patients receiving RCM have no reaction to conventional diagnostic material and 99% have no severe reaction.

Over the years, studies by Greenberger and Patterson [34] have shown that premedication of patients who have a history of reaction to RCM but must receive RCM again has reduced the chances of a subsequent anaphylactoid reaction from 30% to less than 10% using conventional RCM and to as little as 0.5% using low-osmol, nonionic RCM in the next diagnostic procedure.

This premedication protocol has been used successfully for over a decade, and involves the principal use of oral prednisone and diphenhydramine. Since 1991, it also involves the use of low-osmol, nonionic RCM instead of conventional nonionic RCM for the next diagnostic procedure (Table 18-6) [2]. Some experts advocate adding either cimetidine or ephedrine sulfate to the premedication protocol [2,3••,31•,34].

INSULIN ALLERGY

Most, if not all, allergic reactions to insulin molecule are due to anti-insulin IgE antibodies directed against the insulin [35]. Noninsulin contaminants and other additives to commercial insulin preparations are rarely identified as causative agents in allergic reactions [3••,35]. Usually, this sensitivity does not interfere with diabetes management. Insulin from animal sources differs from the human insulin molecule and is more allergenic. Approximately 40% of patients treated with bovine/porcine insulin are expected to develop insulin-specific IgE and will have positive immediate-reactive skin tests, if tested [3••]. Allergic reactions to human recombinant insulin are unusual but possible [35,36•]. Documented allergic reactions to endogenous human insulin are rare [36•]. Alvarez-Thull et al. [36•] described a patient who was sensitive to her own insulin. This well–worked-up case demonstrated the complexity of insulin allergy and its management.

Systemic anaphylaxis to insulin is very uncommon and usually occurs after interruption and resumption of therapy with bovine/porcine insulin [2]. The approach to managing this type of situation, possibly involving a desensitization protocol, can be found in the literature [24].

ALLERGIC-LIKE REACTIONS TO ANGIOTENSIN-CONVERTING ENZYME INHIBITOR MEDICATIONS

Angiotensin-converting enzyme inhibitor antihypertensive medications block the metabolism of angiotensin,

Table 18-6. PREMEDICATION PROTOCOL FOR INDIVIDUALS WITH A PREVIOUS REACTION TO RADIO CONTRAST MEDIA WHO REQUIRE RADIO CONTRAST MEDIA PROCEDURES

Time	Medication	Dose, *mg*
13 hours before procedure	Prednisone*	50
7 hours before procedure	Prednisone*	50
1 hour before procedure	Prednisone*	50
	Diphenhydramine hydrochloride	50‡
	Cimetidine†	300‡
	Ephedrine sulfate†	25
Diagnostic procedure	Low-osmol nonionic radio contrast media	

* 200 mg intravenous hydrocortisone may be substituted for prednisone.
† Use of either/both cimetidine and ephedrine is optional.
‡ May be given intravenously.

bradykinin, and substance P [3••]. Angioedema occurs in 0.1% to 0.2% of patients taking these drugs, and of these, up to 25% may have life-threatening episodes of laryngeal edema. A separate group of patients may develop a chronic cough while taking these medications. ACEI administration may also increase the risk of anaphylaxis from any cause in these patients [3••].

Usually, the symptoms of angioedema occur within the first week of administration of the ACEI. Cough may also occur early, but has been found to begin six months into therapy. Late angioedema reactions have been reported as uncommon. However, a retrospective review by Anderson *et al.* [37•] of records involving 156 cardiac transplant patients compared with 341 renal transplant patients, identified six patients (five from the cardiac transplant group) who had ACEI angioedema late in onset. These reactions occurred from several months to over 1 year after starting the medication. Some patients had multiple reactions before the drugs were discontinued. The prevalence of these reactions in the cardiac group were 24 times that in the general population, and usually involved African-Americans. Allergic-like reactions in patients taking ACEI medication should be a matter of concern even if the patients have been taking these medications for an extended period of time without problems.

CONCLUSIONS

Most adverse reactions to drugs are due to nonimmunologic or unknown reasons. Those allergic (IgE antibody–mediated) or allergic-like (symptoms similar to allergic reactions) to β-lactam antibiotics, other antimicrobial agents (*eg*, sulfa antibiotics), aspirin or NSAID agents, local anesthetics, RCM, insulin, and ACEI medications are of current concern to the allergy

and immunology specialist. Most IgE-mediated allergic reactions to β-lactam antibiotics are directed towards the β-lactam ring, found in all classes of these antibiotics. A few cases of individuals who are sensitive only to the side chains or other components of amoxicillin and cephalosporin antibiotics have been found in isolated groups around the world, but fewer have been found in North America. Although skin testing to penicillin metabolites can help the allergy- and immunology-specialty physicians identify the true β-lactam allergy, all of these skin test reagents are not commonly available to the majority of physicians. Thus, patients who have had a severe previous reaction to β-lactam antibiotics or have had an equivocal or negative skin test to some of the β-lactam metabolites may still be at risk of having a reaction on subsequent antibiotic administration. Therefore, in these cases, an incremental oral drug challenge under controlled conditions is advised. In cases of other antibiotic reactions, an incremental oral drug challenge is the only test to assess for the risk of subsequent exposure to the patients. In both β-lactam antibiotic sensitivity and other antibiotic sensitivity (*eg*, sulfa) where known sensitivity exists and precludes safe subsequent challenge, desensitization is advised.

Recent studies have shown that patients with penicillin allergy may not be any more likely to develop adverse reactions to other antibiotics than the general population.

Aspirin and other NSAIDs have been associated with a group of allergic-like reactions. In addition to the respiratory group of patients (nonallergic rhinitis, nasal polyps, and asthma), and urticaria/angioedema anaphylaxis group, a new group of patients with isolated periorbital edema as the single manifestation of sensitivity has been described. Although some patients in the respiratory group can be helped with aspirin desensitization, patients with either dermal or anaphylactoid reactions usually do not respond to desensitization. Aspirin-sensitive patients with either dermal or anaphylactoid reactions usually do not respond to desensitization.

Allergic-like reactions to local anesthetics are rare. An incremental subcutaneous challenge with the local anesthetic of choice, however, can assist the specialist in advising the dentist or surgeon as to a safe local anesthetic to administer in a patient with a history of reaction.

Re-administration of conventional RCM in a patient with a history of allergic-like reaction can result in another reaction in up to 30% of patients. This risk can be reduced to as little as 0.5% on re-exposure if the patients are premedicated 13 hours with prednisone and antihistamine plus the use of low-osmol, nonionic RCM in the subsequent diagnostic procedure.

Insulin allergy has been less of a problem with the use of human recombinant insulin in diabetic management. However, some diabetics developed true IgE-mediated allergy to the human insulin molecule and rare patients reacted even to their own endogenous insulin.

With the use of ACEI as antihypertensive medication, some patients have developed angioedema and others developed a cough—both of which are allergic-like reactions. Although these reactions usually start early (eg, 1 week of therapy) some patients have now been identified as having late reactions (over 1 year). Furthermore, a few patients using ACEI medications have been found to have a higher risk of true allergic reactions to other substances.

REFERENCES AND RECOMMENDED READING

Recently published papers of particular interest have been highlighted as:
- Of interest
- • Of outstanding interest

1. Anderson JA, Adkinson NF Jr.: Allergic reactions to drugs and biological agents. *JAMA* 1987, 258:2891–2899.

2. Anderson JA: Allergic reactions to drugs and biological agents. *JAMA* 1992, 268:2845–2857.

3.•• deShazo RD, Kemp SF: Allergic reactions to drugs and biological agents. *JAMA* 1997, 278:1895–1906.
Approximately every 5 years the American Academy of Allergy, Asthma, and Immunology sponsors an allergy/immunology primer for all physicians. This 1997 issue of the primer is the fourth edition and features a comprehensive, yet suscient review of allergic and allergic-like reactions to drugs and biological agents.

4. Bianca NL, Vega JK, Garcia J, et al.: New aspects of allergic reactions to β-lactams: cross-reactions and unique specifications. *Clin Exp Allergy* 1994, 24:407–415.

5.•• Macy E, Richter PK, Falkoff R, Zeiger R: Skin testing with penicilloate and penilloate prepared be an improved method: amoxicillin oral challenge in patients with negative skin-test responses to penicillin reagents. *J Allergy Clin Immunol* 1997, 100:586–591.

This study confirms the reliability of a minor determinant group of antigens produced with improved extraction methods. It also validates previous studies, using elective penicillin skin tests to determine the true prevalence of β-lactam allergies.

6. Bianca K, Vega JM, Garcia J, et al.: Allergy to penicillin with good tolerance to other penicillin: study of the incidence in subjects allergic to β-lactams. *Clin Exp Allergy* 1990, 20:475–481.

7. Pham NH, Baldo BA: β-Lactam drug allergens: fine structural recognition patterns of cephalosporin-reactive IgE antibodies. *J Mol Recognit* 1996, 9:287–296.

8. Sastre J, Quijano LD, Novalbos A, et al.: Clinical cross-reactivity between amoxicillin and cefadroxil in patients allergic to amoxicillin and with good tolerance of penicillin. *Allergy* 1996, 51:383–386.

9•• Webber EA: Cefazolin-specific side chain hypersensitivity. *J Allergy Clin Immunol* 1996, 98:849–850.
This paper describes a rare case in which a patient was found allergic only to cefazolin and negative to other β-lactams based on skin test and oral challenge.

10. Warrington LK, McPhillips S: Unpredictable anaphylaxis to cefazolin without allergy to other β-lactams [abstract]. *J Allergy Clin Immunol* 1995, 95:284.

11. Castro SM, Swartz RH, Nazafian LF: Ampicillin- and amoxicillin-delayed hypersensitivity: side-chain–specific allergic reactions in a child. *Ped Asthma Allergy Immunol* 1996, 10:197–203.

12.•• Romano A, Torres MJ, Fernandez J, et al.: Allergic reactions to ampicillin: studies on the specificity and selectivity in subjects with immediate reactions. *Clin Exp Allergy* 1997, 27:1425–1431.
Patients in Spain and Italy with a history of reactions to ampicillin were tested with a battery of β-lactam antibiotic metabolites; 48 patients were skin tested and had in-vitro IgE antibody studies. Most patients (73%) reacted to β-lactam metabolites derived from penicillin, 10 were sensitive to ampicillin/amoxicillin, and three to ampicillin alone.

13. Patterson R, DeSwarte RD, Greenberger PA, Granimar LC: Drug allergy and protocols for management of drug allergies. *NER Allergy Proc* 1986, 7:325–342.

14. Sanz ML, Garcia BE, Prieto I, et al.: Specific IgE determination in the diagnosis of β-lactam allergy. *J Invest Allergol Clin Immunol* 1996, 6:89–93.

15. Mendelson LM, Ressler C, Rosen JP, Selcow JP: Routine elective penicillin-allergy skin testing in children and adolescents: a study of sensitization. *J Allergy Clin Immunol* 1984, 73:76–81.

16. Lopez-Serrano MC, Calballero MT, Barranco P, Martinez-Alzamora F: Booster responses in the study of allergic reactions to β-lactam antibiotics. *J Investig Allergol Clin Immunol* 1996, 6:30–35.

17. Levine BB, Redmond AP: Minor haptenic determinate-specific reagins of penicillin hypersensitivity in man. *Int Arch Appl Immunol* 1969, 35:445–455.

18. Lin RY: A perspective on penicillin allergy. *Arch Intern Med* 1992, 152:930–937.

19. Sogn DD, Evans R III, Shepard GM, et al.: Results of NIAID collaborative clinical trial to test the predictive value of skin testing with major and minor penicillin derivatives in hospitalized adults. *Arch Intern Med* 1992, 152:1025–1032.

20. Smith JW, Johnson JE III, Cliff LE: Studies on the epidemiology of adverse drug reactions: an evaluation of penicillin allergy. *N Eng J Med* 1996, 274:998–1002.

21. Mosely EI, Sullivan TJ: Allergic reactions to antimicrobial drugs in patients with a history of prior drug allergy [abstract]. *J Allergy Clin Immunol* 1991, 87:226.

22.•• Koury L, Warrington R: The multiple drug allergy syndrome: a matched-controlled retrospective study in patients allergic to penicillin. *J Allergy Clin Immunol* 1996, 98:462–464.
Koury and Warrington studied 44 consecutive patients with a history of penicillin allergy who had a positive penicillin skin test compared to 44 age- and sex-matched patients with a prior history of penicillin sensitivity but a negative penicillin skin test and 44 controls. There were no more reactions to other antibiotics in the proven-penicillin–allergic group than in other groups.

23. Patriatrca G, Schiavino D, Nuccera E, NElana A: Positive allergological tests may turn negative with no further exposure to the specific allergen: a long-term, prospective follow-up in patients allergic to penicillin. *Invest Allergol Clin Immunol* 1996, 6:162–165.

24. Anderson JA: *Drug Desensitization: Provocation Testing in Clinical Practice.* Edited by Spector SL. New York: Marcel Dekker; 1995:761.

25.• Beal G, Sanwo K, Hussain H: Drug reactions and desensitizations in AIDS. *Immunol Allergy Clin North Am* 1997, 17:319–337.
This paper presents a very current and extensive review of issues relating to drug reactions in patients with HIV infection and AIDS.

26.• Caumes E, Guen-Nonprez G, Lacomte C, *et al.*: Efficacy and safety of desensitization with sulfamethoxazole and trimethoprim in 48 previously hypersensitive patients infected with human immunodeficiency virus. *Arch Den Natol* 1997, 4:465–469.
This paper describes the outcome of a 2-day outpatient desensitization to sulfamethoxazole-trimethoprim in 48 HIV-infected patients with a previous history of reaction When evaluated at 16 months, 37 patients were still tolerating the drug, and of the 11 desensitization failures, eight occurred during the 2-day procedure.

27.• Stevenson DD, Hankammer RN, Mathison DA, *et al.*: Aspirin desensitization treatment of aspirin-sensitive patients with rhinosinusitis-asthma: long-term outcomes. *J Allergy Clin Immunol* 1996, 98:751–758.
In this study, significant decreases in the number of hospitalizations for asthma occurred after a mean 3.1-year desensitization period (median, 0.2 to zero). The average amount of systemic corticosteroids needed to control asthma also decreased (baseline, 7.9 mg per day; 16 months, 1.8 mg per day).

28.•• Quiralte J, Bianco C, Castillo R, *et al.*: Intolerance to nonsteroidal antiinflammatory drugs: results of controlled drug challenges in 98 patients. *J Allergy Clin Immunol 1996, 98:678–685.*
In this elaborate, well-controlled study of 240 consecutive individuals in Spain with a past history of adverse reactions to aspirin and other NSAIDs were evaluated. Of these, 98 patients were identified as sensitive to one or more NSAIDs and four groups of NSAID-sensitive patients were identified: 1) asthma, nonallergic rhinitis, sinusitis, and polyps triad; 2) urticaria; 3) systemic anaphylactoid reactions; and 4) isolated periorbital edema.

29. Katz Y, Goldberg N, Kivity S: Localized periorbital edema induced by aspirin. *Allergy* 1993; 48:366–369.

30.•• Gall I-L, Kaufmann R, Kalveram CM: Adverse reactions to local anesthetics: analysis of 197 cases. *J Allergy Clin Immunol* 1996, 97:933–937.
In this large study from Germany involving 177 patients over 10 years, patients with a history of adverse reactions to local anesthetics were evaluated by skin testing and subcutaneous testing challenge. No positive skin tests were found to any agent. Only three patients responded with objective symptoms to local-anesthetic challenge

31.• Bush RK, Swanson DP: Radiocontrast. *Immunol Allergy Clin North Am* 1995, 15:597–612.
This article represents a recent comprehensive review of adverse reactions to RCM.

32. Lieberman P: Difficult allergic reactions. *Immunol Allergy Clin North Am* 1991;11:213-231.

33. Lang D, Alpren M, Visintainer P, Smith ST: Increased risk of anaphylactoid reaction from contrast media in patients receiving β-adrenergic blockers with asthma. *Ann Intern Med* 1991, 15:270–276.

34. Greenberger PA, Patterson R: The prevention of immediate generalized reactions to radiocontrast media in high-risk patients. *J Allergy Clin Immunol* 1991, 87:867–872.

35. deShazo RD, Galloway JA: Insulin allergy. *Ann Allergy Asthma Immunol* 1996, 76:217–218.

36.• Alvarez-Thull L, Rosenwasser LJ, Brodie TD: Systemic allergy to endogenous insulin during therapy with recombinant (rDNA) DNA insulin. *Ann Allergy Asthma Immunol* 1996, 76:253–256.
This is a unique case report of an individual who developed gestational diabetes, was treated with recombinant human insulin, and then began having generalized urticaria. These allergic reactions were controlled with substantial doses of daily oral corticosteroids.

37.• Anderson JA, Abbosh JK, Levine AB: Increased prevalence of angiotensin-converting enzyme inhibitor (ACEI) drug induced angioedema in cardiac transplant and renal transplant patients. *J Allergy Clin Immunol* 1996, 97:341.
This retrospective study of 156 consecutive cardiac transplant patients and 341 renal transplant patients uncovered six cases of late-onset angioedema to ACEI anti-hypersensitive drug.

Index

Page numbers in *italics* indicate figures; those followed by *t* indicate tables.

Peptide ligands, T lymphocytes and, 27–28
Peptides, in immunotherapy, 32, 58
Perennial nonallergic rhinitis, vasomotor rhinitis as, 103
Pheochromocytoma, anaphylaxis *versus,* 140
Phospholipase, in immunotherapy, 58
  in mast cell/basophil secretion, *17, 18t–19t,* 19–20
Plasmapheresis, in urticaria, 153
Pneumovax, in sinusitis, 129
Poison ivy dermatitis, 163
Pollen, allergen characteristics of, *54t*
  angiotensin-converting enzyme inhibitors in allergy to, 137–138
  cross-reactivity of, *56t*
Pollution, nonallergic rhinitis from, 108
Polyps, nasal *See* Nasal polyps
Postnasal drip, in sinusitis, 128
Pranlukast, in asthma, 73
Prednisolone, in asthma, 29
Pregnancy, nonallergic rhinitis in, 106–107
Prostaglandins, in mast cells and basophils, 14
Protein kinase C, in mast cell/basophil secretion, *17, 18t–19t,* 18–19
Proteoglycans, in mast cells and basophils, 14
Pruritus, in atopic dermatitis, 167
  in conjunctivitis, 184
  in urticaria, 146, 152, 157–158, *159t*
Psychomotor function, antihistamines and, 92, *92t, 93,* 94

- R -
Racemic albuterol, in asthma, 82
Radio contrast media, 191, 199, *200t,* 201
Ragweed allergy, allergen characteristics of, *54t*
  cross-reactivity in, *56t*
  studies of, 58, 88–89, *89*
Rash, in antibiotic allergy, 193, 196–197
Reagin, immunoglobulin E formerly known as, 39
Rebound nasal congestion, 106
β-Receptor genetics, in asthma, 83
Recombinant allergens, in allergic diseases, 55–58, *56t–57t*
  cloning of, 55
Renin-angiotensin system, in anaphylaxis, 136–138, *137*
Rhinitis, allergic *See* Allergic rhinitis
  cost of, 125
  differential diagnosis of, *127t*
    sinusitis in, 127–128, *128t*
  nonallergic *See* Nonallergic rhinitis
  occupational, 108–109, *109t*
  prevalence of, 125
  vasomotor, 103–104, 128–129
Rhinitis medicamentosa, 106
Rush immunotherapy, 117

- S -
Salmeterol, in asthma, 80–81
  cost of, *6t,* 82
  theophylline *versus,* 81–82
Scombroid fish poisoning, 140, 179
Secretagogues, in urticaria, 158–159
Sedation, antihistamine-induced, 4, 91–92
Sedatives, driving restrictions and, 92, *93*
Self-management training programs, in asthma, 8
Shellfish allergy, 133–134, *174t*
Sinus anatomy, 125, *126*

Sinusitis, 125–132
  acute, 125–127, *126, 126t–127t*
  chronic, 104, *104t,* 127–132 *See also* Chronic sinusitis
  cost of, 125
  prevalence of, 125
  recurrent, 128
  rhinitis *versus,* 127–128, *128t*
  signs and symptoms of, 126, *126t*
Sjögren's syndrome, nonallergic rhinitis from, 110
Skin biopsy, in urticaria, 152, 161
Skin disorders *See also* specific conditions
  allergic, 157–170, 196–198
Skin testing, in contact dermatitis, 163
  in drug allergy, 191, 193–199, *194t–195t*
Slow-reacting substance of anaphylaxis, cysteinyl leukotrienes formerly known as, 70
Smell sense, in sinusitis, 128
Solar urticaria, 147, *148t*
Soybean allergy, *54t, 174t*
Spinhaler, in asthma, 83
Spiros inhaler, in asthma, *84t*
STAT6 activation, immunoglobulin E and, 40, *40–41*
Stem cell factor, in mast cell development, 11–12
Stevens-Johnson syndrome, 196–197
Strawberry-induced urticaria, 160
Sulfonamide reactions, 196–197, *197t*
Surgical treatment, of nasal obstruction, 105
  of sinusitis, 131–132
  of vasomotor rhinitis, 103–104
Syncope, in anaphylaxis, 135

- T -
T cell hypothesis, 33, *34*
T cell tolerance, 31–33
T cells, 25–34 *See also* T lymphocytes
T helper cells, in allergic responses, 25–33, *26, 27t, 33–34,* 51–52
  in asthma, 61–62
  in dermatitis, 163, *165,* 167–168
  in immunotherapy, 114, 120
  regulation of, 32, *34*
T helper cytokines, in asthma, 29–31, *31*
T lymphocytes, 25–34
  epitopes of, 55, 114
  in immunotherapy, 32–33
  in asthma, 33, *34*
  inactivation of, 31–32
Tear film breakup time, in conjunctivitis, 186
Terbutaline, in asthma, 7
Terfenadine, in asthma, 96
  cardiotoxicity of, 94
  chlorpheniramine combined with, 96
  cost of, 4, *4t*
  drug interactions with, 94
  efficacy of, *90t,* 91
  interaction with zileuton of, 75
  pharmacokinetics of, 87–89, *88t*
  psychomotor effects of, *93,* 94
  topical agents *versus,* 95
Theophylline, in asthma, β-agonists *versus,* 81–82
  cost of, *6t,* 82
  interaction with zileuton of, 75
Thyroid carcinoma, anaphylaxis *versus,* 140
Thyroid disease, chronic urticaria and, 148
Thyroid hormone, in urticaria, 150–152
Tolerance, infectious, 32

Topical antihistamines, 94–95
Toxoplasma gondii, leukotrienes and, 70
Transforming growth factor–β, 32, *33*
Trantas' dots, *186t,* 188–189
Triamcinolone, in allergic rhinitis, *4t,* 4–5
  in asthma, *6t*
Tricyclic antidepressants, in urticaria, 162
Trimethoprim-sulfamethoxazole, 197
Triple response of Lewis, in urticaria, 157–158
Tryptase, in anaphylaxis, 135, 138–139
  in mast cells, *13t,* 13–14
  in urticaria, 158
Tumor necrosis factor-α, in asthma, 63, *63t*
  in mast cells and basophils, 14
Tumor necrosis factor receptor, immunoglobulin E and, 41
Tumors, nonallergic rhinitis from, 109
Turbuhaler, in asthma, *82, 82–83, 84t*
Tyrosine kinase, in mast cell/basophil secretion, *17, 17–18, 18t–19t*

- U -
Urticaria, 145–154, 157–162, 198
  acute, 146
  cholinergic, 147–148
  chronic, 146–151, *147,* 161, *161t*
  classification of, 145–146, *146t, 158t*
  differential diagnosis of, 146–150, *147, 148t, 149*
  evaluation of, 151–152
  idiopathic, *159*
  pathobiology of, 150–151, *151t*
  treatment of, 152–153, 161–162

- V -
Vaccines, allergen, 56–58
  in sinusitis, 129
Vascular cell adhesion molecule 1, in asthma, 63, *63t*
Vasculitis, chronic urticaria *versus,* 148
  nonallergic rhinitis from, 110
  zafirlukast associated with, 75
Vasoconstriction, from cysteinyl leukotrienes, 71
Vasomotor rhinitis, nonallergic, 103–104, 128–129
Vernal conjunctivitis, *185t,* 188
Viral infection, in asthma pathophysiology, 61–62
  conjunctivitis from, *185t, 187, 187*
  urticaria in, 146
Visual analog scale, antihistamines and, 92, *93*

- W -
Warfarin, interaction with zafirlukast of, 75
Wheal and flare reactions, in antihistamine efficacy, *88t, 89, 90t,* 91
Work-related injury, antihistamines and, 4

- Z -
Zafirlukast, adverse effects of, 75
  in asthma, *6t,* 7, 73, 96
    experimental, 71
  drug interactions with, 75
  in sinusitis, 131
Zileuton, adverse effects of, 74–75
  in asthma, 72–73, 75
  cost of, *6t*
  experimental, 72
  drug interactions with, 75
  in sinusitis, 131
  in urticaria, 162